RADIOTHERAPY

A MEDICAL DICTIONARY, BIBLIOGRAPHY,
AND ANNOTATED RESEARCH GUIDE TO
INTERNET REFERENCES

JAMES N. PARKER, M.D.
AND PHILIP M. PARKER, PH.D., EDITORS

ii

ICON Health Publications
ICON Group International, Inc.
4370 La Jolla Village Drive, 4th Floor
San Diego, CA 92122 USA

Printed in the United States of America.

Last digit indicates print number: 10 9 8 7 6 4 5 3 2 1

Publisher, Health Care: Philip Parker, Ph.D.
Editor(s): James Parker, M.D., Philip Parker, Ph.D.

Publisher's note: The ideas, procedures, and suggestions contained in this book are not intended for the diagnosis or treatment of a health problem. As new medical or scientific information becomes available from academic and clinical research, recommended treatments and drug therapies may undergo changes. The authors, editors, and publisher have attempted to make the information in this book up to date and accurate in accord with accepted standards at the time of publication. The authors, editors, and publisher are not responsible for errors or omissions or for consequences from application of the book, and make no warranty, expressed or implied, in regard to the contents of this book. Any practice described in this book should be applied by the reader in accordance with professional standards of care used in regard to the unique circumstances that may apply in each situation. The reader is advised to always check product information (package inserts) for changes and new information regarding dosage and contraindications before prescribing any drug or pharmacological product. Caution is especially urged when using new or infrequently ordered drugs, herbal remedies, vitamins and supplements, alternative therapies, complementary therapies and medicines, and integrative medical treatments.

Cataloging-in-Publication Data

Parker, James N., 1961-
Parker, Philip M., 1960-

Radiotherapy: A Medical Dictionary, Bibliography, and Annotated Research Guide to Internet References / James N. Parker and Philip M. Parker, editors
        p.   cm.
Includes bibliographical references, glossary, and index.
ISBN: 0-497-00927-7
1. Radiotherapy-Popular works.   I. Title.

Disclaimer

This publication is not intended to be used for the diagnosis or treatment of a health problem. It is sold with the understanding that the publisher, editors, and authors are not engaging in the rendering of medical, psychological, financial, legal, or other professional services.

References to any entity, product, service, or source of information that may be contained in this publication should not be considered an endorsement, either direct or implied, by the publisher, editors, or authors. ICON Group International, Inc., the editors, and the authors are not responsible for the content of any Web pages or publications referenced in this publication.

Copyright Notice

Acknowledgements

The collective knowledge generated from academic and applied research summarized in various references has been critical in the creation of this book which is best viewed as a comprehensive compilation and collection of information prepared by various official agencies which produce publications on radiotherapy. Books in this series draw from various agencies and institutions associated with the United States Department of Health and Human Services, and in particular, the Office of the Secretary of Health and Human Services (OS), the Administration for Children and Families (ACF), the Administration on Aging (AOA), the Agency for Healthcare Research and Quality (AHRQ), the Agency for Toxic Substances and Disease Registry (ATSDR), the Centers for Disease Control and Prevention (CDC), the Food and Drug Administration (FDA), the Healthcare Financing Administration (HCFA), the Health Resources and Services Administration (HRSA), the Indian Health Service (IHS), the institutions of the National Institutes of Health (NIH), the Program Support Center (PSC), and the Substance Abuse and Mental Health Services Administration (SAMHSA). In addition to these sources, information gathered from the National Library of Medicine, the United States Patent Office, the European Union, and their related organizations has been invaluable in the creation of this book. Some of the work represented was financially supported by the Research and Development Committee at INSEAD. This support is gratefully acknowledged. Finally, special thanks are owed to Tiffany Freeman for her excellent editorial support.

About the Editors

James N. Parker, M.D.

Dr. James N. Parker received his Bachelor of Science degree in Psychobiology from the University of California, Riverside and his M.D. from the University of California, San Diego. In addition to authoring numerous research publications, he has lectured at various academic institutions. Dr. Parker is the medical editor for health books by ICON Health Publications.

Philip M. Parker, Ph.D.

Philip M. Parker is the Eli Lilly Chair Professor of Innovation, Business and Society at INSEAD (Fontainebleau, France and Singapore). Dr. Parker has also been Professor at the University of California, San Diego and has taught courses at Harvard University, the Hong Kong University of Science and Technology, the Massachusetts Institute of Technology, Stanford University, and UCLA. Dr. Parker is the associate editor for ICON Health Publications.

About ICON Health Publications

To discover more about ICON Health Publications, simply check with your preferred online booksellers, including Barnes&Noble.com and Amazon.com which currently carry all of our titles. Or, feel free to contact us directly for bulk purchases or institutional discounts:

ICON Group International, Inc.
4370 La Jolla Village Drive, Fourth Floor
San Diego, CA 92122 USA
Fax: 858-546-4341
Web site: **www.icongrouponline.com/health**

Table of Contents

FORWARD

In March 2001, the National Institutes of Health issued the following warning: "The number of Web sites offering health-related resources grows every day. Many sites provide valuable information, while others may have information that is unreliable or misleading."[1] Furthermore, because of the rapid increase in Internet-based information, many hours can be wasted searching, selecting, and printing. Since only the smallest fraction of information dealing with radiotherapy is indexed in search engines, such as **www.google.com** or others, a non-systematic approach to Internet research can be not only time consuming, but also incomplete. This book was created for medical professionals, students, and members of the general public who want to know as much as possible about radiotherapy, using the most advanced research tools available and spending the least amount of time doing so.

In addition to offering a structured and comprehensive bibliography, the pages that follow will tell you where and how to find reliable information covering virtually all topics related to radiotherapy, from the essentials to the most advanced areas of research. Public, academic, government, and peer-reviewed research studies are emphasized. Various abstracts are reproduced to give you some of the latest official information available to date on radiotherapy. Abundant guidance is given on how to obtain free-of-charge primary research results via the Internet. **While this book focuses on the field of medicine, when some sources provide access to non-medical information relating to radiotherapy, these are noted in the text.**

E-book and electronic versions of this book are fully interactive with each of the Internet sites mentioned (clicking on a hyperlink automatically opens your browser to the site indicated). If you are using the hard copy version of this book, you can access a cited Web site by typing the provided Web address directly into your Internet browser. You may find it useful to refer to synonyms or related terms when accessing these Internet databases. **NOTE:** At the time of publication, the Web addresses were functional. However, some links may fail due to URL address changes, which is a common occurrence on the Internet.

For readers unfamiliar with the Internet, detailed instructions are offered on how to access electronic resources. For readers unfamiliar with medical terminology, a comprehensive glossary is provided. For readers without access to Internet resources, a directory of medical libraries, that have or can locate references cited here, is given. We hope these resources will prove useful to the widest possible audience seeking information on radiotherapy.

The Editors

---

[1] From the NIH, National Cancer Institute (NCI): **http://www.cancer.gov/cancerinfo/ten-things-to-know**.

CHAPTER 1. STUDIES ON RADIOTHERAPY

Overview

In this chapter, we will show you how to locate peer-reviewed references and studies on radiotherapy.

The Combined Health Information Database

The Combined Health Information Database summarizes studies across numerous federal agencies. To limit your investigation to research studies and radiotherapy, you will need to use the advanced search options. First, go to **http://chid.nih.gov/index.html**. From there, select the "Detailed Search" option (or go directly to that page with the following hyperlink: **http://chid.nih.gov/detail/detail.html**). The trick in extracting studies is found in the drop boxes at the bottom of the search page where "You may refine your search by." Select the dates and language you prefer, and the format option "Journal Article." At the top of the search form, select the number of records you would like to see (we recommend 100) and check the box to display "whole records." We recommend that you type "radiotherapy" (or synonyms) into the "For these words:" box. Consider using the option "anywhere in record" to make your search as broad as possible. If you want to limit the search to only a particular field, such as the title of the journal, then select this option in the "Search in these fields" drop box. The following is what you can expect from this type of search:

- **Phase II Trial of Concurrent Paclitaxel, Carboplatin and Radiotherapy in State III/IV Resectable Cancer of the Oral Cavity and Oropharynx**

  Source: International Poster Journal. 4(1), Poster 112. 2002.

  Contact: Available from Quintessence Publishing Co, Inc. 551 Kimberly Drive, Carol Stream, IL 60188-9981. (800) 621-0387 or (630) 682-3223. Fax (630) 682-3288. E-mail: quintpub@aol.com. Website: www.quintpub.com.

  Summary: In the treatment of head and neck cancer, chemotherapy used to be limited to metastatic or recurrent settings. During the last twenty years, the addition of chemotherapy to aggressive local treatment has been investigated to overcome high local relapse rates. This article reports on a phase II trial of the use of concurrent Paclitaxel, Carboplatin and **radiotherapy** in patients with stage III (n = 6) or IV (n = 22) resectable cancer of the oral cavity and oropharynx. One early death was reported due to septic neutropenia. Clinical response was as follows: Carboplatin and **radiotherapy** (CR), 14 of 27 patients (52 percent); Paclitaxel and **radiotherapy** (PR), 13 of 27 patients (48 percent). Mucositis occurred in all patients. The follow up of this ongoing study shows that 88 percent of the patients were alive at the 1 year mark. 3 figures. 5 tables. 8 references.

- **Quality of Life and Oral Function Following Radiotherapy for Head and Neck Cancer**

  Source: Head and Neck. 21(1): 1-11. January 1999.

  Contact: Available from John Wiley and Sons, Inc. 605 Third Avenue, New York, NY 10158. (212) 850-6645.

  Summary: Multiple oral complaints occur following radiation therapy for oral or pharyngeal cancer, but the frequency and severity of symptoms of dysfunction and discomfort are not well understood. This article reports on a study undertaken to assess the quality of life, oral function, and oral symptoms following radiation therapy. A general quality of life survey, with an added oral symptom and function scale was mailed to 100 patients more than 6 months following radiation therapy. Sixty-five patients responded. Difficulty chewing or eating was reported by 43 percent of respondents. Dry mouth was reported by 91.8 percent, change in taste by 75.4 percent, dysphagia by 63.1 percent, altered speech by 50.8 percent, difficulty with dentures by 48.5 percent, and increased tooth decay by 38.5 percent of dentate patients. Pain was common (58.4 percent) and interfered with daily activities in 30.8 percent. Mood complaints were reported by approximately half the patients and interference with social activities was reported by 60 percent. The frequency of oral side effects correlated with radiation treatment fields and dose. The authors conclude that oral complications following radiation therapy for head and neck cancer are common and negatively affect quality of life. 6 tables. 34 references. (AA-M).

- **Necrotizing Stomatitis After Radiotherapy in a Patient with AIDS: Case Report**

  Source: Journal of Oral and Maxillofacial Surgery. 60(1): 100-101. January 2002.

  Contact: Available from W.B. Saunders Company. Periodicals Department, P.O. Box 629239, Orlando, FL 32862-8239. (800) 654-2452. Website: www.harcourthealth.com.

  Summary: Necrotizing stomatitis (NS) is recognized as an opportunistic disease associated with AIDS. NS is often described as beginning as an aggressive necrotizing ulcerative gingivitis (inflammation of the gums with ulcering) that then invades the surrounding tissues and ultimately exposes the underlying bone. This article reports a case of NS that developed in a patient with full blown AIDS after craniofacial **radiotherapy** for treatment of a pharyngeal nonHodgkins lymphoma (NHL). The authors present the case report, then discuss NS in the HIV infected patient. In this case, no significant periodontal disease was detected. The initial signs of the disease were related to irradiation of the head and neck; the side effects of radiation therapy provoked colonization of the orofacial tissues and the consequent necrotizing infection. However, radiation therapy is reported to be the only curative treatment for pharyngeal NHL in immunosuppressed HIV patients. The authors caution that the management of NS in the full blown AIDS patient has a poor prognosis because it is impossible to achieve a disease free state and NS is just one of the multiple disorders associated with immunosuppression. A conservative attitude must prevail, with sensibly adapted antibiotic therapy, local debridement, improved oral hygiene, lavage with antiseptic agents, and analgesic (painkillers) medication. Periodontal curettage, dental extraction, and aggressive surgical procedures are to be avoided. Even severely immunosuppressed patients are sometimes able to arrest the destructive process; however, the final outcome in the majority of cases is death after a short period because of the compromised clinical situation. 2 figures. 9 references.

- **Influence of Pre-Radiation Salivary Flow Rates and Radiation Dose on Parotid Salivary Gland Dysfunction in Patients Receiving Radiotherapy for Head and Neck Cancers**

  Source: SCD. Special Care in Dentistry. 18(3): 102-108. May-June 1998.

  Contact: Available from Special Care Dentistry. 211 East Chicago Avenue, Chicago, IL 60611. (312) 440-2660. Fax (312) 440-2824.

  Summary: Radiotherapy used for head and neck cancers causes permanent salivary gland dysfunction (SGD). Previous short-term studies have demonstrated that pre-radiotherapy salivary flow rates and the amount of radiation exposure to parotid glands influence the amount of radiotherapy-induced SGD. This article reports on a study undertaken to determine which variables are related to the development of long-term post-radiotherapy SGD. Parotid flow rates (PFR) were assessed prior to and 1 year after completion of **radiotherapy** in spared parotid glands from 24 patients from 2 parotid-sparing protocols. The results reveal that spared PFR were not significantly higher 1 year post-radiotherapy in patients who had high pre-radiotherapy PFR, when compared with patients with low pre-radiotherapy PFR. However, patients who received higher doses of **radiotherapy** to spared parotid glands had lower PFR 1 year post-radiotherapy, compared with patients who had received lower doses of **radiotherapy**. These one-year findings suggest that high pre-radiotherapy PFR do not provide protection against radiotherapy-induced salivary gland dysfunction. Conversely, reduced **radiotherapy** dosages to contralateral parotid glands are protective of PFR after completion of **radiotherapy**. 2 figures. 4 tables. 21 references. (AA).

- **Aggressive Ameloblastoma Treated With Radiotherapy, Surgical Ablation, and Reconstruction**

  Source: JADA. Journal of the American Dental Association. 129(1): 84-87. January 1998.

  Summary: The ameloblastoma is a benign, slow growing, rare, odontogenic (arising from the dentition, or teeth) neoplasm. The solid or multicystic ameloblastoma has a tendency to be locally invasive and has a high incidence of recurrence if not adequately removed. This article presents a case report of an aggressive ameloblastoma treated with **radiotherapy,** surgical ablation, and reconstruction. Surgical resection of aggressive solid or multicystic ameloblastoma is a well documented and accepted treatment modality. Controversies exist, however, with regard to the extent of operative intervention. Unresectable lesions have been treated with radiation or combined radiation and chemotherapy. The authors present a case report of a patient with recurrent ameloblastoma who underwent simultaneous hard and soft tissue reconstruction. The patient had been treated with external beam radiation for a recurrent ameloblastoma with direct extension to the cranial base. Significant hard and soft tissue defects developed. Twenty two years after the initial treatment, the 40 year old patient developed an infection of the right mandible with a draining extraoral fistula. This led to a nontraumatic pathological fracture of the posterior mandible (lower jaw). In addition, pronounced soft tissue atrophy was present on the irradiated side of the face. The patient's postoperative course was uneventful and intermaxillary fixation was released at six weeks. Bony union was evident and no motor nerve deficit was observed. Fourteen months after surgery, the patient remained free of tumor and symptoms. 5 figures. 15 references.

- **Radiotherapy for Metastases to the Mandible in Children**

  Source: Journal of Oral and Maxillofacial Surgery. 60(3): 269-271. March 2002.

  Contact: Available from W.B. Saunders Company. Periodicals Department, P.O. Box 629239, Orlando, FL 32862-8239. (800) 654-2452. Website: www.harcourthealth.com.

Summary: This article presents a retrospective review of all children treated since 1979 at the authors' institution with radiation therapy for symptomatic metastases (spread of cancer) that involved the mandible (lower jaw). Nine children were treated with 1 or more courses of **radiotherapy** for symptomatic metastases that involve the mandible. Six children had a neuroblastoma, 1 had angiosarcoma of the liver, 1 had adenocarcinoma of the rectum, and 1 had peripheral primitive neuroectodermal tumor (Ewing's sarcoma) of the spine. In 3 children, the mandible was the first bone involved by metastases. Seven children were treated with short intensive courses of **radiotherapy** consisting of 1 to 3 fractions to a total dose of 400 to 1,200 cGy. One child received 2,400 cGy in 6 fractions, and another child received 3,000 cGy in 10 fractions. Three children were treated with second courses of **radiotherapy** at 1, 2, and 5 months, respectively, from the initial course of **radiotherapy.** All children had received chemotherapy. All children died of disseminated disease at 5 to 59 months from their initial diagnosis, 5 to 29 months from the detection of metastases to bone, and only 6 days to 17 months (median, 20 months) from the first treatment of metastases to the mandible. The authors conclude that the outlook for children with metastases that involve the mandible is very poor, and the authors recommend short intensive courses of **radiotherapy** consisting of 1 to 3 treatments to total doses of 400 to 1,200 cGy for palliation of pain. 1 table. 7 references.

- **Radiotherapy and Oral Sequelae: Preventive and Management Protocols**

  Source: Journal of Dental Hygiene. 71(1): 23-29. January-February 1997.

Summary: This article provides background information on **radiotherapy** and presents dental hygiene protocols for the treatment of head and neck radiation patients. These patients experience specific oral complications or sequelae that require specialized care. To assist dental hygienists in understanding the genesis of these complications, the authors include a brief history of the use of **radiotherapy** and its effects on mammalian tissue. Complications may include mucositis, candidiasis, xerostomia, loss of taste, trismus, severe caries, nutritional deficit, and osteoradionecrosis. The authors present management protocols for the prevention and treatment of these complications. They caution that maximum protocol effectiveness and long-term success may only be attained by educating and communicating with the patient. The authors conclude that, as the number of head and neck radiation patients increases, a thorough understanding of the disease and treatment process is becoming more necessary for all oral health care providers. 5 figures. 1 table. 25 references. (AA-M).

- **Prospective Study of Salivary Gland Function in Patients Undergoing Radiotherapy for Squamous Cell Carcinoma of the Oropharynx**

  Source: Oral Surgery Oral Medicine Oral Pathology. 97(2): 173-89. February 2004.

Summary: This article reports on a study of the impact of head and neck cancer treatment on salivary function. The study was conducted on 54 patients with advanced squamous cell carcinoma with confirmed (n = 50) or suspected (n = 4) primary oropharyngeal localization who were treated with radiation alone or in combination with surgery or chemotherapy, or both. Results showed that head and neck surgery, particularly when submandibular gland resection was performed, had a negative impact on salivary flow rates but did not influence pH or buffering capacity. Nonetheless, the effect of surgery on salivary flow rates decreased progressively and disappeared at 3 to 6 months after **radiotherapy.** More than two thirds of the salivary output was lost during radiation treatment. All patients were experiencing salivary dysfunction at 1 year after completion of **radiotherapy.** The results of this study confirm that cancer treatment involving full-dose **radiotherapy** (RTH) to all major salivary glands for locally advanced squamous cell carcinoma of the oropharynx induces severe hyposalivation with alteration of salivary pH and buffering capacity. Head and neck surgery has a negative impact on salivary flow rates, especially when the submandibular gland is removed. However, surgery before irradiation is not a factor aggravating hyposalivation when postoperative **radiotherapy** includes all the major salivary glands. 3 figures. 4 tables. 55 references.

- **Artificial Urinary Sphincter for Post-Prostatectomy Incontinence in Men who had Prior Radiotherapy: A Risk and Outcome Analysis**

  Source: Journal of Urology. 167(2 Part 1): 591-596. February 2002.

  Contact: Available from Lippincott Williams and Wilkins. 12107 Insurance Way, Hagerstown, MD 21740. (800) 638-3030 or (301) 714-2334. Fax (301) 824-7290.

  Summary: This article reports on a study that retrospectively reviewed the authors' experience with the artificial urinary sphincter for postprostatectomy incontinence (involuntary loss of urine following removal of the prostate), comparing the outcome of those patients who did and did not receive previous radiation therapy. A total of 86 patients with postprostatectomy incontinence treated with implantation of artificial urinary sphincter includes 58 who did not (group 1) and 28 who did (group 2) receive prior radiation therapy during treatment of prostate carcinoma. In group 2, radiation was the primary treatment, followed by salvage prostatectomy in 5 patients, adjuvant after radical retropubic prostatectomy in 20 patients, and after transurethral prostatic resection (TURP) in 3 patients. Mean patient age plus or minus standard deviation was 68.3 plus or minus 6.6 years (group 1) and 69.7 plus or minus 6.6 years (group 2). Reoperation was required in 13 patients (22.4 percent) in group 1 and in 7 patients (25 percent) in group 2. Urethral atrophy or inadequate compression was seen in 8 patients (14 percent) and 4 patients (14 percent), and urethral erosion was observed in 1 patient (2 percent) and 2 patients (7 percent) in groups 1 and 2, respectively. Infection of the device was observed in 4 patients (7 percent) in group 1 but none in group 2. Continence status was similar in both groups (around 60 percent). Urgency with or without urge incontinence was reported after implantation of artificial urinary sphincter in 47 percent and 44 percent of patients in groups 1 and 2, respectively. The authors conclude that the artificial urinary sphincter has a similar outcome in patients with postprostatectomy incontinence whether or not they have received previous radiation therapy. 5 tables. 12 references.

- **Overview of the Oral Complications of Adult Patients with Malignant Haematological Conditions Who Have Undergone Radiotherapy or Chemotherapy**

  Source: Journal of Advanced Nursing. 22(6): 1085-1091. December 1995.

  Summary: This review article covers mouth care in adult patients with malignant hematological (blood) conditions and, in particular, those with disturbed immunity or bone marrow depression due to **radiotherapy** (radiation) or chemotherapy. The oral assessment tools available are discussed. The author describes different products used and the research that supports their use, as well as staging systems used to introduce such products to the patient's schedule. The author focuses on the nursing care involved in this provision of care. The author notes that patient education has been found to be the most important aspect of mouth care in these patients. Topics include chemotherapy agents, maintaining hydration (avoiding xerostomia), infections, mouth washes, and toothbrushes. Chlorhexidine mouthwashes, professional scaling (if the patient's white cell count allows it), elimination of possible sources of oral infection and irritation, and relief of pain form the basis of care for these patients. 47 references. (AA-M).

Federally Funded Research on Radiotherapy

The U.S. Government supports a variety of research studies relating to radiotherapy. These studies are tracked by the Office of Extramural Research at the National Institutes of Health.[2] CRISP (Computerized Retrieval of Information on Scientific Projects) is a searchable database of federally funded biomedical research projects conducted at universities, hospitals, and other institutions.

Search the CRISP Web site at **http://crisp.cit.nih.gov/crisp/crisp_query.generate_screen**. You will have the option to perform targeted searches by various criteria, including geography, date, and topics related to radiotherapy.

For most of the studies, the agencies reporting into CRISP provide summaries or abstracts. As opposed to clinical trial research using patients, many federally funded studies use animals or simulated models to explore radiotherapy. The following is typical of the type of information found when searching the CRISP database for radiotherapy:

- **Project Title: 3D IMAGE GUIDED PATIENT SYSTEM FOR STEREOTACTIC RADIOTH.**

  Principal Investigator & Institution: Zhuang, Ping; Genex Technologies, Inc. 10605 Concord St, Ste 500 Kensington, Md 20895

  Timing: Fiscal Year 2002; Project Start 15-AUG-2002; Project End 31-JUL-2003

  Summary: (provided by applicant): With rapid development in 3D conformal radiation therapy and stereotactic **radiotherapy,** which tends to treat small and highly tailored clinical targets with very high doses, increasingly stringent setup accuracy become more important. Currently, many researches in early tumor detection use imaging techniques such as CT, MRI, and SPECT, treatment plan optimization using inverse planning, and beam management using IMRT and SRT. There are lack of development in patient refixation technique. The primary objective of the SBIR effort proposed herein is to develop a novel patient refixation technique feasible for daily treatment of fractionated **radiotherapy.** The technique can achieve a high accuracy and precision within 1-mm by using a novel high-speed three-dimensional (3D) video camera. The precise 3D-surface images of patient can be captured following the patient positioned on the treatment couch. The surface images are compared with the reference 3D image that is created

---

[2] Healthcare projects are funded by the National Institutes of Health (NIH), Substance Abuse and Mental Health Services (SAMHSA), Health Resources and Services Administration (HRSA), Food and Drug Administration (FDA), Centers for Disease Control and Prevention (CDCP), Agency for Healthcare Research and Quality (AHRQ), and Office of Assistant Secretary of Health (OASH).

from the previous CT scans or 3D-video image with the patient in the planned treatment position. The 3D surface fitting and frame subtraction techniques will generate quantitative parameters regarding patient?s positioning error in all six degree-of-freedom, facilitating the re-position adjustment. Because the video image is acquired instantly, this frame-less patient refixation system also provides a solution for the real-time detection and correction of patient motion relative to the treatment machine in a single fraction. In the proposed Phase 1 effort, we will (1) Design an accurate patient refixation system using a 3D video camera; (2) Build prototype hardware of the 3D video camera and assess the clinical feasibility; (3) Develop the proposed 3D image subtraction and comparison algorithms to unfold patient positioning error; (4) Improve the software tools to interactively visualize and rapidly quantify 3D positioning errors; and (5) Perform patient reposition experiments. PROPOSED COMMERCIAL APPLICATION: The proposed 3D imaging technology adds one more dimension (literally and figuratively) to fractional radiation treatment repositioning applications, and will lead to a new generation of commercial products of patient repositioning systems for **radiotherapy**. With hundreds of radiation treatment machines in USA and many more in Europe, the market for a clinically acceptable 3D-camera-based refixation system is significant. If it succeeds, it will have a significant impact on biomedical research and will revolutionize many current practices in rafixation during cancer treatment. It would find utility in reconstructive surgery due to cancer, body deformities, orthotics, rehabilitation, resident training and education.

Website: http://crisp.cit.nih.gov/crisp/Crisp_Query.Generate_Screen

- **Project Title: 99MTC AND 188RE COMPLEXES FOR CONJUGATION TO PEPTIDES**

  Principal Investigator & Institution: Francesconi, Lynn C.; Associate Professor; Hunter College Room E1424 New York, Ny 10021

  Timing: Fiscal Year 2004; Project Start 01-APR-2004; Project End 31-MAR-2008

  Summary: (provided by applicant): Targeted technetium (99m Tc) and rhenium (188 Re) radiopharmaceuticals consist of a targeting vector that determines the specificity for the target (receptor, biochemical process) and is linked to an organic ligand that forms a complex (or chelate) with the radiometal. Our long-range goal is to design new conjugates consisting of the 99m Tc/ 188 Re chelate and the targeting vector (Figure 1) that will have exceptional stability, targeting ability and rapid elimination of unbound radioactivity. The objective of this proposal is to design, synthesize and test simple Tc/Re complexes (chelates) based on two Tc/Re "cores", [M v =O] 3+ and M I (CO)3 + , M= 99m Tc, 188 Re, and complementary peptide ligand systems. (Aims 1 and 2) The peptide ligands are chosen to provide an understanding of the factors (structure, lipophilicity, stereochemistry) that lead to 1) the formation of one major product (two, in the case of stereoisomers) upon radiolabeling, 2) the metal chelates remaining intact in in vivo and in vitro assays (high stability) and 3) elimination of the intact metal chelates in the urine via the kidneys (renal system). This understanding is key to the design of targeted 99m Tc and 188 Re radiopharmaceuticals because we hypothesize that the metal chelate has a profound effect on the stability of the radiometal and the biodistribution of the entire molecule. The chelates designed in this project can be easily conjugated to target vectors (biomolecules) by standard solid phase peptide synthesis (SPPS) techniques for further in vivo testing for specificity to the target and application as imaging or **radiotherapy** agents. Aim 3, a collaborative effort with New York University School of Medicine proposes to conjugate the best chelates from Aims 1 and 2 to a 13 amino acid peptide that is the active site of the HU177 antibody. Both the peptide and the antibody bind to an antigen of collagen type IV that is exposed when collagen unravels in the vicinity of tumors as part of angiogenesis. The 99m Tc and 188 Re conjugates will be tested for in vivo tracking of the peptide and antibody and for applications in imaging and therapy.Our proposed study differs from other Tc and Re radiopharmaceutical studies because we will work with both the tracer (99m Tc, 188 Re, [10[-10] -10[-12] M]) and the macroscopic (99 Tc and Re [10[-2] -10[-3] M]) species. This is critical to gain a complete understanding of the structure, speciation and chemistry of the radiopharmaceutical. In this effort we employ techniques that have not been used for 99m Tc and 188 Re radiopharmaceutical studies and will provide important information on structures and chemistry. These techniques include, but are not limited to, preparative HPLC to prepare the 99 Tc macroscopic analogs, that can be related to the tracer species, and the use of Circular Dichroism and 17 O NMR Spectroscopy.

Website: http://crisp.cit.nih.gov/crisp/Crisp_Query.Generate_Screen

- **Project Title: ADULT HODGKIN'S DISEASE AND EPSTEIN BARR VIRUS**

Principal Investigator & Institution: Ambinder, Richard F.; Professor; Oncology; Johns Hopkins University 3400 N Charles St Baltimore, Md 21218

Timing: Fiscal Year 2002; Project Start 05-APR-2002; Project End 31-MAR-2007

Summary: (PROVIDED BY APPLICANT): Successes in the treatment of Hodgkin's disease (HD) highlight the long-term consequences of chemotherapy and radiation therapy in the management of this disease. The current inter-group trial reflects the improvement in failure free survival as it pays increasing attention to reducing the late effects of therapy in survivors. The presence of Epstein-Barr virus (EBV) in a significant proportion of HD tumors offers the opportunity to develop the use of virus-specific tumor markers and virus-specific immune therapy. The Eastern Cooperative Oncology Group (ECOG) and Southwestern Oncology Group (SWOG) trial E2496 offers an unparalleled opportunity to address these questions. Through evaluation of this large group of patients, the determination of whether EBV detection in biopsy specimens identifies a poor risk group (particularly in patients over the age of 45 years) should be possible. In addition, the validation of the utility of tissue arrays in the detection of EBV in HD will allow the development of this important and cost-efficient resource. A careful analysis will be performed to determine whether EBV detection studies in tissue arrays or in plasma by real-time PCR yield results parallel to those achieved with detection studies applied to conventional tissue sections. In parallel, the determination of the rate of viral DNA clearance in plasma and the effect of different treatment regimens on this clearance will be performed using real-time PCR. The rate of clearance as well as the persistence of viral DNA in plasma will analyzed to determine if they predict resistant disease or relapse. The relationship between plasma IL-10 levels, IL-10 promoter polymorphisms, and the EBV status of the tumor will be evaluated. Finally, we seek to characterize the cytotoxic T-cell response to EBV antigens expressed in HD (in the context of response to other EBV antigens and antigens from other viruses) and to assess the impact of chemotherapy/radiotherapy on these responses. This work should lay the groundwork for future viral antigen targeted therapies.

Website: http://crisp.cit.nih.gov/crisp/Crisp_Query.Generate_Screen

- **Project Title: AMORPHOUS SELENIUM IMAGING FOR TOMOTHERAPY**

Principal Investigator & Institution: Fang, Guang M.; Tomotherapy 2228 Evergreen Rd Middleton, Wi 53562

Timing: Fiscal Year 2003; Project Start 05-SEP-1998; Project End 31-JUL-2005

Summary: (provided by applicant): TomoTherapy Incorporated was founded in 1997 to develop and commercialize a new type of radiation therapy device for improving cancer treatment. TomoTherapy's first FDA cleared product, the HiArt System, combines, for the first time, the means to accurately plan, deliver, verify and review treatments for cancer therapy, and as a result, to greatly improve treatment results and lifestyles of cancer patients because of the better targeting of irradiation to the tumor and the sparing of normal tissue. This "entire **radiotherapy** department in a machine" integration and automation greatly reduces the need for human intervention, thus reducing staff needs for cancer treatment. The HiArt System employs image-guided radiation delivery, enabling tumors to be irradiated more effectively while saving the critical organs surrounding the tumor. Central to the capability of image-guided **radiotherapy** is a detector system that efficiently detects high energy x-rays employed in cancer therapy. The objective of the proposed project is to develop a new type of megavoltage detector system that meets all the requirements of tomotherapy imaging applications. The proposed design combines i) amorphous selenium (a-Se) material which has seen extensive research and development in applications ranging from imaging and display, to radiology and astronomy, with ii) TomoTherapy's patented technology for improving detection efficiency for high energy x-rays. This new detector system will improve the detection efficiency, a key requirement for an imaging detector, over the existent technology by an order of magnitude, thus offering great improvement in resolving power on the images. When employed, the multi-row approach and the improved detection efficiency and readout speed of the new detector will improve the tomotherapy imaging quality and throughput significantly, and offers great potential for imaging the patient in real-time during treatment, a key element for further improving cancer treatment where organ motion is a significant obstacle to improved precision. It is expected that the proposed detector will also save $10 to $20 million in tomotherapy manufacturing cost yearly. This technology also has potential applications in other areas as well, including security inspections at ports, forest inspections and orthopedic imaging where there are implanted metal devices or joints.

Website: http://crisp.cit.nih.gov/crisp/Crisp_Query.Generate_Screen

- **Project Title: ANTI-ANGIOGENIC TETRATHIOMOLYBDATE +XRT IN NSCLC-PHASE 1**

Principal Investigator & Institution: Khan, Mohamed K.; Radiation Oncology; University of Michigan at Ann Arbor 3003 South State, Room 1040 Ann Arbor, Mi 481091274

Timing: Fiscal Year 2003; Project Start 05-SEP-2003; Project End 31-MAY-2004

Summary: (provided by applicant): This is a phase I trial that will seek to determine the acute toxicity that occurs when the anti-angiogenic copper reduction agent Tetrathiomolybdate (TM), is combined with standard **radiotherapy** treatment in patients with stages II, IIIA, or IIIB non-small cell lung cancer (NSCLC). TM is a copper reduction agent shown to be anti-angiogenic in humans, and to affect multiple proteins involved in angiogenesis via the copper depletion mechanism. Preclinical experiments demonstrate that TM can be successfully combined with **radiotherapy** to improve the treatment of local tumors in mice, and that the effect is additive and non-toxic. This trial will test whether a multi-target anti-angiogenic agent can be combined with **radiotherapy** in the treatment of cancer. The specific aims of this proposal are: 1) to determine the acute toxicity that occurs when anti-angiogenic copper reduction therapy with tetrathiomolybdate (TM) is combined with standard **radiotherapy** in stage II-IIIB NSCLC. 2) To determine whether non-invasive markers of the effect of TM on angiogenesis can be found in these irradiated patients. The measurement of biological markers (VEGF, bFGF, TGF-?, IL-6, IL-8), and imaging studies with 99mTc-MIBI scanning will be used for this. Both have previously been shown to be important in angiogenesis. 3) To assess the late toxicity that occurs when TM is combined with standard **radiotherapy** in stage II-IIIB NSCLC. 4) To record the tumor response, recurrence, and survival data. Patients will begin on an induction regimen of TM that will rapidly deplete their copper down to ranges where angiogenesis is inhibited. The patients will be placed into one of four possible pre-assigned ranges of copper depletion and then standard **radiotherapy** will then be delivered. They will then continue at their assigned range of copper reduction for a total of one year using maintenance dosages of TM. The dose of TM will be determined by empiric (ceruloplasmin, Cp) measurements of each individual's copper chelation state. Serum collection and measurements of pro-angiogenic factors (shown to be affected by TM or radiotherapy), and 99mTc-MIBI scanning (shown to correlate with angiogenesis in tumors) will be done to non-invasively assess angiogenesis at different time points. Chest CT and Chest x-ray will be taken to record tumor response, and to compare with 99mTc-MIBI scans.

Website: http://crisp.cit.nih.gov/crisp/Crisp_Query.Generate_Screen

- **Project Title: AUTOLOGOUS DENDRITIC CELL VACCINES IN NSCLC**

Principal Investigator & Institution: Hirschowitz, Edward A.; Medicine; University of Kentucky 109 Kinkead Hall Lexington, Ky 40506

Timing: Fiscal Year 2004; Project Start 19-APR-2004; Project End 31-MAR-2006

Summary: (provided by applicant): Clinical outcomes of unresectable stage III NSCLC are universally poor. Survival with combination chemo-radiotherapy is 11-18 months. Investigation of additional therapies is warranted. Immunotherapies, specifically cancer vaccines, have therapeutic potential. Preliminary data indicate that autologous dendritic cells, pulsed with allogeneic tumor antigens can induce measurable immune responses in individuals with NSCLC. Responses have been seen irrespective of stage or prior therapy, and the spectrum includes responders and nonresponders. The host environment appears to play a significant role in regulating T cell responses to vaccines. We postulate that physiologic (inducible) and pathologic (constitutive expression by NSCLC tumor cells) COX-2 activity can mediate immune regulation. COX-2 is the enzyme responsible for PGE-2 production, a prominent immunosuppressive cytokine with numerous direct and indirect effects that polarize the immune response towards suppression or tolerance. Specifically, PGE-2 and monocyte-derived IL 10 induced by PGE2 may significantly suppress antigen presentation and proliferation of NSCLC specific T cells, as well as lead to premature death of DCs. Modifying the host environment with COX-2 inhibitors is feasible and a rational strategy to enhance T cell responses to DC vaccines. Literature and preliminary data support these precepts. Thus, studies are designed to test the routine effectiveness of DC vaccines in unresectable stage III NSCLC and further evaluate the immune modulating effects of COX-2 inhibitors used in concert with tumor vaccines. Postulating an inverse relationship between COX-2 activity and immunologic response to vaccines, biomarkers of COX-2 activity will be evaluated as correlative markers of immune reactivity. Markers will also be used to track biologic effects of the COX-2 inhibitor Celebrex in NSCLC.

Website: http://crisp.cit.nih.gov/crisp/Crisp_Query.Generate_Screen

- **Project Title: AUTOMATIC IMAGE REGISTRATION FOR PROSTATE RADIOTHERAPY**

Principal Investigator & Institution: Duncan, James S.; Professor; Diagnostic Radiology; Yale University 47 College Street, Suite 203 New Haven, Ct 065208047

Timing: Fiscal Year 2002; Project Start 03-FEB-2000; Project End 31-JAN-2004

Summary: The effectiveness of externam beam radiation treatment for prostate cancer is decreased due to a variety of uncertainties in the treatment setup, including the physical characteristics of the treatment beam, patient positioning issues, patient organ motion and operator non-reproducibility. The development and administration of a treatment plan using image- guided techniques to account for some of these uncertainties can positively impact its effectiveness. However, the use of these techniques to date has been limited by i.) a lack of accuracy, robustness and reproducibility in the registration of the high resolution 3D computed tomographic (3DCT) or simulator images acquired in a reference)or planning) frame to the highly noisy and blurry portal images, acquired in the treatment environment and ii.) the difficulty in measuring organ motion and relating it to these data. Thus, we first propose to develop a new automated, accurate, and robust system for performing bony anatomy- based 3DCT- to- multiple- (2D) portal image registration by simultaneously incorporating portal image segmentation. The system will rely on a combination of dense field (region-based) and sparse field (gradient/boundary features) information and will use information- theoretic metrics in an optimization framework to solve for the mapping parameters. This approach will be validated using a gold standard developed from serial CT acquisitions taken each week during the treatment. Next, we will study the relationship between setup variation due to bony structure movement and that due to organ motion in preparation for the design of a future complete system that can acquire treatment- environment images of the prostate using an ultrasound probe attached to an articulated arm in an external- skin-marker-based frame, and the 3DCT-to-multiple portal registration algorithm described above. The feasibility of using external markers to relate portal and ultrasound information will be a key part of this study as well. Finally, we will evaluate the utility of the 3DCT-to-multiple portal registration approach by applying it to the problem of quantitatively studying the sensitivity of errors in the delivery of an optimal dose distribution for a particular patient on a particular day to variations in patient-positioning-related setup for treatment plans of different complexity. These studies will help us understand the utility of more complex treatment plans and planning systems in today's health care environment.

Website: http://crisp.cit.nih.gov/crisp/Crisp_Query.Generate_Screen

- **Project Title: BIOIMAGING IN RADIOTHERAPY FOR LUNG CANCER**

Principal Investigator & Institution: Choi, Noah C.; Massachusetts General Hospital 55 Fruit St Boston, Ma 02114

Timing: Fiscal Year 2003; Project Start 30-SEP-2003; Project End 31-JUL-2008

Summary: (provided by applicant): The long-term goal of this study is to develop a biomarker, measurable 10 days after **radiotherapy** (RT) or chemoradiotherapy (CRT), which is capable of estimating the probability of tumor control (TCP) at 12 months (m) in non-small cell lung carcinoma (NSCLC). Accelerated glucose transport is a hallmark of biochemical changes that occur with malignant cellular transformation. Cessation of glucose uptake in response to RT or CRT may be an early biochemical event that may be a sign for eventual cell death leading to tumor control. The glucose analog, 2-fluoro-2-deoxy-D-glucose (FDG) allows a measurement of glucose metabolic rate (MRglc) by quantitative 18F-FDG and positron emission tomography (PET). MRglc 10 days after RT or CRT may vary depending upon the presence or absence of residual tumor, and the amount of residual tumor. There may be a correlation between the levels of residual MRglc 10 days after RT or CRT, representing the amount of residual tumor, and the rate of subsequent clinical tumor control at 12 m. We propose an in vivo assay in which the rate of tumor control at 12 m will be correlated with the levels of residual MRglc 10 days after RT or CRT. MRglc will be measured with simplified kinetic method of 18F-FDG PET at the primary lesion before and 10 days after RT or CRT, and at 3, 6, and 12 m follow-up. Patients with medically inoperable stage I and II, and locally advanced stage III NSCLC will be accrued for this study. Tumor control is defined as (1) absence of regrowth by computed tomography (CT) and (2) absence of an increase in MRglc from the nadir value after RT or CRT. Specific Aims of this study are: (1) To determine the levels of residual MRglc 10 days after RT or CRT and the rate of tumor control at 12 m at the corresponding levels of residual MRgtc, (2) To generate dose-response relationship between the gradient of residual MRglc and corresponding TCP from the above data, (3) To determine the level of residual MRglc that corresponds to the probability of tumor control (MRglc-TCP) >95% at 12 m, and (4) To plan for a phase II clinical study in which RT dose schedule and tumor volume for RT are guided by MRglc-TCP >95% with study endpoints of improved tumor control and survival over that of the current standard CRT or RT.

Website: http://crisp.cit.nih.gov/crisp/Crisp_Query.Generate_Screen

- **Project Title: BIOLOGICAL MAPPING OF BRAIN TUMORS USING MRI**

Principal Investigator & Institution: Mcmillan, Kathryn M.; Medical Physics; University of Wisconsin Madison 750 University Ave Madison, Wi 53706

Timing: Fiscal Year 2004; Project Start 01-JUN-2004; Project End 31-MAY-2007

Summary: (provided by applicant): Integrating advanced magnetic resonance imaging (MRI) methods should better describe and delineate glioblastoma multiforme (GBM) brain tumors in preparation for radiation therapy treatment. We hypothesize that the use of these imaging modalities will result in more precise **radiotherapy** treatment planning. The proposed research is based upon extensive preliminary data indicating chemical shift imaging (CSI), perfusion and diffusion imaging and MR-based hypoxia mapping add additional information about tumor physiology that can be incorporated into a treatment pJan with the goal of decreasing the rate of tumor recurrence. Although regions of abnormality on T2 MRI are known to correlate with microscopic spread of tumor, some of this abnormality represents edema without malignant cells while other areas may contain a high concentration of malignant cells that should be incorporated into the treatment boost volume. While most malignant brain tumors recur within the radiation treatment fields, 20-25% of recurrences occur outside of these fields. Thus, the imaging techniques will be used to identify "high-risk subvolumes" within each tumor, which may be at high risk of recurrence. After completing **radiotherapy,** patients will be followed with serial advanced MRI scans; the study endpoint being the first recurrence. The location of the recurrence will test the prediction of the advanced imaging methods.

Website: http://crisp.cit.nih.gov/crisp/Crisp_Query.Generate_Screen

- **Project Title: CANCER AND LEUKEMIA GROUP B**

Principal Investigator & Institution: Fleming, Gini F.; Associate Professor of Clinical Medicine; Medicine; University of Chicago 5801 S Ellis Ave Chicago, Il 60637

Timing: Fiscal Year 2002; Project Start 30-SEP-1986; Project End 31-MAR-2003

Summary: (adapted from the applicant's abstract): The University of Chicago has had a major commitment to both laboratory and clinical cancer research since 1930. As part of the clinical translation of that research, the University of Chicago and its Cancer Research Center joined the Cancer and Leukemia Group B (CALGB) in 1985, and has subsequently strongly supported the CALGB both scientifically and clinically. Numerous protocols, committees, and programs are lead by Chicago faculty. Over the past five years the University of Chicago has increased its accrual from 184 patient points to 294 patient points, and in 1996 27 percent of the main member's patient accrual was African American. These accomplishments occurred by disciplined activity at the main member and also by supporting seven dedicated affiliated institutions in northern Illinois, Michigan and Indiana. Chicago is in the process of adding three new affiliates in the next year and remains very involved with the training and quality control of all its affiliate institutions. The goals of this application are: (1) increase the patient accrual to 300-350 patients/year; (2) to lead and assist CALGB scientific activities in the disease-related committees of respiratory (Drs. Vokes and Olak), prostate (Drs. Vogelzang, Steinberg and Vijaykumar), breast (Dr. Fleming), leukemia (Dr. Larson) and GI (Dr. Mani); (3) to lead and assist and participate in the CALGB committees such as psycho/oncology (Marcy List, Ph.D.), pharmacology and experimental therapeutics (Dr. Ratain), transplantation (Dr. Williams), genetics (Dr. Olopade), AIDS related malignancies (Dr. Liebowitz), surgical oncology (Dr. Michelassi) and pathology (Dr. Vardiman); (4) to encourage Chicago faculty to be protocol chairs for future protocols; and (5) to actively assist and participate in the CALGB committees of audit, minority issues, oncology nursing, cancer control, and **radiotherapy.** The University of Chicago proposes to accomplish these goals by the following methods: (1) to increase accrual from the main member with the assistance of new energetic physicians in colorectal, breast, surgery, leukemia and prostate cancer and by generating new ideas for phase I, II and III protocols; (2) to maintain the high accrual from the affiliate hospitals and increasing accrual by adding new qualified affiliates; (3) to maintain the strong leadership roles of Drs. Vogelzang, Vokes, Larson, Schilsky, Ratain, Williams, Olopade, List, Vardiman and Michelassi within the CALGB; (4) to recruit new young investigators to CALGB leadership roles (Drs. Manni, Leibowitz and Daugherty); especially those with a specific laboratory expertise which can be correlated with clinical treatment or outcome; and (5) to provide volunteers for numerous CALGB administrative committees. The University of Chicago and its affiliates remain firmly committed to serving all members of their respective communities, especially serving the needs of women and minorities.

Website: http://crisp.cit.nih.gov/crisp/Crisp_Query.Generate_Screen

- **Project Title: CD1D REACTIVE T CELLS IN BONE MARROW TRANSPLANTATION**

Principal Investigator & Institution: Exley, Mark A.; Assistant Professor; Beth Israel Deaconess Medical Center St 1005 Boston, Ma 02215

Timing: Fiscal Year 2002; Project Start 01-FEB-2001; Project End 31-JAN-2004

Summary: (Applicant's Abstract) There are two distinct populations of CD1d-reactive T cells currently recognized, the 'classical' CD161+ (NK1) invariant TCR-alpha positive 'NK T cells' and 'non-invariant' polyclonal T cells. Murine bone marrow (BM) T cells are dominated by CD4/CD8-double negative (DN) non-invariant CD1d-reactive CD161+ T cells. BM DN CD161+ T cells can suppress both graft versus host disease (GvH) in vivo following bone marrow transplantation (BMT), and mixed lymphocyte reactions (MLR) in vitro. BMT following high dose chemo-/radiotherapy is used for a range of cancers.

High dose cytotoxic treatments achieve better tumor clearance, but are myeloablative. BMT results in long term hematopoietic cell reconstitution, and activated T lymphocytes in the BMT graft can contribute to therapy ('graft versus tumor', GvT). However, allo-reactive T cells can also cause acute graft versus host disease (GvH), a serious complication of BMT. There is emerging evidence that it is possible to separately influence these two effects of BMT. The applicant has found that human CD161+ invariant T cells recognize CD1d on diverse targets. In contrast, a large fraction of mature T cells in human BM preferentially recognize CD1d on lymphoid cells and are "non-invariant". Peripheral blood progenitor cell (PBPC) product also contains substantial numbers of non-invariant CD1d-reactive T cells. His preliminary data with human CD1d-reactive T cells show overall similarity to results in the mouse and considerable potential for protection against GvH. Therefore, this application is to determine whether human BM and PBPC-derived CD1d-reactive T cells taken at harvest can be expanded in vitro to therapeutically relevant numbers whilst retaining the phenotype potential to ameliorate MLR/GvH. These preclinical studies are necessary to evaluate the hypothesis that human CD1d-reactive T cells have the therapeutic potential to selectively suppress acute GvH in the context of conventional BM and PBPC transplants for cancer.

Website: http://crisp.cit.nih.gov/crisp/Crisp_Query.Generate_Screen

- **Project Title: CERVICAL CANCER--PREDICTIVE ASSAY BY MR IMAGING**

Principal Investigator & Institution: Mayr, Nina A.; Radiological Sciences; University of Oklahoma Hlth Sciences Ctr Health Sciences Center Oklahoma City, Ok 73126

Timing: Fiscal Year 2003; Project Start 21-SEP-1998; Project End 31-JUL-2005

Summary: Radiotherapy is the principal treatment modality for advanced cervical cancer, but local control is frequently not achieved. The failure rate may be reduced by treating high-risk patients with more intense therapies including higher doses of radiation, chemotherapy, and/or surgery. However, there is no well-established predictor to identify patients whose high risk for failure justified the increased morbidity of more aggressive therapy. The investigators seek to identify those at high risk early, such that more aggressive treatment can be rendered that may improve outcome. Quantitative tumor volume and enhancement pattern analysis based on sequential MRI examination were shown to provide very early signals of failure in plot studies. Tumor size and dynamic enhancement pattern judged by the MRI prior to radiation therapy and temporal changes during the early course of radiation therapy appear to be sensitive predictors of tumor response; consistent with the notion that tumor blood supply and or oxygenation status strongly influence radiation response. The overall goal of this project is to test the hypothesis that MR-based measurements predict the likelihood of tumor control in patients with advanced cervical cancer treated by conventional radiation therapy. This will be achieved by three specific aims: (1) further develop, test, and refine predictive metrics of advanced cervical cancer radio-responsiveness based on contrast enhanced MRI and MR-based tumor volumetry, (2) apply MRI in a clinical population through their course of therapy and correlate tumor response with image-based metrics, and (3) determine predictive value (positive and negative) of MRI-based metrics. On completion, this project will provide a clinically validated MR protocol for prediction of tumor radio-responsiveness in advanced cervical carcinoma treated with radio-therapy. A prognostic index using MRI in a clinical setting to identify the high-risk patients who require more aggressive multi-modality therapy will be developed. The pixel signal distribution within the entire tumor between the radiosensitive and resistant groups will be further defined using multi-spectral and multi- temporal analysis, and characterized to discern subgroups contributing to treatment failure within the heterogeneous tumor.

Website: http://crisp.cit.nih.gov/crisp/Crisp_Query.Generate_Screen

- **Project Title: CHARACTERIZATION OF THE P53 APOPTOTIC TARGET GENE PERP**

  Principal Investigator & Institution: Attardi, Laura D.; Radiation Oncology; Stanford University Stanford, Ca 94305

  Timing: Fiscal Year 2002; Project Start 01-JAN-2002; Project End 31-DEC-2006

  Summary: The p53 tumor suppressor is mutated in at least half of all human cancers, and mice deficient in p53 develop cancer at 100 percent frequency, underscoring the critical role of p53 in preventing tumorigenesis. p53 exerts its tumor suppressive function by sensing cellular stress and inducing cells to undergo either G1 arrest or apoptosis to limit their proliferation. Although the mechanism by which p53 activates G1 arrest is becoming clearer, there is considerably less understanding of the mechanism by which it induces apoptosis. To identify genes specifically activated during apoptosis, we performed a subtractive hybridization screen in which G1-arrested cell RNA populations were subtracted from apoptotic cell RNA populations. In this screen, we isolated a novel gene, PERP (p53 apoptosis effector related to PMP-22), that is preferentially expressed in apoptotic cells. PERP encodes a novel tetraspan membrane protein related to the PMP-22/gas3 protein commonly implicated in human hereditary peripheral neuropathies such as Charcot Marie Tooth disease. PERP is induced during p53-dependent but not p53- independent apoptosis, and expression of PERP in cells is sufficient to induce cell death, together suggesting it is a strong candidate mediator of p53 function in apoptosis. The role of PERP in p53 function will be investigated in this proposal. To conclusively determine the importance of PERP in p53 function, a PERP knockout mouse has been generated. Through analysis of various cell types derived from PERP-deficient mice, the importance of PERP for p53-mediated apoptosis will be defined. Furthermore, by studying PERP null mice, the role of PERP in normal development as well as in p53-mediated tumor suppression will be elucidated. If there is an embryonic lethal phenotype of the PERP null mice, we will utilize a conditional PERP knockout mouse we have also generated to specifically inactivate PERP in certain tissues and determine its role as a tumor suppressor in those contexts. In addition, the mechanism by which PERP induces cell death will be examined through cell biological approaches, to clarify the link between p53 and the apoptotic machinery. Together, these approaches will define the role of PERP in mediating p53 function in apoptosis and tumor suppression. As activation of the p53-dependent apoptotic response is thought to determine the response of at least some tumor types to **radiotherapy** and chemotherapy, an understanding of the pathway also has important clinical implications, both for prognosis and therapy.

  Website: http://crisp.cit.nih.gov/crisp/Crisp_Query.Generate_Screen

- **Project Title: CHILDRENS NATIONAL MEDICAL CENTER**

  Principal Investigator & Institution: Packer, Roger J.; Children's Research Institute Washington, D.C., Dc 20010

  Timing: Fiscal Year 2002; Project Start 01-APR-1999; Project End 31-MAR-2004

  Summary: As a member of the Pediatric Brain Tumor Clinical Trials Consortium, the CNMC Neuro-Oncology Program proposes to develop, facilitate, and participate in innovative hypothesis-driven, technically challenging, clinical research designed to improve the survival and quality of life of children with primary central nervous system tumors. It is anticipated that these investigations will include, but will not be limited to: the use of novel chemotherapeutic agents; means to overcome the blood-brain barrier, immunotherapeutic approaches; modifications of radiation therapy; and new neurobiologic approaches, such as gene therapy, maturation agents, and anti-angiogenesis agents. The CNMC Neuro-Oncology Program plans on participating in research investigations which will improve the means to diagnose and characterize childhood brain tumors and to develop and participate in carefully monitored innovative diagnostic and therapeutic studies which will lead to future Phase III studies for children with such tumors. Over the past five years, the CNMC Neuro-Oncology Program has evaluated and managed 442 children (new to the institution) with primary central nervous system tumors and has entered over 189 children on Phase I, Phase II, and Phase III clinical investigations. Investigations have been done over this period of time, in concert with private industry and working groups, evaluating novel approaches such as gene therapy, immunotherapy, and approaches to overcome the blood-brain barrier; as well as evaluations of new chemotherapeutic agents, intensification of chemotherapy, and means to increase the efficacy of **radiotherapy.** The CNMC Neuro-Oncology Program has a well-developed multidisciplinary clinical core which includes a weekly neuro-oncology clinic, a quarterly groupwide neuro- oncology planning meeting, and a regional referral system. The program has a well-designed data management system, and an established system for specimen accrual. State-of-the-art neuroradiologic, neuropathologic, neurosurgical and radiation-oncologic facilities are available. In addition, innovative neurobiologic investigations in childhood brain tumors have been successfully completed and are underway at CNMC. The well-developed program structure, expertise of the CNMC Neuro-Oncology Program, proven commitment to performance of clinical trials, and available facilities should ensure the ability of the CNMC Neuro-Oncology Program to effectively participate in the proposed Pediatric Brain Tumor Clinical Consortium.

Website: http://crisp.cit.nih.gov/crisp/Crisp_Query.Generate_Screen

- **Project Title: CIRCULATING INHIBITORS OF ENDOTHELIAL CELL GROWTH**

Principal Investigator & Institution: Folkman, Judah Judah.; Director; Children's Hospital (Boston) Boston, Ma 021155737

Timing: Fiscal Year 2002; Project Start 16-MAY-1995; Project End 31-DEC-2003

Summary: (Adapted from the investigator's abstract) The long term objectives of this grant and its Specific Aims are: 1) To elucidate the molecular mechanisms of action of two endogenous inhibitors of angiogenesis previously identified in this laboratory, and 2) To discover other proteins which make up a family of natural angiogenesis inhibitors in the body. The first Aim will focus on the following questions: 1) What is the effect of angiostatin on endothelial cell cycle progression? 2) How does glycosylation effect angiostatin function? 3) How is collagen XVIII processed to endostatin? And 4) What is the molecular mechanism of the specificity of endostatin as an inhibitor of vascular endothelial cells? The second Aim will involve purification and sequencing of a new angiogenesis inhibitor that has recently been detected. They will employ a double tumor model in mice, also called the "concomitant resistance" model. One of these inhibitors is generated by human bladder cancer cells. Endostatin is already in clinical trial. They believe that these inhibitors along with others, yet to be identified and fully characterized, may eventually be added to conventional chemotherapy or to **radiotherapy** or to immunotherapy to improve efficacy of anti-cancer therapy, to decrease toxicity, and to reduce the development of acquired drug resistance. A study of mechanism of endogenous inhibitors may enlarge their understanding of the family of proteins which operate to suppress angiogenesis under physiological conditions.

Website: http://crisp.cit.nih.gov/crisp/Crisp_Query.Generate_Screen

- **Project Title: CLINICAL INVESTIGATION IN HODGKIN'S DISEASE**

Principal Investigator & Institution: Horning, Sandra J.; Professor of Medicine; Medicine; Stanford University Stanford, Ca 94305

Timing: Fiscal Year 2002; Project Start 07-FEB-1992; Project End 31-MAR-2006

Summary: (Provided by applicant): The long-term objectives of this application are to maintain or improve the efficacy ofHodgkin's disease (HD) therapy while reducing late effects through a series of clinical trials in which novel, abbreviated chemotherapy is combined with reduced volumes and doses of radiation therapy. The specific aims in this proposal represent the evolution of prospective clinical trials conducted at Stanford University Medical Center continuously since 1962. During that period of time, the influence of advances in diagnostics, staging, multi-modality therapeutics and appreciation of the late effects of treatment has extended from HD management to that of other neoplasms. Although the cure rate of HD is high relative to other cancers, morbidity and mortality in excess of that expected on the basis of age and gender, primarily due to second cancers and ischemic heart disease provides a strong rationale for continued clinical investigations. In Aim 1, a risk-adapted Phase II trial is proposed for favorable, early stage disease in which patients will receive 12 weeks of chemotherapy alone or 8 weeks of chemotherapy and low dose **radiotherapy.** Following the success of Stanford V chemotherapy with or without **radiotherapy** and international consensus in prognostic factors in advanced HD, a Phase III Intergroup trial comparing this approach with ABVD is proposed in patients with 0-2 risk factors in Aim 2. For higher risk patients, those with 3 or more adverse factors, a Phase II trial of a novel chemotherapy regimen based upon Stanford V and introducing the new active agents, gemcitabine and vinorelbine, is planned in Aim 3. Aim 4 relates to the continued follow-up of patients enrolled in HD clinical trials at Stanford since 1962 and the provision of information management and statistical support to analyze efficacy and long-term morbidity and mortality. The ability to chronicle the late effects of treatment at Stanford has been made possible by a dedicated group of investigators, use of standardized diagnostics and treatments, and maintenance of a database now containing information on more than 3000 HD patients. Identification and notification of patients at risk is important for follow-up care and screening, where appropriate. Continued follow-up of HD patients and maintenance of the Stanford HD database, which can be considered a national resource, has never been more important as the time period after treatment of patients receiving lower doses and volumes of **radiotherapy** as well as novel combinations of chemotherapy approaches 10-15 years, a critical latency for second cancers.

Website: http://crisp.cit.nih.gov/crisp/Crisp_Query.Generate_Screen

- **Project Title: COGNITIVE BEHAVIORAL ASPECTS OF CANCER RELATED FATIGUE**

Principal Investigator & Institution: Jacobsen, Paul B.; Professor and Director, Health Outcomes; Psychology; University of South Florida 4202 E Fowler Ave Tampa, Fl 33620

Timing: Fiscal Year 2002; Project Start 01-SEP-1999; Project End 31-MAY-2004

Summary: It is estimated that 178,700 American women will be diagnosed with breast cancer in 1998. A large proportion of these women will receive adjuvant chemotherapy,

radiotherapy, and/or hormonal therapy based on evidence indicating that such treatment extends disease-free survival as well as overall survival. As more women receive adjuvant treatment, there is growing recognition of the potential for long-term side effects. Along these lines, it has been shown that administration of adjuvant chemotherapy can result in secondary leukemia, cardiotoxicity, and ovarian failure. Clinical observations and a limited number of research reports suggest that persistent fatigue may also be a long-term side effect of adjuvant chemotherapy. Although fatigue has been identified as one of the most frequent and distressing symptoms affecting breast cancer patients treated with adjuvant chemotherapy, relatively little is known about its characteristics, etiology, or treatment. We propose to address these issues by conducting the first controlled, longitudinal study of fatigue in breast cancer patients before, during, and after adjuvant chemotherapy and **radiotherapy** treatment. Women with early stage breast cancer scheduled to receive adjuvant treatment will be recruited and undergo a baseline assessment before the start of chemotherapy. Additional assessments will be performed during the course of chemotherapy and before and during a subsequent course of **radiotherapy.** Following completion of **radiotherapy,** patients will continue to be monitored for six months. An age-matched sample of women with no history of cancer will be recruited and monitored over a six-month period for comparison purposes. These data will be used: 1) to determine the severity, chronicity, and course of fatigue associated with adjuvant treatment of breast cancer; 2) to characterize the cognitive, affective, and behavioral manifestations of fatigue that persists following completion of adjuvant treatment; and 3) to test the utility of a cognitive-behavioral model designed to explain the perpetuation of fatigue following completion of adjuvant treatment. Preliminary analyses of study data are expected to provide empirical support for adaptation and pilot testing, during the final months of funding, of a cognitive-behavioral intervention originally developed for chronic fatigue syndrome for use with breast cancer patients experiencing persistent fatigue related to adjuvant treatment.

Website: http://crisp.cit.nih.gov/crisp/Crisp_Query.Generate_Screen

- **Project Title: COMBINED RADIOIMMUNOTHERAPY WITH RADIOTHERAPY**

Principal Investigator & Institution: Humm, John L.; Associate Member; Sloan-Kettering Institute for Cancer Res New York, Ny 100216007

Timing: Fiscal Year 2002; Project Start 01-APR-1999; Project End 31-JAN-2004

Summary: This grant application examines the hypothesis that radiolabeled antibody heterogeneity is the principal source of failure of radioimmunotherapy (RIT). It proposes that this limitation can be overcome by the combination of RIT with external beam **radiotherapy** (XRT). This study will investigate the interaction between XRT with RIT, and determine the optimum combination of these two modalities for maximum tumor efficacy. The hypothesis will be tested with the murine SW1222 colorectal xenograft model system using intact A33 IgG monoclonal antibody as the targeting agent and its single chain hypervariable sFv fragment. There are four specific aims: (1) To determine the 3D microdistribution of radiolabeled A33 IgG within the SW1222 tumor xenograft system using phosphor plate autoradiography. The dependence of the distribution will be investigated with respect of the antibody/antigen molar ratio, the effect of molecular weight, by concomitant administration of the single chain hypervariable fragment sFv A33 with the parent A33 IgG, and following pre-external beam irradiation. (2) To determine how radiation tissue damage facilitates/impedes the penetration of antibody into the tumor. This will be achieved by conventional histological and immunohistochemical stains designed to ascertain the effects of radiation damage on tumor blood supply, tumor cell density, as well as antigen density and inflammatory response. These changes will be used to provide a scientific rationale for the measured radiolabeled antibody distribution from specific aim 1. In addition, this aim will attempt to quantitate changes in tumor cell response by determining the fraction of cells undergoing apoptotic cell death, (by the tunel assay), as well as changes in the fraction of cycling cells, (determined by IUdR incorporation and Ki67 and PCNA immunohistochemistry), as a surrogate of mitotic cell death. (3) To determine the therapeutic efficacy by tumor growth delay and cure after treatment with XRT and RIT alone and then in combination. Experiments will be performed in which tumors are treated with XRT followed by RIT, XRT and RIT simultaneously, and RIT prior to XRT, in order to determine the optimum combination therapy. Variations in the tumor response will be correlated with the results from aim 1 and 2. (4) To develop a radiobiological model, which determines the therapeutic effectiveness from a heterogeneous activity distribution. The model will be tested using information from the source distribution from autoradiographic data (aim 1) to predict overall tumor response measured by specific aim 3.

Website: http://crisp.cit.nih.gov/crisp/Crisp_Query.Generate_Screen

- **Project Title: CORE: CHEMISTRY / MOLECULAR IMAGING CHEMISTRY**

  Principal Investigator & Institution: Piwnica-Worms, David R.; Professor of Radiology; Washington University Lindell and Skinker Blvd St. Louis, Mo 63130

  Timing: Fiscal Year 2002; Project Start 31-MAY-2002; Project End 31-MAR-2007

  Summary: (provided by applicant) The MICC will serve as a crucial interface for various interdisciplinary projects proposed in this P50 grant. In addition to ensuring the timely availability of chemical reagents necessary for bioassays proposed by various investigators, the core will also provide a training environment for students and post-doctoral fellows in chelation chemistry, radiopharmaceutical synthesis, optical probe conjugation and preparation of MR relaxivity agents. To meet these needs, the MICC will supply information, reagents, and effort in three important areas: 1) PET and SPECT radiopharmaceuticals for molecular imaging of reporter gene expression, 2) Peptide-based radiopharmaceuticals for imaging and **radiotherapy,** and 3) Near infrared probes for molecular imaging applications.

  Website: http://crisp.cit.nih.gov/crisp/Crisp_Query.Generate_Screen

- **Project Title: DEVELOPING LIGAND/RECEPTOR SYSTEM WITH INFINITE AFFINITY**

  Principal Investigator & Institution: Chmura, a J.; Lexrite Labs Box 473, 100 N 1St St Dixon, Ca 95620

  Timing: Fiscal Year 2002; Project Start 01-APR-2002; Project End 31-MAR-2004

  Summary: (provided by applicant): Developing technology to target therapeutic agents to cancer cells, while sparing normal cells, is a promising approach to improved treatment. The specific targeting reagents of choice are monoclonal antibodies and their derivatives. Currently there is a good selection of such molecules that bind to highly expressed tumor antigens. The anticancer antibodies Rituxan and Herceptin have been approved by the FDA for use as therapeutic drugs, and several more antibody-based drugs are expected to be approved soon. The binding affinities of many antibodies to characteristic cancer antigens are strikingly low; they depend on multivalent binding for their practical utility. For this reason, the utility of engineered proteins with single binding sites-such as single chain Fv molecules or Fab fragments-is limited. The use of modern combinatorial genetic techniques has led to improvements in the antigen-binding properties of engineered proteins, but further advances are needed. We propose a combined genetic/chemical approach to radically improve one such ligand/receptor interaction to the point of specific, irreversible binding. This research will ultimately lead to products that are themselves therapeutic drugs, or that serve as the first step in targeting drugs, radionuclides, or other effectors, to sites of disease. PROPOSED COMMERCIAL APPLICATION: Target-selective, irreversibly bindig platform for drug delivery, suitable for use in targeted therapy, **radiotherapy,** prodrug delivery, and other applications where long-lived specific binding is preferred.

Website: http://crisp.cit.nih.gov/crisp/Crisp_Query.Generate_Screen

- **Project Title: DEVELOPMENT OF NEW HYPOXIC CYTOTOXINS FOR CANCER THERAPY**

Principal Investigator & Institution: Brown, J Martin.; Professor and Director; Radiation Oncology; Stanford University Stanford, Ca 94305

Timing: Fiscal Year 2002; Project Start 25-APR-2000; Project End 31-MAR-2004

Summary: Improvements in the cure rate of cancer by current treatments, including **radiotherapy** and chemotherapy, depend on exploiting some difference between normal and malignant tissues. One such difference is their level of oxygenation: human solid tumors are on average poorly oxygenated compared to normal tissues because of their inadequate vascularization to tumors is currently a negative prognostic factor, it could also be exploited if a drug that is activated to a cytotoxic species only under low oxygenation could be added to standard therapy. Tirapazamine (TPZ), a drug preferentially metabolized under hypoxia, is the first drug to enter clinical trials to test this rationale. Importantly, it has proven effective in Phase II and II clinical trials when combined with the ant-cancer drug, cisplatin. However, the efficacy of TPZ is limited by its systemic toxicity, particularly when combined with **radiotherapy.** We have recently discovered a number of features of the enzymology and toxicity of TPZ as well as developed new assays that could potentially be exploited in development of analogs of TPZ designed to maximize anti- tumor efficacy and minimize systemic toxicity. This Program Project combines the efforts of three laboratories with extensive experience in the design, synthesis and testing of hypoxia-activated cytotoxic compounds, including TPZ. The goal of the collaboration will be apply these newly discovered features and assays, as well as the extensive knowledge gained of factors affecting the efficacy and toxicity of hypoxic cytotoxins, to develop optimum second generation TPZ analogs for use with fractionated radiation and for use with cisplatin-based chemotherapy.

Website: http://crisp.cit.nih.gov/crisp/Crisp_Query.Generate_Screen

- **Project Title: DEVELOPMENT OF NEW PEPTIDE-PEPTIDE NUCLEI ACID CONJUGATES: FOR IMAGING OF BCL-XL**

Principal Investigator & Institution: Lewis, Michael R.; University of Missouri Columbia 310 Jesse Hall Columbia, Mo 65211

Timing: Fiscal Year 2003; Project Start 01-AUG-2003; Project End 31-JUL-2008

Summary: (Revised Abstract) (provided by applicant): The overall goal of the proposed research is to develop new radiolabeled peptide-peptide nucleic acid (peptide-PNA) constructs for molecular imaging of proto-oncogene expression in cancer. The hypotheses to be addressed in this application are 1) that overexpression of bcI-XL in non-Hodgkin's lymphoma (NHL) can be detected in vivo by radiolabeled antisense PNAs conjugated to peptides for intracellular delivery, and 2) that in vivo imaging of bcI-XL overexpression correlates with poor response to conventional chemotherapy in canine lymphoma patients. The bcI-XL gene is a member of a new category of cellular oncogenes involved in blocking tumor cell apoptosis, which is a major cytotoxic response to chemotherapy and **radiotherapy.** Furthermore, bcl- XL overexpression is involved in blocking anoikis, or anchorage-dependent apoptosis, and may play a role in tumor invasion and metastasis. The objective of this research application is to synthesize peptide-antisense-PNA conjugates labeled with the diagnostic imaging radiometal 111In and evaluate these radiopharmaceuticals for bcl- XL mRNA targeting in vitro and in vivo. These goals will be accomplished by synthesizing new bcI-XL antisense PNAs conjugated to peptides for intracellular delivery (Specific Aim 1), evaluating the bcI-XL mRNA binding properties of the peptide-PNA conjugates by Northern blot analysis (Specific Aim 2), performing in vitro cell uptake, internalization, efflux, and fluorescence microscopy studies of the peptide-PNA conjugates in bcI-XL -positive and -negative lymphoma cell lines in culture (Specific Aim 3), performing biodistribution and microSPECT imaging studies in SCID mice bearing human NHL xenografts, in order to select the optimal tumor targeting conjugate (Specific Aim 4), and evaluating the optimal 111In- labeled anti-bcI-XL peptide-PNA construct by performing gamma scintigraphy studies in canine lymphoma patients receiving conventional chemotherapy, in order to determine whether in vivo bcI-XL imaging correlates with treatment outcome (Specific Aim 5).

Website: http://crisp.cit.nih.gov/crisp/Crisp_Query.Generate_Screen

- **Project Title: ENHANCING RADIATION THERAPY: VASCULAR TARGETING AGENTS**

Principal Investigator & Institution: Siemann, Dietmar W.; Professor and Associate Chair for Resear; Radiation Oncology; University of Florida Gainesville, Fl 32611

Timing: Fiscal Year 2004; Project Start 01-APR-2004; Project End 31-MAR-2008

Summary: (provided by applicant): The aberrant vascular morphology, spatial heterogeneity in vessels, and metabolic microenvironments associated with solid tumors, are major factors contributing to treatment failures in **radiotherapy.** Since all of these may be affected by treatment with vascular targeting agents (VTAs), the combination of such agents with **radiotherapy** is likely to improve treatment outcomes. Indeed, we previously have shown that combining a VTA with **radiotherapy** would allow the two treatments to act in a complimentary fashion in tumors at the microregional level resulting in an overall amplification of the antitumor effects of radiation. Though clearly promising, many questions regarding the successful application of this new approach to cancer treatment remain. The central goal of the present application is to develop new insights into the underlying mechanisms of vascular targeting therapy and to explore new avenues to maximize its therapeutic potential. One of the issues to be addressed in this research program is whether at lower doses than have typically be used pre-clinically, but closer to those attainable in the clinic, enhancement of radiation response by VTAs is still feasible. Secondly, we propose to examine whether post VTA treatment conditions provide a favorable setting for the application of antiangiogenic therapies. This strategy is based on the observation that cells surviving VTA treatment at the tumor periphery aggressively promote neovascularization in order to achieve the rapid regrowth that occurs from the viable rim. A third component of the program is focused on the evaluation of new emerging second generation compounds as current VTAs progress through early clinical trial evaluations. Specifically the antitumor potency and potential superiority of a recently identified lead candidate analog of combretastatin will be examined. Finally, based on the hypothesis that targeting the tumor neovasculature should offer the possibility of inducing responses in all tumors with an established vessel network, we will examine whether in addition to their activity in primary tumors, VTAs can impact the management of metastatic disease.

Website: http://crisp.cit.nih.gov/crisp/Crisp_Query.Generate_Screen

- **Project Title: EXPERIMENTAL RADIOTHERAPY--CARCINOGENESIS, AND PROTECTOR**

  Principal Investigator & Institution: Grdina, David J.; Professor; Radiation & Cellular Oncology; University of Chicago 5801 S Ellis Ave Chicago, Il 60637

  Timing: Fiscal Year 2002; Project Start 30-SEP-1983; Project End 31-MAY-2004

  Summary: While the ultimate goal of this investigation continues to be the characterization of chemopreventive strategies to reduce the genotoxic damage to normal tissues by ionizing radiation during the treatment of potentially curable neoplastic disease, the focus of this application is directed to the investigation of the inhibitory effects of thiols on the process of spontaneous metastasis development. This study will utilize the SA-NH sarcoma that is capable of being grown in C3H mice as a model of spontaneous metastasis formation. SA-NH cell lines are also available for growth under in vitro conditions. The thiols chosen for study are amifostine, N-acetylcysteine (NAC), and captopril because each is currently in clinical use and each has been observed to have an inhibitory effect on metastases development in rodent tumor models. It is anticipated that if any or all of these thiols are found effective in inhibiting metastases formation in mice, their use as anti-metastatic agents could rapidly be translated to clinical protocols for cancer treatment. This study will focus only on thiol related properties that can affect certain well characterized steps in the metastatic process. Three hypotheses will be tested. First, because thiols are sulfhydryl doners they can stimulate the intracellular production of angiostatin, an inhibitor of angiogenesis, from plasminogen. Second, by virtue of their ability to chelate zinc, thiols can inhibit zinc binding to the zinc requiring matrix metalloproteinases (MMPs). In this manner MMP activities required for tumor cell invasion into normal tissues are inhibited. And third, thiols can enhance gene expression and enzyme activity of MnSOD in tumor cells which in turn leads to a reduced metastatic phenotype. Techniques to be used include Northern blot analysis to assess MnSOD gene expression; Western blot analysis to assess angiostatin production; zymogram analysis to measure MMP activities; a spontaneous metastases assay involving the assessment of pulmonary metastases formed following the surgical removal of the primary tumor; and an artificial metastasis assay involving the assessment of pulmonary tumors formed following the injection of viable tumor cells treated under in vitro conditions and then injected into the lateral tail veins of recipient animals.

  Website: http://crisp.cit.nih.gov/crisp/Crisp_Query.Generate_Screen

- **Project Title: FIBER DELIVERY OF CO2 LASERS FOR LARYNGEAL CARCINOMA**

  Principal Investigator & Institution: King, Wesley A.; Omniguide Communications, Inc. 1 Kendall Sq, Bldg 100, 3Rd Fl 02139, Ma 02139

  Timing: Fiscal Year 2004; Project Start 07-MAY-2004; Project End 31-OCT-2004

  Summary: (provided by applicant): The objective of this SBIR proposal is to improve the treatment options for laryngeal carcinoma by developing a fiber enabled CO2 laser system for laryngeal minimally invasive surgery. Current treatments involve **radiotherapy,** chemotherapy, and surgical procedures either through open surgery or through a laryngoscope. The surgeon has several operating tools at his disposal. These include cold steel surgical instruments, as well as laser beams, which can be used through the laryngoscope. The CO_2 laser is the predominant laser tool for these types of surgeries. There is currently no adequate fiber for delivering CO_2 laser for these medical procedures. Accordingly, CO_2 laser systems utilize rigid lens and mirror systems to deliver the laser beam to the treated tissue. Introduction of a fiber enabled CO_2 laser system will enable tangential cutting, easier manipulation of tissue, higher precision, and most importantly, the ability to reach previously inaccessible tissue, for example in the lower airway. While several different fibers have been tried for CO_2 laser delivery, including chalcogenide, polycrystalline and hollow-core metal-coated fibers, none of them have been able to fulfill the entire set of specifications for this application. OmniGuide Communications (OGCI) has developed a new approach for the fabrication of photonic bandgap fibers, based on technology it has exclusively licensed and transferred from MIT. In this Project (Phase I and II) OGCI will leverage its unique technology to develop a fiber that will meet the specifications for laryngological surgery. Phase I will focus on the development of a prototype fiber. Phase II will focus on system integration. Our commercial front, OGCI will collaborate with Lumenis, the world leader in medical laser systems. Our academic partners include both MGH and MEEI. The final goal of this Project is to bring a fiber enabled CO_2 laser system for laryngology to market.

Website: http://crisp.cit.nih.gov/crisp/Crisp_Query.Generate_Screen

- **Project Title: FLT PET TO PLAN THE BEST THERAPY FOR LUNG CANCER**

Principal Investigator & Institution: Vesselle, Hubert J.; Assistant Professor; Radiology; University of Washington Office of Sponsored Programs Seattle, Wa 98105

Timing: Fiscal Year 2004; Project Start 01-APR-2004; Project End 31-MAR-2009

Summary: (provided by applicant): Approximately 45,000 new patients are diagnosed with locally advanced non-small cell lung cancer (stage III NSCLC) each year in the United States. Such disease extent precludes a primary resection for most and at the present time, the best survival rates are achieved by administering concurrent chemotherapy and **radiotherapy** followed by surgical resection for some or by additional chemotherapy for others. However, definite criteria to select patients for either therapeutic approach are not established. Furthermore, the optimal therapy for stage III NSCLC is not yet known and the search for it remains empirical. These limitations result in part from an inability to assess the response of these tumors to chemoradiotherapy with standard anatomically based imaging as Computed Tomography (CT) often overestimates or underestimates residual tumor after therapy. These difficulties are compounded by the lack of tumor markers able to predict or track tumor response. The proposed study plans to develop a novel and more accurate measure of tumor response by evaluating stage III NSCLC patients with FDG PET and FLT (3'-deoxy-3'-[F-18]fluorothymidine) PET prior to and at the conclusion of chemoradiotherapy. PET imaging findings will be compared to clinical and pathological tumor response and to patient outcome. Although FDG PET has demonstrated its usefulness and accuracy as a staging tool in untreated patients, its efficacy in the evaluation of the primary tumor and lymph node response is limited. However, FDG PET will provide valuable information regarding the development of distant metastatic disease outside of **radiotherapy** ports, an important aspect of the overall response assessment. The new tracer FLT has shown its potential as a tracer of cellular proliferation in lung cancer making it ideally suited to evaluating NSCLC response to chemoradiotherapy. We also propose to make comparisons of these dual tracer studies with tumor specimen-derived markers of proliferation and tumor resistance to validate the significance of FLT uptake in tumor response. Finally, we propose to develop a model to predict the outcome of stage III NSCLC patients treated with chemoradiotherapy by using PET-derived measures of response and specimen-derived measures of resistance. This study will constitute the initial validation of FLT as a PET imaging agent to assess tumor response to therapy. At the conclusion of this study, the insight gained in the response of stage III NSCLCs will allow clinicians to plan the best therapy for these patients.

Website: http://crisp.cit.nih.gov/crisp/Crisp_Query.Generate_Screen

- **Project Title: FUNCTION DOMAINS OF KU PROTEINS AS MOLECULAR TARGETS**

Principal Investigator & Institution: Chen, Fanqing; Molecular Biology; University of Calif-Lawrenc Berkeley Lab Lawrence Berkeley National Laboratory Berkeley, Ca 94720

Timing: Fiscal Year 2002; Project Start 26-APR-2002; Project End 31-MAR-2004

Summary: (provided by applicant): Radiation is one of the most efficient therapeutic agents for certain types of cancer. However, cytotoxicity induced by ionizing radiation limits the radiation dosage that can be administrated to patients. Alternatively, several DNA modification agents and other adjunct treatments have been utilized as "radiosensitizers" to combine with the standard **radiotherapy,** thus enhancing the radiosensitivity of the targeted cancer cells. Because of the inherent nonspecificity of current radiosensitizers, the enhancement ratio is relatively moderate, and the applicable range clinically, is limited by side effects. Meanwhile, it has become clear that disruption of DNA repair might dramatically increase radiosensitivity. In this research, we propose to explore the possibility of using DNA double-strand break repair proteins as novel molecular targets for the development of radiosensitizers. Specifically, we will focus on the Ku70 and Ku80 proteins (Ku70/80 heterodimers), which are critical components in the repair of ionizing radiation-induced double-strand breaks in mammalian cells. We plan to identify and validate specific domains of the Ku70/80 heterodimer as novel protein targets for identifying effective radiosensitizers. This study proposes to dissect Ku functional domain using genetic, biochemical, proteolytic digestion/mass spectrometry data, and to express the domains in soluble protein form. Using the expressed recombinant protein domains, we will demonstrate the validity of Ku domains as a molecular target with in vitro biochemical assays, and in vivo dominant negative phenotyping. We also intend to use the combinatorial phage display technique to screen for high-affinity peptides for the interested domains. In viva inhibition studies will be performed by introducing the peptide into cancer cells in a retroviral vector. We will also analyze the structural relationship between the peptide inhibitors and their affected functional domains by NMR. The ultimate goal for this study is to identify the Ku domains that can be used as molecular targets for inhibitory radiosensitizers, and to generate more specific inhibitors/effectors that direct more distinct damages to the cancer cells under inadiation.

Website: http://crisp.cit.nih.gov/crisp/Crisp_Query.Generate_Screen

- **Project Title: GENE METHYLATION AND THERAPEUTIC RESPONSE IN LUNG CANCER**

Principal Investigator & Institution: Belinsky, Steven A.; Director Lung Cancer Program; Lovelace Biomedical & Environmental Res Albuquerque, Nm 87108

Timing: Fiscal Year 2002; Project Start 01-JUN-2001; Project End 31-MAY-2006

Summary: Lung cancer is responsible for approximately one-third of all cancer-related deaths in the U.S. each year. Chemotherapy has been largely ineffective in producing complete responses or cures in the advanced disease setting. Therefore, investigation of new paradigms, including novel therapeutic approaches and early detection, has become an urgent priority for the oncology community. Key to early detection is the development of biomarkers that are found in primary tumor and can be detected in biological fluids prior to advanced disease. These biomarkers may also be useful for predicting therapeutic response during clinical trials. In support of these critical needs, our laboratory has identified two excellent biomarkers, the p16 tumor suppressor gene and the O6-methylguanine-DNA methyltransferase (MGMT) repair gene, whose inactivations through aberrant CpG island promoter hypermethylation occur frequently and early in the development of NSCLC. Furthermore, inactivation of these genes has been detected in exfoliated cells from sputum and shown to precede clinical diagnosis of squamous cell carcinoma (SCC). Aberrant methylation of p16, MGMT, and death-associated protein (DAP) kinase has also been detected in serum from NSCLC patients irrespective of tumor stage. Utilizing specimens and patients on ECOG study E3598, "A Phase III trial of Carboplatin, Paclitaxel and **Radiotherapy,** With or Without Thalidomide, in Patients With Stage III NSCLC," these advances in cancer biology will be translated into the clinic to address several important questions. First, can the detection of gene dysfunction in critical genes through analysis of sputum and/or serum be used for screening or as prognostic factors? This question will be addressed by determining the predictive power of sputum and serum to detect NSCLC through analysis for aberrant methylation of the p16, MGMT, DAP-kinase, and TIMP-3 genes within these biological fluids. Second, does inactivation of genes such as p16, DAP-kinase, or TIMP-3 in NSCLCs affect survival? A recent study demonstrated that median survival was shorter for patients with adenocarcinoma in which the p16 gene was inactivated. Thus, this question will be addressed by determining whether inactivation of p16, DAP-kinase, or TIMP-3 genes can be used to predict survival for patients on E3598. Finally, can detection of methylation markers in serum be useful for cancer diagnosis and/or have predictive value for survival? This will be addressed with patients on E3598. Results could have a profound impact on defining the utility of sputum and serum for detecting NSCLC, predicting survival from these therapeutic regimens, and delineating whether the presence of these tumor markers in serum affect survival. The validation of these genes as biomarkers of lung cancer risk and their detection in sputum and/or serum could ultimately support chemoprevention trials for preventing lung cancer.

Website: http://crisp.cit.nih.gov/crisp/Crisp_Query.Generate_Screen

- **Project Title: GENE MODIFIED CELL LINES AS VACCINE FOR PANCREAS CANCER**

Principal Investigator & Institution: Laheru, Daniel A.; Oncology; Johns Hopkins University 3400 N Charles St Baltimore, Md 21218

Timing: Fiscal Year 2002; Project Start 14-SEP-2002; Project End 31-JUL-2007

Summary: (provided by applicant): Pancreatic cancer is the fourth leading cause of cancer related deaths in the US. Although surgical resection is the only curative option, the median survival is only 15-19 months for resectable stage 1,2 and 3 disease. For patients who present with metastatic disease, the median survival is 3-6 months. The addition of chemotherapy and/or radiation therapy in select settings have resulted in only modest clinical benefits. Therefore, more effective therapies are urgently needed. The central theme of this grant proposal is to optimize immunotherapy for pancreatic cancer by designing and conducting clinical trials using genetically modified pancreatic tumor cell lines as vaccine that would improve on the outcome of: (1) patients with pancreatic adenocarcinoma following surgical resection when given in combination with chemoradiation (Specific Aim #1); and (2) patients with primary metastatic or relapsed disease when given in sequence with immune modulating doses of Paclitaxel or with cytoreductive doses of Gemcitabine (Specific Aim #2). We hypothesize that: (1) Biologic endpoints that include the measurement of post vaccination delayed type hypersensitivity (DTH) responses to autologous tumor (adjuvant study) or to mutated k-ras peptides (metastatic study) and the measurement of the immune infiltration at the vaccine site can correlate with clinical endpoints such as overall and disease-free survival. (2) Measurement of serum GM-CSF levels as a measure of longevity of the vaccine cells following each vaccination can provide an improved understanding of the in vivo kinetics of the allogeneic cells at the vaccine site and will allow for the optimization of the vaccine boosting schedule. (3) The vaccine is associated with minimal toxicities and can be safely integrated with chemotherapy and radiation therapy. The design of Specific Aim #1 is a single institution Phase II study of vaccine in combination with adjuvant chemoradiotherapy for the treatment of pancreatic adenocarcinoma following surgical resection. The study will enroll 60 patients over 2 years. The design of Specific Aim #2 is a single institution randomized study of vaccine in sequence with Gemcitabine or with Paclitaxel in patients with primary metastatic or relapsed pancreatic adenocarcinoma. This study will enroll 120 patients over 2 years. If these studies demonstrate anti-tumor immunity that is associated with prolongation of disease free survival, they will lead to the design and conduction of multi-center phase III studies. Ultimately, these studies could lead to the approval of a new therapeutic option for pancreatic cancer, which is currently fatal in most patients. In addition, data from these studies could contribute to a better understanding of how to schedule multiple vaccine boosts. Finally, these data will provide valuable information on how to best integrate the vaccine with other therapeutic modalities including surgery, **radiotherapy** and chemotherapy.

Website: http://crisp.cit.nih.gov/crisp/Crisp_Query.Generate_Screen

- **Project Title: GENETIC AND PHYSICAL ANALYSIS OF RECOMBINATION REPAIR**

Principal Investigator & Institution: Nickoloff, Jac A.; Professor and Chair; Molecular Genetics & Microbiol; University of New Mexico Albuquerque Controller's Office Albuquerque, Nm 87131

Timing: Fiscal Year 2002; Project Start 01-JUL-1992; Project End 31-DEC-2003

Summary: The goals of the proposed research are to clarify the mechanisms, genetic consequences, and interrelationships of recombination and mismatch repair in the model eukaryote, Saccharomyces cerevisiae. Additional goals are to clarify the genetic control of spontaneous and double-strand break (DSB)-induced recombination, and the effects of transcription on mismatch repair, recombination, and mutagenesis. In many of the proposed studies, HO nuclease will be used to cleave unique, defined genomic sites in yeast chromosomes; this is a controlled system for modeling DNA damage-induced recombination by genotoxic agents such as radiation. DNA repair and genetic recombination are ubiquitous and fundamental cellular processes that are involved, for example, in gene regulation, immune system development, and genetic instability associated with cellular transformation and tumor progression. Recombination is stimulated by many agents that damage DNA, such as ionizing radiation and radiomimetic chemicals; these agents are also known to be mutagenic and carcinogenic.

Mismatch repair defects are common in many forms of cancer. Five Aims are proposed. Aim 1 focuses on the role of mismatch repair during DSB-induced gene conversion. We will determine whether allelic gene conversion is mediated by mismatch repair; whether conversion on opposite sides of a DSB is mediated by independent mismatch repair tracts; and whether one or more heterozygosities increase conversion tract lengths. Aim 2 focuses on the repair of loop mismatches. Loop mismatch repair varies among organisms, it differs from single-base mismatch repair, and it is influenced by loop structure. We will determine whether unpaired bases in a stem-loop influence repair efficiency, and the efficiency of nonpalindromic loop repair. Aim 3 focuses on donor choice during DSB-induced gene conversion, including the effects of donor proximity and transcription levels, and the minimum length of a donor locus required for efficient DSB-induced gene conversion. Aim 4 focuses on the genetic control of spontaneous and DSB-induced recombination. We will employ both knock-out and overexpression strategies to investigate the roles of XRS2, RAD51, and RAD52 in recombinational repair. An overexpression strategy will also be used to identify new genes involved in spontaneous and/or DSB- induced recombination. Aim 5 focuses on transcriptional effects on DNA dynamics. We will determine whether transcription influences single-base mismatch repair, gene conversion tract directionality, allele conversion preference for spontaneous events; and mutagenic loss of palindromic sequences. These studies will provide insight into mechanistic aspects of DSB repair, transcription, recombination, and mismatch repair. These DNA dynamic processes are important in cancer etiology and cancer therapy (e.g., radiotherapy), and in technical aspects of gene therapy. Studies of transcriptional effects on DNA dynamics will provide insight into the different genetic consequences of DNA damage, repair, and recombination during development and during different stages of the cell cycle.

Website: http://crisp.cit.nih.gov/crisp/Crisp_Query.Generate_Screen

- **Project Title: GENOMIC AND PROTEOMIC ANALYSIS OF PROSTATE CANCER**

Principal Investigator & Institution: Sadar, Marianne D.; British Columbia Cancer Agency 600 W 10Th Ave Vancouver, Bc

Timing: Fiscal Year 2004; Project Start 01-APR-2004; Project End 31-MAR-2009

Summary: (provided by applicant): Localized prostate cancer can be treated surgically or by **radiotherapy.** However, a large percentage of men will already have metastatic disease upon initial diagnosis. The only effective systemic therapy available for metastatic prostate cancer is androgen deprivation. The inability of androgen deprivation to completely and permanently eliminate all prostate cancer cell populations is manifested by the predictable pattern of initial response and relapse with the ultimate progression to androgen independence. Androgen deprivation is associated with a gradual transition of prostate cancer cells through a spectrum of androgen dependence, androgen sensitivity and ultimately androgen independence. There is mounting evidence supporting the concept that prostate cancer progression is accompanied by a shift in reliance on endocrine controls to paracrine and eventually autocrine controls and that this complex process is the result of changes, which occur at molecular levels of cellular control. However, the molecular mechanisms involved in the development of androgen independent prostate cancer are unknown. Investigation of these molecular mechanisms has been impeded by problems related to cell heterogeneity of biopsy material and the lack of an ideal in vivo model. Available human xenograft models that progress to androgen independence after castration of the host yield tumors that are highly contaminated with host cells. Therefore, we have developed an in vivo model that encompasses the use of hollow fibers to retrieve uncontaminated packages of prostate cancer cells (tumors) that can be used for subsequent molecular biology analyses of the progression of prostate cancer to androgen independence. We propose to characterize gene expression in cells harvested from animals both prior and subsequent to the onset of androgen independent tumor progression. Specific Aim 1 will employ serial analysis of gene expression technology (SAGE) and Affymetrix GeneChips, while in Aim 2, ICATLC/ MC/MS and two-dimensional gel electrophoresis (2D gels) will be used to identify changes in protein expression in during progression of prostate cancer cells to androgen independence. A double pronged approach is required to identify global changes in expression in the transcriptome and proteome during progression to androgen independence. The results of Aims 1 and 2 will be confirmed using in situ hybridization and/or immunohistochemistry in clinical samples from prostate cancer patients before and after xenografting into hosts. We are in a unique position, having both access to the only model available that provides uncontaminated (by host cells) sources of RNA and protein during the stages of progression of prostate cancer cells to androgen independence, proven expertise and facilities for SAGE library construction, sequencing, bioinformatic analysis, and a novel human xenograft model. The data obtained from these studies will be used to identify important pathways and molecular mechanisms involved in the progression of prostate cancer to androgen independence. Only through the identification of these pathways and mechanisms can new targets and therapeutics be developed that may potentially delay or avert the progression of prostate cancer to androgen independent disease.

Website: http://crisp.cit.nih.gov/crisp/Crisp_Query.Generate_Screen

- **Project Title: GENOMIC PROFILE-BASED PROGNOSTIC MARKERS FOR EPENDYMOMA**

Principal Investigator & Institution: Lau, Ching; Associate Professor; Pediatrics; Baylor College of Medicine 1 Baylor Plaza Houston, Tx 77030

Timing: Fiscal Year 2002; Project Start 27-SEP-2002; Project End 31-JAN-2004

Summary: (provided by applicant): Ependymoma is a neuroepithelial tumor that occurs predominantly in children and young adults, accounting for 8-10 percent of intracranial tumors in children. Despite recent advances in neurosurgery, **radiotherapy** and chemotherapy, nearly half of the children with intracranial ependymoma eventually die of progressive disease. This unsatisfactory prognosis reflects our poor understanding of the biology of this tumor. Current prognostic factors such as age at diagnosis and degree of surgical resection are inadequate predictors of outcome. Despite claims that the outcome of differentiated and anaplastic ependymoma are different, the influence of histology on prognosis remains controversial. Thus there is an urgent need to identify reliable prognostic markers to provide a more objective and accurate way to classify ependymomas for treatment stratification in multi-institutional clinical trials. One strategy to discover such prognostic markers is to identify genetic alterations that determine the malignant behavior in tumor cells. We have recently developed new approaches to perform comprehensive genetic analysis on pediatric brain tumors by using state-of-the-art genomic technologies. One technique, comparative genomic hybridization (CGH), enables us to create complete profiles of chromosome copy number aberrations (CNAs) in tumors with high efficiency and precision. Our preliminary results with a small number of cases suggest that these profiles identify clinically relevant subgroups of ependymomas. This proposal will expand our study to provide enough statistical power to draw definitive conclusions. At the same time, we are making major modifications to the standard CGH technique by converting it into a high throughput and more sensitive format. Instead of analyzing the aberrations at the level of chromosomes, we are substituting an array of mapped clones of DNA fragments for individual chromosomes. This latest modification greatly improves the precision and efficiency of CGH, produces a precise physical map of the genetic abnormality and will allow the analysis of more samples in less time. This proposal will be the biologic study arm of a new COG Phase II trial for ependymoma (ACNS-0121) approved by CTEP. Our goal is to build a molecular classification system for ependymomas to allow objective patient stratification for future clinical trials. In addition, identifying the genetic abnormalities in ependymomas may ultimately lead to the discovery of new therapeutic targets.

Website: http://crisp.cit.nih.gov/crisp/Crisp_Query.Generate_Screen

- **Project Title: GYNECOLOGIC ONCOLOGY GROUP**

  Principal Investigator & Institution: Disaia, Philip J.; Professor and Chairman; American College of Ob and Gyn 409 12Th Street Sw Washington, Dc 20024

  Timing: Fiscal Year 2002; Project Start 01-MAY-1980; Project End 31-MAR-2003

  Summary: The Gynecologic Oncology Group (GOG) is the foremost multi-disciplinary cooperative clinical trial research group devoted to the study of gynecologic malignancies. Since its inception in 1970, the GOG has been a recognized leader in the development of new forms of treatment and has relied on the phase III trial as the design to identify new information. Supporting that major activity are the concerted efforts of modality committees providing recent approaches and procedures in each of the relevant diagnostic and therapeutic disciplines. The GOG has an active, effective program in the study of new chemotherapeutic agents in gynecologic cancers and this program has introduced important findings for study in the Phase III setting. In patients with advanced cervical, endometrial and ovarian cancers, the GOG has defined significant improvement associated with the use of cisplatin. The GOG has performed a series of trials to examine the role of paclitaxel either as a single agent or in combination with other agents. Isofamide was found to be one of the most active single agents in squamous carcinoma of the cervix. The results of Phase III studies by the GOG have provided a new standard of treatment in suboptimal ovarian cancer using platin and taxol. Two recently completed trials of post-operative patients with intermediate risk endometrial and cervical cancer showed a significant improvement with adjuvant **radiotherapy.** The benefit of post-operative adjuvant chemotherapy has been confirmed for patients with totally resected, early stage ovarian cancer. In addition, the GOG has been active in developing new mechanisms to enhance translational research, cancer prevention and control and medical informatics. The Group has collaborative actively with the NCI in evaluating new data management collection and reporting systems. After more than 25 years, the GOG continues to be foremost in developing new strategies in the management of these cancers.

  Website: http://crisp.cit.nih.gov/crisp/Crisp_Query.Generate_Screen

- **Project Title: HEALING TOUCH, IMMUNITY, AND FATIGUE IN BREAST CANCER**

  Principal Investigator & Institution: Lutgendorf, Susan K.; Associate Professor; Psychology; University of Iowa Iowa City, Ia 52242

  Timing: Fiscal Year 2003; Project Start 01-AUG-2003; Project End 31-JUL-2005

  Summary: (provided by applicant): Breast cancer patients use Complementary and Alternative Medicine (CAM) in greater proportions than any other group of cancer patients. The primary reason breast cancer patients cite for use of CAM is strengthening the immune system. Healing touch (HT) is a CAM treatment frequently used by cancer patients to reduce adverse side effects of chemotherapy and radiation and to enhance immunity. HT is classified by NIH as a "biofield" therapy as its effects are proposed to be secondary to manipulation of "energy fields" around the body of a patient. A recent meta-analysis has demonstrated relatively large effects of HT on well being and on physiological parameters, even from brief treatments. However, to date, there are no data on the effects of HT on immune function among breast cancer patients during treatment. This is particularly important as several immune parameters show long-term suppression or alteration, particularly after combined adjuvant chemotherapy and radiation among breast cancer patients. Additionally, there are no data on the effects of HT on the common side effects of breast cancer treatment which can include profound fatigue and radiation-induced skin damage. Physiological mechanisms underlying possible effects of HT are also poorly understood. This study is designed to reduce this knowledge gap by examining how HT affects cellular immune function and biomarkers related to two of the most problematic side effects of breast cancer treatment, fatigue and radiation-induced tissue damage. Effects on the subjective experience of fatigue and clinician rated skin damage will also be noted. Participants will be 42 early stage breast cancer patients who are receiving a standard course of **radiotherapy** following breast conservation surgery and chemotherapy. The significance of this study is that it will provide preliminary data on a) feasibility of this intervention in a breast cancer population, b) the impact, if any, or HT on these intermediate outcome measures, c) information on mechanisms of action, and d) whether the magnitude of the impact is large enough to be sufficient clinical significance to be examined in future Phase II and III dose and efficacy trials.

Website: http://crisp.cit.nih.gov/crisp/Crisp_Query.Generate_Screen

- **Project Title: HIGH-RESOLUTION PROTON BEAM MONITOR**

Principal Investigator & Institution: Ebstein, Steven M.; Lexitek, Inc. 14 Mica Ln, Ste 6 Wellesley, Ma 02481

Timing: Fiscal Year 2004; Project Start 01-JUL-2004; Project End 31-DEC-2004

Summary: (provided by applicant): Proton beam **radiotherapy** holds the promise for improving local control of cancer as it permits improved dose localization compared to perhaps any other radiation technique. The improved dose localization, possible through the dose deposition properties of charged particles, permits higher tumor doses with increased sparing of normal tissue doses. Thus, both an increase in tumor control and a reduction in radiation morbidity are expected. Current and future proton beam facilities require instrumentation to monitor the proton beam in real time for control and safety. Current developments in dynamically controlled scanned proton beams are expected to further improve the therapeutic advantage of protons. These developments, and the comparable developments in conventional X-ray **radiotherapy,** further increase the need for accurate and fast detector instrumentations. We will develop a new scintillator-based detector for the real-time monitoring of a scanned, narrow-focused, proton beam during the irradiation of a patient. This detector will track the position of the proton beam with millimeter and microsecond resolution in real-time in order to verify the relevant spatial and dosimetric beam parameters. The detector can provide feedback into the control system of the scanning beam to dynamically correct for any deviations in the beam parameters. The use of a scintillator minimally affects the proton beam and ensures that delicate instrument components are not unduly exposed to primary or scattered radiation. The only component in the beam, the scintillator, is inherently radiation robust and should show little aging due to radiation exposure, and is inexpensive to replace if needed. In Phase I, we will validate the main detector components and performance, including position response, time response, and accuracy using the proton beam facilities at the Northeast Proton Therapy Center, NPTC, at the Massachusetts General Hospital. In Phase II, we will construct a working detector that can be integrated into the treatment facility at the NTPC, and which can be easily replicated for other proton facilities. A scanning proton beam facility requires a detector system that performs like the one proposed. While many other elements go into a useful proton beam facility, this detector is one essential element of the technology that will promote improved control of cancerous tumors.

Website: http://crisp.cit.nih.gov/crisp/Crisp_Query.Generate_Screen

- **Project Title: INTERNAL PILOTS FOR REPEATED MEASURE ANOVA**

  Principal Investigator & Institution: Muller, Keith E.; Associate Professor; Biostatistics; University of North Carolina Chapel Hill Aob 104 Airport Drive Cb#1350 Chapel Hill, Nc 27599

  Timing: Fiscal Year 2003; Project Start 15-JAN-2003; Project End 31-DEC-2005

  Summary: (provided by applicant): Repeated measures of continuous data often provides the best combination of cost and statistical sensitivity for a wide range of health research in many disciplines. As driving examples, consider comparing methods of displaying digital mammograms, or **radiotherapy** planning films. The limited number and cost of qualified readers encourage choosing a minimum sample size, while scientific goals demand great sensitivity to differences. An accurate sample size analysis allows the scientist to resolve the conflict. Unfortunately, accurate sample size choice requires an accurate value for error variance of Gaussian data. Uncertainty surrounding the variance makes an Internal Pilot design very appealing. Such designs use the first fraction of the data to estimate the variance and then adjust the sample size up or down, as needed to achieve the target power. However, appropriate analysis methods are not available for repeated measures with internal pilots. Our research will meet the need for such new methods. (1) We will develop better statistical power approximations for the "univariate approach" to repeated measures (UNIREP ANOVA), including exact properties and more accurate approximations.(2) We will derive exact and approximate properties of the distribution of final sample size of Internal Pilot designs used with UNIREP ANOVA.(3) We will describe analytic properties of UNIREP ANOVA in Internal Pilot designs, including some exact and large sample distributions, as well as practical algorithms.

  Website: http://crisp.cit.nih.gov/crisp/Crisp_Query.Generate_Screen

- **Project Title: LIMITING CELLULAR INJURY--THE ROLE OF CYTOSOLIC SERPIN**

  Principal Investigator & Institution: Silverman, Gary A.; Associate Professor; Children's Hospital (Boston) Boston, Ma 021155737

  Timing: Fiscal Year 2002; Project Start 08-JAN-2001; Project End 31-DEC-2005

  Summary: The squamous cell carcinoma antigen (SCCA) serves as a diagnostic serum marker for advanced squamous cell carcinomas (SCC) of the uterine cervix, lung, esophagus, and head and neck (HNSCC). For certain tumors, SCCA also serves as a prognostic indicator. Elevated pretreatment SCCA levels portend a bad outcome in stage IB and IIA cervical carcinomas. Moreover, a persistent increase of SCCA after radiation therapy (RT) is the most important negative predictor of disease-free survival in HNSCC. Interestingly, RT induces a rapid increase in both the intracellular and extracellular amounts of SCCA synthesized by SCC cells. These findings suggest that between cellular SCCA content and radioresistance are not understood. To better understand the relationship of SCCA to the pathogenesis of SCC, we undertook a series of molecular and biochemical analyses. Genomic analysis of SCCA reveals the presence of two, tandemly arrayed genes, SCCA1 and SCCA2. The genes encode 390 amino acid proteins with high homology to members of the high molecular weight serine proteinase inhibitor (serpin) family. Although SCCA1 and SCCA2 are nearly identical in their amino acid sequence, biochemical analysis shows that they inhibit distinct classes of proteinases. SCCA1 paradoxically inhibits lysosomal cysteine proteinases, whereas SCCA2 inhibits chymotrypsin-like serine proteinases. Since cysteine and serine proteinases augment intracellular injury, especially that induced by post-irradiation oxidative stress, we hypothesize that increases in intracellular SCCA1 and/or SCCA2 content projects tumors from **radiotherapy** by blocking proteinase-mediated damage. The objective of this proposal is to test this hypothesis while gaining initial insight into the proteolytic cascades that, under certain intracellular conditions, may activate or even supersede caspase-mediated cell death pathways. The specific aims are to: 1) Determine directly whether the expression of SCCA 1/2 protects SCC cells from the lethal effects of ionizing irradiation, 2) identify the potential site of action of SCCA1 and SCCA2 by determining their precise subcellular localization in SCC tumor cell lines before and after irradiation, and 3) identify the cytosolic or nuclear targets of SCCA1/2 in irradiated SCC cells. These studies have broad implications by identifying proteinases from more than one mechanistic class that are capable of mediating radiation-induced injury and by ascribing a biologic activity to members of the serpin family whose function heretofore has been unrecognized. Finally, these studies may establish the presence of a novel intracellular defense mechanism for safeguarding against the consequences (e.g., lysosomal injury and proteinase release) of an overwhelmed antioxidant defense system.

Website: http://crisp.cit.nih.gov/crisp/Crisp_Query.Generate_Screen

- **Project Title: MEASURING CYTOGENETIC DAMAGE IN HUMAN BLOOD**

Principal Investigator & Institution: Dertinger, Stephen D.; Litron Laboratories, Ltd. Suite 207 Rochester, Ny 14620

Timing: Fiscal Year 2002; Project Start 01-APR-2002; Project End 31-MAR-2004

Summary: Humans are exposed to genotoxic agents through a variety of sources. Micronucleus (MN) formation is an endpoint which can be used to detect DNA damage resulting from clastogenic or aneugenic mechanisms. A sensitive and high throughput system to measure human blood for MN would have a myriad of biomonitoring applications. For example, such a system could provide information regarding the chromosome damaging activity of new drugs undergoing clinical trials, chemotherapy regimens, as well as accidental radiation or chemical exposures. A goal of the current application is to optimize methods developed during Phase 1 that allow for the flow cytometric measurement of MN in human reticulocytes (RETs0. Experiments are planned to test whether MN-RET measurements represent a sensitive indicator of cytogenetic damage. To achieve this goal, our Phase II aims are to. 1. COMPLETE optimization of cell staining and handling procedures. 2. DEVELOP biological standards to aid the calibration of flow cytometer parameters. 3. MEASURE the time-course and magnitude of MN-RET induction in **radiotherapy** and radio-plus chemo-therapy patients before and during the course of treatment. 4. MEASURE the time-course and magnitude of MN-RET induction in **radiotherapy** and radio-plus chemo-therapy patients before and during the course of treatment. 5. COLLABORATE with researchers in an environmental biomonitoring study of Chernobyl liquidators, clean-up workers and settlers. PROPOSED COMMERCIAL APPLICATIONS: The successful completion of this research project will enable Litron Laboratories to become an expert facility, capable of performing cytogenetic measurements on human blood samples on a fee-for-fee service basis. Additionally, by developing the necessary reagents into kit format, it will be possible to make this technology available to other laboratories having access to a single-laser flow cytometer. This technologically innovative technique has the potential to become an important clinical tool for measuring DNA damage carried by environmental exposures: radiation and/or chemotherapeutic therapies, aging and a myriad of other possible sources.

Website: http://crisp.cit.nih.gov/crisp/Crisp_Query.Generate_Screen

- **Project Title: METHOD TO GUARANTEE THE QUALITY OF RADIOTHERAPY PLANNING**

Principal Investigator & Institution: Langer, Mark; Professor; Advanced Process Combinatorics 3000 Kent Ave West Lafayette, in 47906

Timing: Fiscal Year 2004; Project Start 04-SEP-2001; Project End 31-MAR-2006

Summary: (provided by applicant): This project will develop a package of planning products for radiation treatment that will introduce a measure of quality assurance now lacking, provide clinicians the opportunity to raise tumor dose, and expose the tradeoffs among the treatment constraints and objectives. The new approach based on mixed integer programming (MIP) will ensure that the dose distributions prepared for patients do not fail to meet the conditions specified because of inferior performance in a planning routine. The result will be a package for picking beams and beam angles, constructing intensity profiles, and evaluating the effect of uncertainties in treatment objectives or in target and organ positions. Constraints can include dose, dosevolume, and homogeneity limits, and restrictions on beam number. Phase I demonstrated the feasibility of using MIP to optimize tumor dose to within a known error of the best possible while enforcing prescribed constraints, and revealed the tradeoffs among the objective and constraints. Phase II aims to speed performance by customizing a proprietary solver to the developed algorithms and adding new formulations, to integrate the processes of intensity optimization and treatment delivery in order to limit the dose distortions users now face, and to engineer displays of the multidimensional tradeoffs present.

Website: http://crisp.cit.nih.gov/crisp/Crisp_Query.Generate_Screen

- **Project Title: MINIMAL-DISEASE RADIOIMMUNOTHERAPY OF COLORECTAL CANCER**

Principal Investigator & Institution: Govindan, Serengulam V.; Immunomedics, Inc. 300 American Rd Morris Plains, Nj 07950

Timing: Fiscal Year 2003; Project Start 01-JUL-2003; Project End 31-DEC-2003

Summary: (provided by applicant): Colorectal cancer accounts for 15% of all cancers, and the 5-year survival rate for patients with metastatic tumors is close to zero. Targeted **radiotherapy** or radioimmunotherapy (RAIT) has the potential to bring about durable clinical responses in small-volume disease of colorectal cancer. The ultimate goal of the proposed work is to produce a clinically useful, commercially viable, radioimmunotherapeutic for treating minimal-disease of colorectal cancer using a humanized anti-CEA monoclonal antibody (MAb), hMN-14, and an intracellularly trapped form ('residualizing') of iodine-131 radionuclide, I-131-IMPR4. The latter is a specially designed radioiodinated peptide, with structural features to aid in residualization after catabolism of the carrier MAb, which solves the problem of in vivo 'deiodination' associated with directly radioiodinated MAbs. The immediate goal of the Phase I research is to obtain preclinical proof that hMN-14 labeled with I-131-IMPR4 (I-131-IMPR4-hMN-14) is significantly better than directly radioiodinated hMN-14 (I-131-hMN-14) in terms of tumor uptake and retention of radioactivity. This will be determined by (i) comparing in vitro bindings and processing of the two labels by four colorectal cell lines, and (ii) by targeting and maximum-tolerated-dose (MTD)/therapy experiments in a human tumor xenograft model of colon carcinoma in nude mice. A concurrent objective is to improve the achievable specific activity of I-131-IMPR4-hMN-14. Criteria of success will be the findings of (1) a 50-200% increase in tumor-cell retention of radioactivity of I-131-IMPR4 label versus direct I-131 label in in vitro experiments, (2) a preliminary evidence of therapeutic advantage for the residualizing I-131 versus direct I-131 label in the preclinical MTD/therapy study, and (3) specific activity enhancement to 10 mCi/mg in radioiodinations with I-131-IMPR4. Successful feasibility study will lead to extended preclinical therapy studies and the initiation of a clinical Phase I RAIT trial in a SBIR Phase II program.

Website: http://crisp.cit.nih.gov/crisp/Crisp_Query.Generate_Screen

- **Project Title: MITIGATING CANCER TREATMENT-RELATED FATIGUE BY EXERCISE**

Principal Investigator & Institution: Mock, Victoria; Associate Professor and Director; None; Johns Hopkins University 3400 N Charles St Baltimore, Md 21218

Timing: Fiscal Year 2002; Project Start 01-JUL-2001; Project End 31-MAR-2005

Summary: Fatigue is the most frequently reported unmanaged symptom of cancer patients receiving chemotherapy or radiation therapy. Despite the prevalence of fatigue and its profoundly negative effect upon functional status and quality of life, little research has been published on interventions to prevent or treat fatigue. The purpose of this randomized controlled clinical trial is to test the effectiveness of a nurse-directed walking exercise program to mitigate fatigue and maintain physical functioning during treatment for prostate, breast, or colorectal cancer. Subjects will be stratified by cancer diagnosis and randomized to exercise (EX) or usual care (UC) groups. Subjects in the EX group will be prescribed an individualized home-based walking exercise program that the patients will maintain throughout their cancer treatment. Subjects in the control group will receive the usual care given during cancer treatment. In addition, both groups will receive a booklet, Managing Fatigue. All subjects will be assessed by treadmill and self- report at pretest (baseline before cancer treatment) and at posttest (end of **radiotherapy** or chemotherapy). In addition, fatigue and other symptoms will be assessed during treatment for both groups. Follow-up symptom assessments and activity levels will be determined at one month, three months, and six months posttreatment. The major outcome variable is fatigue level; additional variables are physical functioning (VO2 max, body composition, muscle strength), emotional distress, difficulty sleeping, and health related quality of life. Groups will be compared by MANCOVA. Multivariate regression procedures will be used to determine the predictors of cancer-related fatigue and of adherence to exercise during cancer treatment. This study is significant as it tests the effectiveness of a low-cost self-care health promotion activity in mitigating fatigue, the most common and distressing symptom of cancer treatment. The biobehavioral outcomes include both subjective self-reported symptoms and objective physiologic changes in functional capacity and performance.

Website: http://crisp.cit.nih.gov/crisp/Crisp_Query.Generate_Screen

- **Project Title: MOLECULAR EPIDEMIOLOGY OF SECONDARY LUNG CANCER**

Principal Investigator & Institution: Shields, Peter G.; Professor and Associate Director for Can; Lombardi Comprehensive Cancer Center; Georgetown University Washington, Dc 20057

Timing: Fiscal Year 2003; Project Start 15-JAN-2003; Project End 31-DEC-2007

Summary: (provided by applicant): Several studies indicate that women with breast cancer who undergo **radiotherapy** are susceptible to secondary lung cancer, whether they are smokers or nonsmokers. However, all studies to date have methodological limitations and have been small. Also, none have used molecular markers, which can improve exposure assessments or elucidate mediating mechanisms. Over time, **radiotherapy** methods have changed and doses to the lung have lessened. On the other hand, prevalence of smoking has increased among women in the western world. The identification of lung cancer risk is important in the context of the debates for benefits of radiation therapy in good prognosis tumors or older women. Thus, a study of breast and secondary lung cancer is needed to improve dosimetry assessments for radiation induced lung cancer, with and without an interactive effect of smoking. Also, studying a unique population of women who have had both breast and lung cancer can provide new insights into carcinogeneis and cancer risk. In order to do this, we are proposing a population-based study using the Swedish Cancer Registry (SCR) and determination of radiation doses to the whole lung and side of the lung where the tumor subsequently develops. Reliable smoking data will be available. Our specific aims are to: 1) determine risk factors for secondary lung cancer in women treated with **radiotherapy** for breast cancer using complementary nested case-control and case-only study designs (n=559 cases and 559 matched controls); 2) to determine p53 inactivation pathways, (i.e., mutational spectra and loss of heterozygosity) in lung tumors of women with a prior history of breast cancer (n=402) and; 3) to determine the frequency of p53 inactivation pathways in breast tumors of women who did and did not develop lung cancer, and compare them to the frequency of p53 inactivation pathways in the lung tumors (n=342 cases and 342 controls). The first aim will allow us to identify risks. The second aim will provide information about the mechanistic relationship of **radiotherapy** to lung cancer and may identify a unique spectrum for radiation-related lung cancer. The third aim considers the combined occurrence of breast and lung cancer in a woman as phenotype of susceptibility for multiple primary cases. This study provides unique opportunities. Using the SCR and the unparalleled ability to obtain tissue blocks dating back to the 1950's, we can provide new data to understand risk in the context of molecular markers, especially because we will be able to retrieve the tumor blocks from both the breast and lung cancer from the same women.

Website: http://crisp.cit.nih.gov/crisp/Crisp_Query.Generate_Screen

- **Project Title: MOLECULAR GENE AND RADIATION THERAPIES FOR CANCER**

Principal Investigator & Institution: Freytag, Svend O.; Division Head; Radiation Oncology; Henry Ford Health System 2799 W Grand Blvd Detroit, Mi 48202

Timing: Fiscal Year 2004; Project Start 01-AUG-2004; Project End 31-JUL-2009

Summary: (provided by applicant): Adenovirus-medicated suicide gene therapy is an investigation cancer therapy that has produced impressive results in preclinical models. Despite these promising results, this approach has shown limited efficacy in the clinic largely due to a low efficiency of gene transfer in vivo. To overcome this limitation, our research program has developed a novel, trimodal approach that utilizes an oncolytic, replication-competent adenovirus to selectively and efficiently deliver a pair of therapeutic suicide genes to tumors. Preclinical studies have demonstrated that the replication-competent adenovirus itself generates a potent anti-tumor effect. The therapeutic efficacy of the adenovirus can be enhanced significantly by invoking two suicide gene systems (CD/5-FC and HSV-1 TK/GCV), which render malignant cells sensitive to specific pharmacological agents and, importantly, sensitizes them to radiation. Two phase I clinical trials that evaluated the safety and efficacy of replication-competent adenovirus-mediated double suicide gene therapy without (BB-IND 8436) and with (BB-IND 9852) three-dimensional conformal **radiotherapy** (3D-CRT) in men with prostate cancer have been completed with excellent results. The results demonstrate that replication-competent adenovirus-mediated double suicide gone therapy can be combined safely with conventional dose 3D-CRT and is showing signs of biological activity. This Program Project builds on our previous preclinical and clinical accomplishments with a single-minded goal- to develop the technology of replication-competent adenovirus-mediated double suicide gene therapy to a point where it will be a safe and effective adjuvant to radiation therapy in the clinic. To accomplish this, we have assembled a highly interactive group of projects and cores that function as a comprehensive and cohesive unit that will advance gone therapy technology on three fronts: 1) by developing better adenoviral vectors and therapeutic genes, 2) by developing better means of vector delivery and monitoring of therapeutic gone expression in vivo, and 3) by evaluating the merit of these preclinical advancements in three Phase I/II clinical trials. The combined basic and clinical science described here will generate new important knowledge and may ultimately lead to more effective cancer treatments.

Website: http://crisp.cit.nih.gov/crisp/Crisp_Query.Generate_Screen

- **Project Title: MONITORING RADIATION THERAPY OF PROSTATE CANCER BY MRSI**

  Principal Investigator & Institution: Kurhanewicz, John; Associate Professor; Radiology; University of California San Francisco 3333 California Street, Suite 315 San Francisco, Ca 941430962

  Timing: Fiscal Year 2002; Project Start 05-FEB-1999; Project End 31-JAN-2004

  Summary: Prostate cancer is an extremely prevalent disease, resulting in the deaths of over 41,800 men annually in the United States. When prostate cancer is confined to the gland, or is minimally invasive into the seminal vesicles and capsule, it has been conventionally treated by surgical removal. An increasing number of patients are now selecting focal radiation therapies (conformal radiation therapy and Brachytherapy) which have demonstrated lower complication rates without survival disadvantage, and are much less intrusive. Selection of appropriate patients, therapeutic planning, and assessment of therapeutic efficacy of focal radiation therapies requires an accurate knowledge of the location, spatial extent and aggressiveness of the cancer prior to and after therapy. Currently available clinical measures (PSA, histology of biopsies) and non-invasive radiologic techniques (transrectal ultrasound, CT, MRI) often cannot reliably provide this information. The goal of the current proposal is to determine whether the metabolic information provided by 3-dimensional 1H spectroscopic imaging (MRSI) can accurately assess the spatial extent and grade of prostate cancer prior to and after conformal radiation therapy and radioactive seed implantation (Brachytherapy). The feasibility of accomplishing this goal is supported by our experience in performing over 800 MRI/MRSI examinations of prostate cancer patients, the large patient population at UCSF, the direct involvement of radiation oncologists and urologists in the project, and the large amount of preliminary MRSI/MRI data which support the biochemical hypotheses which form the basis of this proposal. Specifically, in a 3-D MRSI study of 85 prostate cancer patients prior to radical resection, we demonstrated that choline and citrate levels could assess the presence and spatial extent of prostate cancer prior to therapy with high specificity. In a recently completed study of 62 pre-radical prostatectomy patients with step section histopathology, we demonstrated for the first time that the addition of MRSI to MRI can significantly improve both cancer staging and localization of cancer within the prostate prior to therapy. There is also preliminary evidence that the magnitude of the changes in choline and citrate are correlated with cancer grade, and that MRSI can discriminate cancer from necrosis and other viable tissues after therapy. However, there has not been to date, a serial prospective MRSI study on a clinically significant number of prostate cancer patients receiving **radiotherapy.** The data acquired in this proposal should allow us to determine if combined MRI/MRSI can: 1) improve our understanding of the metabolic effects of radiation therapy on normal and malignant prostatic tissues, 2) improve the selection of patients for radiation therapy, 3) aid in therapeutic planning, and 4) allow a early, more quantitative assessment of therapeutic efficacy.

Website: http://crisp.cit.nih.gov/crisp/Crisp_Query.Generate_Screen

- **Project Title: MR SPECTROSCROPY AND IMAGING IN HEAD AND NECK TUMORS**

  Principal Investigator & Institution: Poptani, Harish; Radiology; University of Pennsylvania 3451 Walnut Street Philadelphia, Pa 19104

  Timing: Fiscal Year 2004; Project Start 01-JUN-2004; Project End 31-MAY-2008

  Summary: (provided by applicant): More than 55,000 Americans will develop cancer of the head and neck (HN) this year accounting for nearly 3% of all cancers in the United States. These cancers are more common in men and in people over age 50. More than 85% of these cancers are related to tobacco and alcohol consumption. Despite aggressive surgery and **radiotherapy** (RT), which may result in significant functional loss, the survival rate of patients with head and neck cancer has remained relatively unchanged over the past three decades. The predictive indices based on tumor morphology or clinical characteristics are generally less accurate in defining outcome of response. Hence, there is an urgent need for a reliable predictor of early response in these tumors. Magnetic resonance spectroscopy (MRS) and imaging (MRI) can non-invasively identify specific metabolic patterns and tissue physiology that may be used as markers for predicting and monitoring early treatment response. Preliminary studies on 41 cases of non-Hodgkins Lymphomas and 12 cases of HN tumors indicate that 31p MRS can predict response prior to initiation of therapy. 1H MRS and MRI provides higher sensitivity and spatial resolution than 31p MRS and would thus facilitate studying smaller tumors and investigating heterogeneous tumor response. The overall goal for this proposal is to test the hypothesis that NMR spectroscopy and imaging can predict and monitor early response to treatment of head and neck tumors. This hypothesis will be tested with the following specific aims: Aim 1: To evaluate the utility of the PME/13 NTP ratio in predicting and detecting treatment response by 31p MRS, Aim 2: To determine if total choline (Cho) and lactate (Lac) levels can predict and monitor treatment response and Aim 3: To use physiological MRI parameters (T2, ADC and DCE) as predictors/monitors of local tumor response to chemotherapy and radiation therapy of HN tumors. 31p MRS studies will be performed using proton decoupled and NOE enhanced 3D CSI sequence. 1H MRS studies will be performed by implementing a selective multi-quantum coherence transfer pulse sequence (Sel-MQC), for detection of lactate (Lac) and total choline (TCho) on the clinical scanner. Standard MRI pulse sequences for implementing dynamic contrast enhanced (DCE), diffusion weighted imaging (DWI) and T2 weighted imaging (T2WI) imaging will be streamlined so that a complete examination consisting of 31p MRS or 1H MRS combined with DCE, DWI and T2WI can be implemented on human HN patients within one hour.

Website: http://crisp.cit.nih.gov/crisp/Crisp_Query.Generate_Screen

- **Project Title: NABTC MEMBER INSTITUTION GRANT (UCSF PROJECT LEADER)**

Principal Investigator & Institution: Lieberman, Frank S.; Neurological Surgery; University of Pittsburgh at Pittsburgh 350 Thackeray Hall Pittsburgh, Pa 15260

Timing: Fiscal Year 2002; Project Start 18-MAR-1994; Project End 31-DEC-2003

Summary: (Applicant's Description) Malignant brain tumors are highly lethal cancers. Despite considerable efforts at improving treatment through advances in neurosurgical technique, neuroimaging, **radiotherapy,** and chemotherapy, the overall prognosis of patients with malignant brain tumors remains grim. To improve outcome, coordinated clinical research is required to evaluate promising new treatment approaches. Laboratory studies of basic brain tumor biology are needed to develop more effective and better tolerated therapeutic strategies. The North American Brain Tumor Consortium (NABTC) was established four years ago for the broad purpose of stimulating cooperative efforts among multidisciplinary teams of clinical and laboratory researchers to improve treatment for patients with brain tumors. To accomplish the long term goal of developing more effective therapies for patients with brain tumors, we specifically propose to: 1. Share expertise with brain tumor clinicians and researchers in multiple disciplines. 2. Conduct joint Phase I and 11 clinical trials for patients with brain tumors, providing adequate patient populations for their timely completion. 3. Share brain tumor specimens and data that will be useful in the conduct of clinical pharmacologic and correlative laboratory studies. This proposal describes the neuro-oncology activities at the University of Pittsburgh, and reviews the resources available through the University of Pittsburgh Cancer Institute (UPCI), an NCI-designated Comprehensive Cancer Center, and the University of Pittsburgh Medical Center (UPMC), qualifying it for continuing participation in the North American Brain Tumor Consortium. The Central Operations Office/Coordinating Center for the NABTC will remain at the University of California, San Francisco. The UPCI and UPMC will provide essential support for all NABTC-related trials through such facilities as the General Clinical Research Center, the Clinical Core Facility, and the Tumor Tissue Bank. The University of Pittsburgh will collaborate with other members of the NABTC to rapidly evaluate new treatments by enrolling patients in Phase I and 11 NABTC clinical trials and to develop promising new therapeutic strategies through translational laboratory studies of brain tumor specimens.

Website: http://crisp.cit.nih.gov/crisp/Crisp_Query.Generate_Screen

- **Project Title: NOTCH-1 IN REGULATION OF APOPTOSIS IN TUMOR CELLS**

Principal Investigator & Institution: Miele, Lucio; Associate Professor; Pharmaceutics/Pharmacodynamics; University of Illinois at Chicago 1737 West Polk Street Chicago, Il 60612

Timing: Fiscal Year 2002; Project Start 13-JAN-2000; Project End 31-DEC-2004

Summary: Notch genes encode transmembrane receptors that control cell differentiation in numerous cell types during development. Humans and mice have 4 homologous notch genes. Mutations causing constitutive activation of notch-1,-2 and 4 are oncogenic in vivo and in vitro. Clinically, constitutive activation of notch-1 is associated with T-cell acute lymphoblastic leukemia (T-ALL), and strikingly increased expression with altered intracellular distribution of notch-1 have been demonstrated in various human malignancies and pre-neoplastic lesions (uterine cervix, colon and lung). We and others have recently discovered that notch-1 has anti-apoptotic activity in vitro in transformed cells in various experimental models. Additionally, we found that downregulating the expression of notch-1 in murine erythroleukemia (MEL) cells in the presence of differentiation- inducing hybrid polar drugs leads to massive apoptosis. Whether notch-1 affects apoptosis in non-transformed cells which do not overexress it remains unknown. Our hypothesis is that notch-1 plays an important role in regulating apoptosis susceptibility in notch-1 expressing tumor cells. This implies that interfering with notch-1 expression or signaling may be used to enhance the efficacy of chemotherapy or **radiotherapy** in human malignancies expressing notch-1. Our long term objective is the development of therapeutic regimens targeting notch-1 using gene therapy, recombinant notch-1 antagonists or notch-1 monoclonal antibodies for clinical testing in human malignancies expressing notch-1. We have generated experimental agents in each of these catagories. Our Aims our as follows: 1. To determine if notch-1 participates in apoptosis regulation in normal cells, by studying its role in thymocyte apoptosis using notch-1 antagonists and novel transgenic mice we have developed. 2. To elucidate the mechanism(s) through which notch-1 protects MEL cells from apoptosis, by investigating signaling pathways known to be linked to notch-1 which participate in regulating apoptosis. 3. To conduct pre-clinical studies of notch-1 inducible antisense retrovirus vectors, a recombinant notch-1 antagonists and a notch-1 blocking monoclonal antibody in mouse tumor models. The experimental agents will be studied alone and in combination with antineoplastic drugs. Studies will be conducted in both immunodeficient animals with human cervical cancer cells and immunocompetent animals with syngeneic murine tumor cells transformed by human papillomavirus 16 (HPV16). These experiments will elucidate the possible uses of notch-1 as a target for cancer treatment and the mechanisms of notch-1 targeting agents. Additionally, they will provide information on the safety profile of these agents and initial proof of concept for clinical trials of notch-1 targeting agents in notch-1 expressing malignancies.

Website: http://crisp.cit.nih.gov/crisp/Crisp_Query.Generate_Screen

- **Project Title: P53 TARGETS AND CHEMO/RADIOSENSITIVITY**

Principal Investigator & Institution: El-Deiry, Wafik S.; Associate Professor; University of Pennsylvania 3451 Walnut Street Philadelphia, Pa 19104

Timing: Fiscal Year 2003; Project Start 25-AUG-2003; Project End 31-MAY-2008

Summary: p53 is a major determinant of tumor response to chemo/radiotherapy in part through regulation of cell cycle checkpoints and apoptosis. Recent evidence suggests that transcriptional activation by p53 is critical for apoptosis and tumor suppression. A number of p53 downstream target genes have been identified, including p21WAF1, KILLER/DR5, Fas/APO1, Bax, Bak, Noxa, PUMA, Bid, Caspase 6, and PIDD. Our recent studies have uncovered distinct patterns of p53 target gene transcriptional induction in vivo, both in magnitude of induction and location within tissue compartments, as well as a wide range of cell death induction in various tissues. We hypothesize these patterns dictate the phenotype of p53-induced death in vivo. We have also recently proposed a novel molecular mechanism of chemo/radiosensitivity that relies on the upregulation of a novel class of pro-apoptotic p53 targets which can lower the cell death threshold following exposure of cells to chemotherapy or radiation. Using microarray screens we have identified polo-like kinase 2 as a candidate p53 target gene and have found that RNA-interference with its expression can remarkably sensitize cancer cells to microtubule active chemotherapeutics. In the next funding period we propose to extend our findings through completion of the following specific aims: Aim 1: Identify and characterize candidate p53 target genes that regulate tissue radiosensitivity. Aim 2: Investigate the molecular basis of tissue and cell-specific p53 activation and p53 target gene regulation. Aim 3: Investigate the relative importance of specific p53 targets to irradiation-induced cell death of normal and tumor tissues using in vitro and in vivo strategies. Aim 4: Investigate the role of polo-like kinase 2 as a p53 target in control of a G2/M checkpoint and therapeutic response to radiation. Additional studies interacting with other projects include analysis of irradiation-induced foci (Tim Yen), analysis of defective apoptotic responses during metastases and p53 targets restricted in induction by cell cycle phase (Ruth Muschel) and analysis of pro-survival signals downstream of Ras and Akt in inhibition of radiosensitivity (Gillies McKenna and Eric Bernhard). Our studies are expected to further our understanding of the molecular basis of irradiation-induced apoptosis, the role of p53, and may lead to novel strategies for protection of tissues from toxicity and/or for enhanced tumor cell killing.

Website: http://crisp.cit.nih.gov/crisp/Crisp_Query.Generate_Screen

- **Project Title: PEDIATRIC BRAIN TUMOR RESEARCH CENTER**

Principal Investigator & Institution: Blaney, Susan; Assistant Professor; Pediatrics; Baylor College of Medicine 1 Baylor Plaza Houston, Tx 77030

Timing: Fiscal Year 2002; Project Start 01-APR-1999; Project End 31-MAR-2004

Summary: The Texas Children s Cancer Center(TCCC) Brain Tumor Program (BTP) is a multidisciplinary, highly integrated program of clinical and laboratory research dedicated to improving survival rates of children with central nervous system(CNS) tumors. The Program is one of the largest of its kind in the United States, each year evaluating more than 50 children. The BTP is composed of clinical and laboratory investigators whose research encompasses the entire spectrum of pediatric neuro-oncology. They are exceptionally qualified to design, conduct, and monitor clinical trials for children with brain tumors. In national cooperative group clinical research and in numerous studies sponsored by the National Cancer Institute and private industry, the BTP has led new approaches to the treatment of infants with brain tumors, introduced new agents against brain tumors through Phase I and Phase II clinical trials, and pioneered the use of highly conformal radiation therapy (RT) to decrease toxicity to normal structures surrounding brain tumors. The BTP works closely with the Gene Therapy Program, Molecular Neuro-Oncology Program, and Clinical Pharmacology Group, all within TCCC, to translate advances in laboratory and pre-clinical science to treatment of children with brain tumors. Examples of ongoing clinical trials include those seeking to determine the impact of intrathecal chemotherapy and highly conformal radiation therapy on the survival of infants with brain tumors, the activity of various new agents against leptomeningeal disease, the activity of various agents against malignant glioma, the use of bone marrow transplant for recurrent medulloblastoma, and the efficacy of gene therapy for children with refractory brain tumors. The BTP utilizes the most modern diagnostic neuroimaging modalities and innovative technologies such as functional MR, MR spectroscopy, and 18F imaging. Its neurosurgeons utilize state- of-the-art operating microscopes and guidance systems. RT is delivered through the most technically advanced conformal system. The BTP neuropathologists have complete diagnostic capabilities to classify tumors according to

WHO criteria. The BTP maintains a storage bank of tumor specimens for institutional and cooperative group correlative studies. The BTP has an innovative molecular neuro-oncology program that uses high-throughput technologies to study differential gene expression in pediatric brain tumors. BTP investigators are committed to utilizing their resources for the Pediatric Brain Tumor Clinical Trial Consortium (PBTCTC) studies. The TCCC BTP serves a culturally and ethnically diverse population. It receives considerable research support from Texas Children s Hospital, the largest children s hospital in the United States and from Baylor College of Medicine, one of the top ten medical schools in the country. The unique expertise of the TCCC BTP make it ideally suited to be a Participating Member of the PBTCTC. It offers leadership in the development of new agents, in new uses of sophisticated **radiotherapy,** and in the application of new approaches to brain tumor therapy.

Website: http://crisp.cit.nih.gov/crisp/Crisp_Query.Generate_Screen

- **Project Title: PEROXIREDOXIN 1 IN RADIOTHERAPY OF LUNG CANCER**

Principal Investigator & Institution: Park, Young-Mee; Roswell Park Cancer Institute Corp Buffalo, Ny 14263

Timing: Fiscal Year 2004; Project Start 01-AUG-2004; Project End 31-JUL-2008

Summary: (provided by applicant): **Radiotherapy** remains the major treatment modality for lung cancer. The therapeutic effect of radiation is primarily mediated by the generation of reactive oxygen species (ROS) and ROS-driven oxidative stress. Peroxiredoxins (Prxs) are an expanding family of antioxidant proteins. Prxs are expressed at high levels in all cells and constitute 0.1-0.8% of the soluble protein in mammalian cells. Two highly homologous members of this protein family, Prx1 and Prx2, have been shown to affect cell proliferation/apoptosis and increase the therapy resistance of cancer cells. Most studies to date have been restricted to observations of the elevated expression of Prxs in various cultured cell systems and some human tissues. However, the effects of Prx expression in human cancers, their influence on cancer therapy, and the regulatory basis for their expression in cancer have not been well investigated. The research proposed in this application emanates from our recent studies of Prx1 and Prx2 function and expression in human lung cancer. First, the expression profiles of Prx1 and Prx2 are clearly distinct in human lung cancer tissues. While Prx1 is significantly elevated in lung cancer cells, Prx2 is not and appears to be primarily expressed in the vascular endothelial cells of the tumor periphery. Second, we have found that the upstream regulatory regions of Prx1 and Prx2 display striking differences and that the levels of Prx1 message are much greater than of Prx2 in various human lung cancer cell lines. Thirdly, the expression of Prx1, but not Prx2, is up regulated at the message level in human lung cancer cells by oxidative stress-inducing conditions including exposure to ionizing radiation. Lastly, our studies have shown that over-expression of Prx1 in human lung cancer cells leads to an increase in clonogenic survival and a reduction in apoptosis in vitro following radiation treatment. These findings led us to postulate that Prx1 may possess unique functions and regulatory mechanisms in human lung cancer. Our hypothesis is that environmental and pathophysiological ROS and ROS-driven oxidative stress increase the level of Prx1 expression by activating redox-sensitive transcription factors and that Prx1 provides a cell survival advantage, in part by directly reducing ROS levels and oxidative damage and also by its ability to control the oxidation/function of redox-sensitive molecules that mediate cell proliferation/apoptosis. We propose 4 Specific Aims to test this hypothesis. In Aim 1, we will determine the functional consequences of Prx1 elevation and its potential role in the radiation resistance of human lung cancer. In Aim 2, we will investigate the regulatory mechanisms for the inducible regulation of Prx1 expression by radiation. In Aim 3, we will identify important redox-sensitive target/effector molecules that might mediate Prx1 function in response to radiation. In a translational extension of the above aims, we will test the predictive value of Prx1 in progression and therapy response of lung cancer in Aim 4 using human lung cancer specimen. In summary, the proposed research is highly translational in nature yet addresses important scientific questions on the role of Prx1 in the **radiotherapy** of lung cancer. These studies will define the role of Prx1 in the **radiotherapy** of lung cancer and provide a sound scientific basis upon which the regulation and function of Prx1 in lung cancer cell survival and radioresistance can be evaluated in lung cancer and other human malignancies.

Website: http://crisp.cit.nih.gov/crisp/Crisp_Query.Generate_Screen

- **Project Title: POSITION EMISSION TOMOGRAPHY IN CERVICAL CANCER**

Principal Investigator & Institution: Miller, Tom R.; Professor; Radiology; Washington University Lindell and Skinker Blvd St. Louis, Mo 63130

Timing: Fiscal Year 2002; Project Start 03-APR-2001; Project End 31-MAR-2005

Summary: (Verbatim from the Applicant's Abstract): The overall goal of this project is improved **radiotherapy** treatment of patients with cervical cancer with use of positron emission tomography (PET). PET with F-18 fluorodeoxyglucose (FDG) will be used to provide three-dimensional definition of the primary tumor volume and regional spread of disease to more accurately administer brachytherapy. PET-based prognostic indicators will be developed. The first step will be verification of the ability of PET to accurately define tumor volume and to differentiate recurrent tumor from radiation-induced inflammation. Tumor size and extent of disease will be correlated with the results of magnetic resonance imaging in patients receiving **radiotherapy** with evaluation of FDG uptake before, during and after **radiotherapy.** Techniques will be developed to accurately determine the position of the brachytherapy applicator in relation to the tumor volume. FDG-PET images showing the primary tumor and regional spread of disease will-be spatially registered with the position of the brachytherapy applicator after placement of the applicator in the patient, thus permitting modification of the source loading in the future to optimize the dose to the tumor while minimizing radiation of the adjacent normal structures. The dose to the tumor and normal structures will be evaluated and follow-up will be performed to assess the rate of recurrence and complications in relation to the calculated doses the patients actually received. The potential impact of PET-guided alterations in source loading and treatment duration will be evaluated. To determine the prognostic value of PET, the volume of the primary tumor and the tracer uptake and heterogeneity of uptake within the tumor, obtained from FDG-PET images, will be correlated with the rate of tumor recurrence to determine PET markers that will identify patients at high risk for early recurrence who may need more aggressive initial treatment.

Website: http://crisp.cit.nih.gov/crisp/Crisp_Query.Generate_Screen

- **Project Title: PRE-CLINICAL TRIALS FOR FEMALE FERTILITY PRESERVATION**

Principal Investigator & Institution: Tilly, Jonathan L.; Director; Massachusetts General Hospital 55 Fruit St Boston, Ma 02114

Timing: Fiscal Year 2004; Project Start 01-JAN-2004; Project End 31-DEC-2008

Summary: (provided by applicant): Early ovarian failure and infertility are well-known side effects of anti-cancer treatments. While the need for tumor eradication is clear, the long-term consequences of these treatments on non-target tissues, such as the ovaries, are substantial. Unfortunately, attempts to preserve fertility and ovarian function in female cancer patients have met with little success. In studies with mice, we have shown that sphingosine-1- phosphate (S1P), a metabolite of the pro-apoptotic stress sensor ceramide, completely protects the ovaries from radiation-induced damage in vivo. Long-term in vivo mating trials have further shown that S1P preserves a normal level of fertility in irradiated female mice, and that offspring conceived with oocytes protected from radiation by S1P in vivo show no evidence of transgenerational genomic damage. With the use of a human ovarian-mouse xenograft model, we have also shown that injecting S1P directly into ovarian tissue can prevent radiation-induced loss of human primordial and primary follicles in vivo. Although these findings support that S1P-based strategies could be developed to combat infertility and ovarian failure, two major points still need to be addressed. The first is to establish the safety and efficacy of S1P for preserving ovarian function and fertility in non-human primates exposed to anti-cancer treatments. The second is to validate technologies to deliver S1P only to the ovaries, thereby preventing systemic availability of S1P that could benefit the tumor cells targeted for destruction. To accomplish these goals, the following Specific Aims are proposed: (1) to determine if S1P can be administered directly into the rhesus monkey ovary as a means to protect the gonads from radiotherapy-induced damage in vivo; (2) to evaluate the competency of the oocytes protected from **radiotherapy** by S1P in the non-human primate ovary for fertilization and embryogenesis; and (3) to assess if offspring conceived from non-human primate oocytes protected from **radiotherapy** by S1P in vivo show evidence of propagated genomic damage. The goal of our work is to develop safe and effective strategies for protecting human ovaries in vivo from the side-effect damage caused by anti-cancer therapies. We believe that the published and preliminary data discussed herein strongly support the need for now evaluating the efficacy of, as well as the delivery mechanisms for, S1P in this regard using the non-human primate as a model.

Website: http://crisp.cit.nih.gov/crisp/Crisp_Query.Generate_Screen

- **Project Title: PRETARGETED RADIOIMMUNOTHERAPY WITH IRREVERSIBLE MAB**

Principal Investigator & Institution: Goodwin, David A.; Lexrite Labs Box 473, 100 N 1St St Dixon, Ca 95620

Timing: Fiscal Year 2002; Project Start 01-SEP-2002; Project End 31-DEC-2003

Summary: (provided by applicant): The objective of drug targeting, especially for cancer chemotherapy and radioimmunotherapy, is to enhance the effectiveness of the drug by concentrating it at the target site, and minimizing its effects in non-target sites. Lexrite's long-term goals are to create a pretargeted **radiotherapy** system using multivalent target binding followed by irreversible capture of a radionuclide, to achieve high tumor uptake and radiation combined with low normal tissue uptake and radiation toxicity. This combined with long residence time in the tumor and low immunogenicity, will enable repeated therapeutic doses to be given. We will use Lexrite's proprietary new Irreversible Antibody to test the feasibility of a novel 3-step pretargeting protocol using monoclonal antibody B72.3 to image cancer sites. The human LS174T nude mouse xenograft model will be used. B72.3 is a well-studied antibody that has been used clinically for imaging and experimental radioimmunotherapy in TAG-72 positive tumors such as colorectal, breast, prostate and ovarian cancer. Effective treatment of these important cancers is a major goal. In Phase II, this system will be further developed to optimize tumor uptake and reduce background in non-target organs to facilitate pretargeted radioimmunotherapy. Successful accomplishment of the 6 milestones described in this grant application and achievement of the Phase II goals, will lay the groundwork for clinical trials with the optimized pretargeting protocol. The approach described herein will lead to innovations in other areas of targeted imaging and therapy of disease.

Website: http://crisp.cit.nih.gov/crisp/Crisp_Query.Generate_Screen

- **Project Title: PRODERMX: TOPICAL PROTECTOR AGAINST RADIATION DERMATITIS**

  Principal Investigator & Institution: Fahl, William E.; Professor; Procertus Biopharm, Inc. 2800 S Fish Hatchery Rd Madison, Wi 53711

  Timing: Fiscal Year 2003; Project Start 13-AUG-2003; Project End 31-JUL-2004

  Summary: (provided by applicant): Several recent clinical studies have described the side effect of radiation-induced dermatitis that occurs in the majority of cancer patients who receive **radiotherapy.** These same studies also report the lack of effective agents to prevent or treat this dermatitis. In some of these patients, the side effects are severe enough that they withdraw from further **radiotherapy.** Nonetheless, **radiotherapy** remains a standard and essential part of cancer treatment and cure. ProCertus has developed a topically applied treatment to diminish or eliminate the dermatitis associated with **radiotherapy.** In current animal proof of concept studies, ProCertus has shown a >90% reduction in radiation-induced dermatitis by pretreating animals with ProDermX, which is currently a research stage human pharmaceutical. This technology consists of a carrier vehicle that delivers a single active agent to the stem cells of the epidermis. The active agent, a proprietary "chemoprotective polyamine," physically protects cellular DNA while also inducing a G1 phase, cell cycle block. This strategy enables the stem cells within the stratum germinativum of the epidermis to survive the radiation exposure, and to continue to replenish the outer layers of the skin and thus maintain a patent skin surface. Though ProCertus scientists have already carried this product through animal model proof of concept, there remain several biological and pharmacological questions that need to be answered before human studies can be initiated. Three Specific Aims have been designed to address and answer these questions during the course of this Phase I SBIR project, which will then enable initial studies in human populations in future research.

  Website: http://crisp.cit.nih.gov/crisp/Crisp_Query.Generate_Screen

- **Project Title: PROGNOSTIC BIOMARKERS FOR HEAD AND NECK CANCER**

  Principal Investigator & Institution: Ang, K Kian.; Professor and Deputy Chairman; Radiation Oncology; University of Texas Md Anderson Can Ctr Cancer Center Houston, Tx 77030

  Timing: Fiscal Year 2002; Project Start 07-FEB-2000; Project End 31-JAN-2004

  Summary: Efforts to refine therapy have reduced the mortality rate and increased the organ preservation rate in patients with head and neck cancer during the past five years. Further, improvement in therapy outcome would result from identification of biological markers that can predict the probabilities would respond to different therapy modalities. Such an achievement would make it possible to select the best therapy for individual patients based on their distinct tumor features. One potential marker is epidermal growth factor receptor (EGFR), a transmembrane glycoprotein with an intracellular domain possessing intrinsic tyrosine kinase activity. The marker is over-expressed in many tumors including the vast majority of head and neck carcinomas.

Emerging data, mostly from in vitro studies, suggest an association between extent of EGFR over-expression and resistance to some cytotoxic drugs and radiation. Preliminary evidence linking EGFR over- expression and poor relapse-free and overall survival has also been reported. The validity of these interesting leads has not, however, been established in a sufficiently large, well-characterized patient population receiving consistent therapy. We propose to identify correlations between EGFR level and clinical outcome in 973 patients with stage III and IV head and neck carcinomas enrolled in a prospective randomized trial of Radiation Therapy Oncology Group. The original study was designed to assess the relative efficacy of four radiation fractionation regimens. Since treatment consisted of **radiotherapy** only in all patients, the study population is ideal for addressing the value of EGFR expression in predicting tumor response to **radiotherapy** in general and to altered fractionation regimens, particularly accelerated fractionations. Biopsy samples and follow-up data are available for these patients. We hope to find a method for identify patients with tumors most likely to respond to **radiotherapy** so that only those with radio-resistant tumors would be subjected to extensive surgery and its attendant morbidity. Our specific aims are as follows: 1) define the range and distribution of EGFR protein expression in stage III and IV head and neck carcinomas; 2) determine the potential association between EGFR expression and clinical prognostic factors and other biomarkers; 3) test a hypothesis that the basal EGFR expression level is an independent prognostic indicator for local-regional control of stage III & IV head and neck cancer treated with **radiotherapy** alone; 4) test a second hypothesis that the basal EGFR expression level is positively correlated with the extent of in vivo tumor clonogen proliferation during the course of **radiotherapy**; and 5) assess whether the addition of EGFR expression level is positivity correlated with the extent of in vivo tumor clonogen proliferation during the course of **radiotherapy**; and 5) assess whether the addition of EGFR expression level imposes risk assessment by RTOG's recursive partitioning analysis had hence refines patient stratification in future trials.

Website: http://crisp.cit.nih.gov/crisp/Crisp_Query.Generate_Screen

- **Project Title: PROLONG THE SURVIVAL OF NSCL PATIENTS BY A PHYTOMIX**

Principal Investigator & Institution: Sacks, Henry S.; Director; Community and Preventive Med; Mount Sinai School of Medicine of Nyu of New York University New York, Ny 10029

Timing: Fiscal Year 2004; Project Start 01-AUG-2004; Project End 31-JUL-2007

Summary: (provided by applicant): The broad long-term objective of this study is to develop non-toxic anticancer and immune-enhancing dietary supplements for the treatment of cancer and immune-deficiency diseases. The specific objective is to test whether a specific mixture of "Selected Vegetables and Herbs Mix (SV)", which consists of non-toxic botanicals containing known anti-cancer and/or immune enhancing components, may prolong the survival of stage 111B/IV non-small cell lung cancer (NSCLC) patients in a phase 3 clinical trial. NSCLC causes more than 150,000 annual deaths in the US and is the leading cause for cancer-related death in the nation. The efficacy of current therapies is marginal. Tumors respond poorly to chemotherapy, whose toxicity adds misery to patients. The median survival time (MST) of stage IIIB/IV NSCLC patients has remained under 9 months. In 2 recent phase I/II clinical trials, SV was shown to improve MST of stage Ill/IV and IIIB/IV NSCLC patients to 15.5 month and to 33.5 month respectively. SV was shown to be non-toxic, improved the Karnofsky Performance Status (KPS) and better maintained the patients' body weight. These results are encouraging but must be confirmed in a large scale randomized clinical trial. In this study the MST will be evaluated trimonthly up to 36 months after the entry of the last patient. Three hundred twenty stage IIIB/IV NSCLC patients with good performance status (ECOG Performance Status >0 or 1) will be offered chemotherapy treatment (gemcitabine+cisplatin (GC)); and within each of the strata, randomized to add active SV or placebo SV to their daily diet. Local treatments, **radiotherapy** and/or surgery, will be used concurrently if indicated. The primary goal of the study is to test the hypothesis that SV may prolong the survival of stage IIIB/IV NSCLC patients. The tumor response to SV and GC and the quality of life of the patients in each stratum will be evaluated and compared. Given the high incidence and poor prognosis of NSCLC, modest improvements in survival can be translated into many thousands of useful added years for these patients.

Website: http://crisp.cit.nih.gov/crisp/Crisp_Query.Generate_Screen

- **Project Title: PSYCHOIMMUNE OUTCOMES: INTERVENTION IN BREAST CANCER**

Principal Investigator & Institution: Kang, Duck-Hee H.; Associate Professor; None; University of Alabama at Birmingham 1170 Administration Building Birmingham, Al 35294

Timing: Fiscal Year 2002; Project Start 01-MAY-2000; Project End 31-JAN-2004

Summary: The specific aims of this study are (1) to examine immunological, psychosocial, and clinical symptom outcomes of an 8-week integrated support program for patients with newly diagnosed breast cancer, and (2) to determine whether the support program has differential effects on patients with persistently low versus high baseline natural killer cell (NK) activity pattern (below versus above median NK activity x 2). The integrated support program includes weekly stress management and social support programs and exercise training activities three times a week. Background and Significance: Cancer diagnosis and treatment are a major source of significant psychological, emotional, and physical distress. Most previous interventions have been limited by a unidimensional approach (psychosocial or physical support, not both), and by the lack of immunological assessments. Given the importance of mind-body interactions in human functioning, an integrated approach of concurrent psychological and physical support will be most beneficial to assist patients in distress. Further, there is indication that breast cancer patients with lower baseline NK activity pattern have a poorer prognosis than those with higher baseline NK activity pattern. A comprehensive examination of an integrated approach will provide insights to improving quality of life for patients with newly diagnosed breast cancer. Design and Method: Using a longitudinal, experimental design with pretest and posttest, 90 patients with stage I-IV newly diagnosed breast cancer will be stratified by disease stage (I-IIB vs. locally advanced) and randomly assigned to the Experimental (intervention) or Control (wait-list) group. NK activity will be examined twice prior to the beginning of intervention to determine the pattern of NK activity. The intervention will begin at the start of chemo- or **radiotherapy.** Post-intervention data will be collected immediately after intervention and at 6 and 12 months from the initiation of intervention, coinciding with patients' routine clinic visits. Dependent Measures and Analysis: The impact of intervention will be measured on immune responses (NK activity and number, lymphokine activated killer cell activity, IL-1alpha, IL-2 and interferon-gamma), psychosocial well-being (distress, mood states, and quality of life), and clinical symptoms (fatigue, nausea, vomiting, and sleep). Longitudinal data analysis methods will be employed to analyze repeated measures of outcome variables, whereas 2-sample t-test or nonparametric Wilcoxon rank-sum test will be used to perform univariate analysis.

Website: http://crisp.cit.nih.gov/crisp/Crisp_Query.Generate_Screen

- **Project Title: QUALITY OF LIFE--THE COLLABORATIVE OCULAR MELANOMA STUDY**

Principal Investigator & Institution: Melia, B. M.; Ophthalmology; Johns Hopkins University 3400 N Charles St Baltimore, Md 21218

Timing: Fiscal Year 2002; Project Start 01-AUG-1994; Project End 31-JUL-2005

Summary: The Collaborative Ocular Melanoma Study (COMS) is a set of randomized clinical trials sponsored by the National Eye Institute and designed to evaluate the role of **radiotherapy** in the treatment of choroidal melanoma. The primary COMS trial will determine whether enucleation or **radiotherapy** without enucleation provides patients with the longest remaining lifespan. The two treatment approaches under investigation, enucleation versus radiation therapy, are likely to have different psychological and physiological effects on the patients receiving them. In addition to consideration of any survival difference between treatment approaches, the impact of the treatments on the patient's quality of life will be an important consideration in determining the best form of therapy. The COMS does not currently incorporate measures of the disease impact on quality of life, with the exception of an assessment of visual acuity. The purpose of the proposed study is to address the issues of quality of life and the psychological and physical impact of treatment in patients with choroidal melanoma using the existing framework of the COMS. Specifically, the study will: 1. estimate baseline quality of life and its changes over time in choroidal melanoma patients from enrollment into the COMS, with follow-up for 5 years; 2. compare baseline quality of life and its changes over time in patients randomized to receive **radiotherapy** versus enucleation; 3. and compare quality of life cross-sectionally according to treatment assignment in patients previously enrolled in the COMS. To achieve these aims, a health-related quality of life instrument, the SF-36 Health Survey, and a visual functioning assessment instrument, the Activities of Daily Vision Scale, will be incorporated into the patient evaluations performed at baseline and during follow-up for the COMS. This study will provide valuable information about the how patients with choroidal melanoma experience the disease and its treatment. Future patients will benefit from these results, which will help them balance the trade-offs between quantity and quality of life related to choice of treatment for this disease.

Website: http://crisp.cit.nih.gov/crisp/Crisp_Query.Generate_Screen

- **Project Title: RADIATION PROTECTION CANCER THERAPY WITH AN SOD MIMETIC**

Principal Investigator & Institution: Gammans, Richard E.; Incara Pharmaceuticals Corporation Box 14287, 79 Tw Alexander Dr Research Triangle Park, Nc 277094287

Timing: Fiscal Year 2003; Project Start 14-AUG-2003; Project End 31-JAN-2004

Summary: (provided by applicant): Phase I. In the treatment of cancer, radiation therapy has been limited by the tolerance of the surrounding normal tissues, such as lung or mucosa. Until now, there have been no compounds available that protect the normal tissues without reducing the tumor response to radiation therapy. The overall goal of this project is to develop a new approach to radiation therapy for cancer, based on the recently discovered radioprotective effects of novel synthetic catalytic SOD mimetic compounds. These compounds may also independently inhibit tumor growth under certain conditions. In Phase 1 of this SBIR application specific SOD mimetics will have demonstrated effectiveness in animal models of radiation therapy of human cancers. The proposed study will specifically research a selected compound in preparation for human studies directed at enhancing the efficacy of radiation therapy. The goal is to both increase tolerance of normal tissues to radiation therapy and retain or increase the net anti-tumor effects. Well-established functional, radiographic and histopathologic end-points will be used to assess possible mechanisms behind this compound's radioprotective effect in rat and hamster models of radiation-induced injury. Models of both radiation-induced mucositis and radiation-induced lung fibrosis will be studied. The antitumor effect of the selected SOD mimetic given alone or in combination with radiation therapy will be evaluated by using standard tumor growth delay assays. This new strategy of utilizing a single compound with both anti-tumor and radioprotective properties in combination with **radiotherapy** could result in an improvement in patient survival with a concomitant reduction in the risk of complications. The potential of independent tumor growth inhibition by the SOD mimetics would be an additional benefit.

Website: http://crisp.cit.nih.gov/crisp/Crisp_Query.Generate_Screen

- **Project Title: RADIATION THERAPY ONCOLOGY GROUP**

  Principal Investigator & Institution: Curran, Walter J.; Clinical Director, Kimmel Cancer Center; American College of Radiology 1101 Market St, 14Th Fl Philadelphia, Pa 19107

  Timing: Fiscal Year 2002; Project Start 01-FEB-1979; Project End 31-DEC-2007

  Summary: OVERALL (provided by applicant) The Radiation Therapy Oncology Group (RTOG) is a multi-disciplinary cancer research group committed to improving the outcome of adults afflicted with malignancies for which new therapeutic approaches to loco-regional disease are needed. The Group is organized into disease site committees and working groups, scientific core committees, and administrative committees. The Group?s clinical research efforts continue to define new standards of care for patients with a diverse range of malignancies and to contribute to the understanding of the biology of these diseases. The Group consists of both clinical and laboratory investigators from more than 260 institutions across the United States and Canada and includes nearly 90 percent of all of the National NCI-designated comprehensive and clinical cancer centers. The Group?s objectives include: 1) to improve upon the survival of patients with those common forms of cancer for which loco-regional tumor control is an important determinant of outcomes; 2) to enhance such cancer patients? quality of life by optimizing structural and functional organ preservation while improving or maintaining survival results; and 3) to pursue new initiatives in drug development, technology assessment, outcomes methodology research, combined modality integration, and translational research to advance the first two objectives. The RTOG continues as the premiere cancer research organization focused on the systematic study of novel methods of delivering **radiotherapy** and the translational research questions underlying such an effort. In addition, its outstanding efforts in defining new standards for combined modality therapy for patients with advanced malignancies are uniquely facilitated by the Group?s scientific and administrative infrastructure.

  Website: http://crisp.cit.nih.gov/crisp/Crisp_Query.Generate_Screen

- **Project Title: RADIODIAGNOSIS & RADIOTHERAPY OF LUNG CANCER METASTASES**

  Principal Investigator & Institution: Kassis, Amin I.; Professor/Director; Radiology; Harvard University (Medical School) Medical School Campus Boston, Ma 02115

  Timing: Fiscal Year 2002; Project Start 01-JAN-2001; Project End 31-DEC-2004

  Summary: Lung cancer claims approximately 150,000 lives each year in the USA and its incidence is increasing globally. Early diagnosis of this disease is difficult to obtain. The five-year survival rate of patients with lung cancer is approximately 14 percent and has not changed over the past several decades. The purpose of the proposed research is to establish the potential of the thymidine analog 5-iodo-2'-deoxyuridine (IUdR) radiolabeled with the gamma-emitting isotope iodine-123 (I-123) for the scintigraphic detection of lung cancer and radiolabeled with either the Auger electron-emitting isotope iodine-125 or the beta-emitting isotope iodine-131 for the therapy of lung cancer. To this end, experiments have been designed to examine the specific uptake of radiolabeled IUdR in nude mice bearing cancer cells growing within the lungs. The approaches described should provide an opportunity for the selective targeting of dividing cancerous cells within the lungs and lead to methods for scintigraphic detection of lung cancer as well as development of an effective/adjuvant therapeutic approach.

Website: http://crisp.cit.nih.gov/crisp/Crisp_Query.Generate_Screen

- **Project Title: RADIOLOGICAL PHYSICS CENTER**

Principal Investigator & Institution: Ibbott, Geoffrey S.; Radiation Physics; University of Texas Md Anderson Can Ctr Cancer Center Houston, Tx 77030

Timing: Fiscal Year 2002; Project Start 01-SEP-1978; Project End 31-DEC-2004

Summary: (adapted from the applicant's description) The primary responsibility of the Radiological Physics Center (RPC) is to assure the National Cancer Institute (NCI) and the Clinical Trial Cooperative Groups that participating institutions have no major systematic dosimetry errors and that adequate quality assurance (QA) procedures are in place, so that participating institutions **radiotherapy** treatments are clinically comparable. To accomplish this goal RPC monitors the basic machine output and brachytherapy source strength, the dosimetry data used by the institution, the calculational algorithms used in treatment planning, and QA procedures. Both on-site and remote audits are undertaken. During on-site reviews, key personnel are interviewed, physical measurements are made on therapy machines, dosimetry and QA data are reviewed, treatment planning algorithms are tested and patient dose calculations are evaluated. Remote audit tools include mailed thermoluminescent dosimeters (TLD), comparison of data with RPC standard data, evaluation of calculations to verify treatment planning algorithms and review of QA procedures and records. Recently, RPC has also utilized mailed anthropomorphic phantoms to verify treatment doses for specialized techniques. RPC routinely monitors the full range of conventional as well as specialized radiation therapy techniques such as stereotaxic treatment, high dose rate brachytherapy, electron beam treatment, etc. Increasing monitoring of three dimensional (3-D) conformal treatment techniques will be a focus of this grant cycle. The RPC currently monitors 1,218 radiation therapy facilities and an average of 1,500 patient charts are annually reviewed of which approximately clinical evaluation for three Cooperative Groups (GOG, NSABP, NCCTG) and two other Groups have asked the RPC to participate in their QA operations (SWOG, RTOG) in evaluation of selected patient protocols. The RPC physicists and staff also attend Cooperative Group meetings. The RPC serves as a resource in radiation dosimetry and physics to nine Cooperative Groups and collaborates with five **radiotherapy** QA offices that serve these cooperative groups.

Website: http://crisp.cit.nih.gov/crisp/Crisp_Query.Generate_Screen

- **Project Title: RADIOPHARMACEUTICALS FOR BREAST TUMOR IMAGING & THERAPY**

Principal Investigator & Institution: Katzenellenbogen, John A.; Professor; Chemistry; University of Illinois Urbana-Champaign Henry Administration Bldg Champaign, Il 61820

Timing: Fiscal Year 2002; Project Start 01-JAN-1984; Project End 31-DEC-2003

Summary: Most breast tumors contain estrogen receptors (ER) that regulate tumor cell growth and mediate the action of estrogen antagonists such as tamoxifen. Not all breast cancers, however, respond to hormone therapy. Therefore, it is important to have effective prognostic tools that will identify those patients most likely to be hormone responders, so that they can be treated with this well tolerated therapy, whereas those unlikely to respond can promptly begin regimens of radiation of chemotherapy. The presence of ER in most breast tumors provides a mechanism for selective localization of estrogens, which if labeled with suitable radionuclides, could be used for diagnostic imaging or **radiotherapy** or breast tumors. During past periods of support on this project, we have developed a series of estrogens labeled with fluorine-18 and carbon-11, some of which are effective agents of imaging estrogen receptor positive (ER+) tumors. Other investigators have developed other adiohalogenated estrogens for ER-mediated **radiotherapy.** Other investigators have developed other radiohalogenated estrogens for ER-mediated **radiotherapy.** Also, recent investigations have revealed that another estrogen receptor subtype, ERbeta, is present in some target tissues, including breast tissue and tumors. We have three goals of the next phase of this project: (1) We intend to develop ER ligands for breast tumor imaging that are labeled with the readily available radionuclide, technetium-99m, as well as its rhenium congener. To accomplish this, we will investigate novel aspects of technetium organometallic chemistry through the application of three new methods for the preparation of cyclopentadienyl tricarbonyl technetium and related systems. These functionalities will be incorporated are pendant and integral groups into steroidal and non-steroidal ER ligands. (2) Based on emerging differences in the structure-binding affinity relationships for ERalpha and ERbeta ligands, derived in part from our investigations, we will prepare ligands selective for these receptors and develop them as tumor imaging agents. (3) We will utilize several radionuclides (iodine-123, and 124 and bromine-76, 77, the later three available to use through a collaboration to prepare ER ligands for **radiotherapy,** and we will have these tested in appropriate animal tumor model systems. These investigations should lead to substantial advances in the availability of diagnostic imaging gents for ER+ tumors and ER subtype- selective imaging agents, to the evaluation in vivo of radiotherapeutic ER ligands.

Website: http://crisp.cit.nih.gov/crisp/Crisp_Query.Generate_Screen

- **Project Title: RADIOSENSITIZATION WITH RECOMBINANT ANTIBODIES TO EGFR**

Principal Investigator & Institution: Bonner, James A.; Chief, Sec. on Med. Biophysics; Radiation Oncology; University of Alabama at Birmingham 1170 Administration Building Birmingham, Al 35294

Timing: Fiscal Year 2002; Project Start 01-APR-2002; Project End 31-MAR-2006

Summary: It is known that the anti-EGFr monoclonal antibody C225 and its smaller Fab fragment cause growth inhibition and accentuate radiation-induced growth inhibition in vitro and in vivo in cells that overexpress EGFr. This finding has been suggested in the human model as well, and currently a National Phase III trial (J Bonner, PI) is underway to test the efficacy of C225 and **radiotherapy** vs **radiotherapy** alone in advanced head and neck malignancies as almost all head and neck malignancies express EGFr and the majority overexpress it. It is known that monoclonal antibodies are limited by the size of the molecule (with respect to penetration into tumor) and the possibility of immune responses against the antibody. These facts may prevent the monoclonal antibodies from eliciting the best possible response in target tumors. Recently technology has been developed to make human recombinant antibodies that are single chain molecules (scFvs) and contain just the critical variable light and heavy chain regions of the antibody and target antigens of interest. We have constructed these molecules for other antigens and have isolated several candidate clones against EGFr. We have also developed the technology to deliver these agents through an adenoviral vector gene therapy-based approach that allows for the secretion of these agents from the cells by the insertion of appropriate peptides. Therefore, it is hypothesized that this gene therapy-based approach will allow for the delivery of high concentrations of anti-EGFr scFv in close proximity to the antigen of interest in a manner that is not possible with the full antibody. Therefore, it is proposed to derive several recombinant antibodies (scFvs) against EGFr and, 1) maximize the anti-proliferative effects of these scFvs; 2) maximize the radiosensitizing properties of these scFvs; and 3) deliver secretory scFvs through a gene therapy-based approach in a manner that will capitalize on the anti-proliferative and radiosensitizing properties of the agents. Human head and neck carcinoma lines will be used to test these questions in vitro and in vivo with an aim toward understanding viable effects with respect to the cells inherent EGFr expression and radiosensitivity. Preliminary data suggests that monoclonal antibody-induced blockade of EGFr results in growth inhibition and radiosensitization through an apoptotic mechanisms. Additionally, the apoptotic events are associated with a dramatic redirection in the anti-apoptotic protein; phosphorylated STAT-3. Studies will be performed to assess the mechanism of scFv-induced growth inhibition and radiosensitization in the context of the above finding.

Website: http://crisp.cit.nih.gov/crisp/Crisp_Query.Generate_Screen

- **Project Title: RADIOTHERAPY PLANNING VIA AUTOSEGMENTED BRAIN STRUCTURES**

Principal Investigator & Institution: Kaurin, Darryl G.; Radiation Oncology; Vanderbilt University 3319 West End Ave. Nashville, Tn 372036917

Timing: Fiscal Year 2002; Project Start 15-APR-2002; Project End 31-MAR-2003

Summary: The present proposal details an atlas-based methodology to autosegment brain structures using magnetic resonance (MR) images for the purposes of **radiotherapy** treatment. This may decrease the amount of time needed by physicians to segment structures in the brain. With decreased segmenting time, there may be greater incentive to use intensity modulated **radiotherapy** (IMRT) with inverse treatment planning, particularly at non-academic institutions. The use of IMRT may decrease patient morbidity through **radiotherapy** optimization planning which minimizes dose to normal structures while providing uniform dose coverage over the tumor. Dose escalation becomes possible when using IMRT, with the intent of improvement in local tumor control. MR brain images will be acquired from patients scheduled to undergo **radiotherapy.** Structures in thee images will be auto- and manually- segmented. While any structure in the brain could be auto-segmented using this method, the structures that will be segmented in this study include the eyes, optic nerves, optic chiasm, pituitary gland, and brainstem (spinal cord, medulla oblongota, pons, and mid brain). A **radiotherapy** treatment plan will be carried out on the computed tomographic scan fused with the MR scan and dose-volume-histogram data for the auto- and manually-segmented structures will be calculated. We propose to test the hypotheses that there is no difference between auto- and manually-segmented structures in position/shape and no clinical difference in radiation dose deposited. A statistical model will be used to determine factors which significantly impact auto-segmentation accuracy, such as structure size, location, and patient disease. This information will then be used to improve auto-segmentation constraints.

Website: http://crisp.cit.nih.gov/crisp/Crisp_Query.Generate_Screen

- **Project Title: RECONSTRUCTION ALGORITHM FOR MULTI-SLICE SPIRAL X-RAY CT**

  Principal Investigator & Institution: Noo, Frederic; Assistant Professor; Radiology; University of Utah Salt Lake City, Ut 84102

  Timing: Fiscal Year 2002; Project Start 01-AUG-2002; Project End 31-JUL-2005

  Summary: (provided by applicant): This project involves the development of reconstruction algorithms for multislice CT using helical data acquisition. With the recent introduction of multi-row detectors and the ability to acquire data over 360 degrees in less than 500 ms, x-ray CT is undergoing a new phase of rapid innovation. Compared to single-slice CT scanners, CT scanners with multi-row detectors can cover larger volumes, achieve higher axial resolution, avoid motion artifacts due to respiration, and improve the detectability of low-contrast details. These advantages have been identified with 4-row scanners and will become increasingly significant with greater numbers of detector rows. Eventually, a powerful imaging system with the capability of achieving early and reliable diagnosis of numerous diseases will be available for biomedical research. With more than 4 rows it is known that the cone-beam (CB) divergence of the beams cannot be neglected during reconstruction. However, from a mathematical point-of-view, designing an algorithm that accurately accounts for this divergence poses a challenge. The design of helical CB reconstruction algorithms is not a priority for CT manufacturers due to the numerous technological problems hindering the development of scanners with multi-row detectors. However, the future of multi-slice CT depends on progress that can be made in this field. Highly accurate reconstruction algorithms are needed to realize the full potential and development of multi-row scanners. This research project aims to satisfy that need. The specific aims are (1) to implement, characterize, and compare existing helical CB reconstruction algorithms, using a collection of figures-of-merit, and to disseminate the coded algorithms; (2) to derive, implement, and characterize new helical CB reconstruction algorithms that provide 3D images with isotropic spatial resolution and high local temporal resolution (< 300 ms); and (3) to derive, implement and characterize new helical CB reconstruction algorithms that provide 3D images with isotropic spatial resolution and high detectability of low-contrast details (possibly at the expense of temporal resolution). Indirectly, this project will have significant impacts on all aspects of medical imaging - particularly in oncology, angiography, evaluation of infections and cardiac diseases, trauma, and **radiotherapy.**

  Website: http://crisp.cit.nih.gov/crisp/Crisp_Query.Generate_Screen

- **Project Title: RNA DECOYS FOR DNA BINDING PROTEINS**

  Principal Investigator & Institution: Maher, Louis J.; Associate Professor; Mayo Clinic Coll of Medicine, Rochester D/B/A/ Mayo Clinic College of Medicine Rochester, Mn 55905

Timing: Fiscal Year 2004; Project Start 01-FEB-2004; Project End 31-JAN-2008

Summary: There is growing appreciation that small, non-coding RNAs can participate in gene regulation. Can small RNAs inhibit DNA-binding proteins? We have developed an artificial example by performing in vitro genetic selection experiments identifying a small RNA aptamer that competitively inhibits human transcription factor NF-kappaB binding to DNA in vitro. Optimization by yeast in vivo genetic selections resulted in an RNA that inhibits NF-kappaB in living yeast cells. We have solved the X-ray co-crystal structure of this unusual RNA/NF-I<B complex. This structure demonstrates how RNA structural plasticity allows DNA mimicry, suggests a new strategy for engineering RNAs specific for different NF-kappaB dimers, and identifies a novel "open" NF-I<B conformation incompatible with DNA binding. NF-kappaB plays an essential role in regulating genes involved in inflammatory responses and protects tumor cells from apoptosis, thus limiting the effectiveness of chemotherapy and **radiotherapy.** Agents that reduce NF-kappaB activity tend to promote apoptosis and have shown promising anticancer activities. Using NF-kappaB as a model of therapeutic interest, we will optimize and test anti-NF-kappaB RNA aptamers in bacterial, yeast, and human cell culture experiments. We will also determine the structure of the free RNA aptamer to understand conformational changes that occur upon protein binding. Our unprecedented RNA/NF-kappaB crystal structure now allows virtual drug screens and in vitro and in vivo validation assays for novel NF-KappaB inhibitors. Such drugs would act by stabilizing our newly-discovered "open" NF-kappaB conformation that is incompatible with DNA binding. Four specific aims are proposed: Aim 1. Optimize and extend anti-NF-kappaB RNA aptamer function by genetic selections in bacteria and yeast. Aim 2. Analyze the structural basis for NF-kappaB binding by anti-NF-kappaB RNA aptamers. Aim 3. Analyze NF-kappaB inhibition by anti-NF-kappaB RNA aptamers in cultured mammalian cells. Aim 4. Identify small molecules that inhibit DNA binding by NF-kappaB.

Website: http://crisp.cit.nih.gov/crisp/Crisp_Query.Generate_Screen

- **Project Title: SENSITIZATION TO THERMORADIOTHERAPY IN HUMAN XENOGRAFTS**

  Principal Investigator & Institution: Leeper, Dennis B.; Professor; Thomas Jefferson University Office of Research Administration Philadelphia, Pa 191075587

  Timing: Fiscal Year 2003; Project Start 15-JUL-2003; Project End 31-MAR-2007

  Summary: Project 1 serves the program by testing the hypothesis that acute acidification by lactic acidosis will enhance thermosensitization and selectively sensitize melanoma xenografts to **radiotherapy.** Protocols were established for acute acidification to less than or equal too pH3 6.3 and oxygenation of melanoma has uniquely high activity of H+ linked monocarboxylate transporters (MCT, a.k.a. lactate symport) that are the major membrane proton exchange. Although thermosensitization by acidification was demonstrated, radiation must be combined with hyperthermia to achieve local control. Five specific aims will test the hypothesis and investigate mechanisms of melanoma acidification. Aim 1 will investigate inhibition of mitochondrial respiration by meta-iobenzylguanidine (MIBG) on melanoma acidification and oxygenation for sensitization to thermoradiotherapy. Variation in glycolytic/respiratory ratio among frozen melanoma biopsy cell suspensions will indicate relative susceptibility to MIBG. Aim 2 will investigate inhibition of the MCT either by alpha-cyano-4-hydroxy-cinnamic acid (CNCn) or by Ionidamine on acidification of melanoma and sensitization to thermoradiotherapy. The activity of the plasma membrane MCT among stored melanoma biopsy cell suspensions will indicate relative susceptibility to CNCn or

Ionidamine. Aim 3 will identify the utility of combining MIBG and CNCn as a cocktail to acidify and oxygenate all melanomas. Melanomas with high rates of respiration will be sensitive to MIBG, and those with high rates of glycolysis sensitive to CNCn. In each protocol excess glucose must be combined with inhibitors to fuel lactate production. Two different F2 melanomas xenografts in nude mice will be studied that differ in vascularity, radiation sensitivity and expression of heat shock proteins. Tumor growth delay will be compared with tibial bone marrow toxicity to establish therapeutic gain. Cellular radiation response parameters in vitro will be determined in Project 3. Project 1 provides mice with melanoma xenografts to Project 2, so that together with Core A, biological endpoints can be investigated to predict response of melanomas and normal tissues to treatment pH9, pHi, 23Nai, pO2, oxygen consumption, bioenergetics and blood flow. Aim 4 supports Project 3 to determine the effect of acute acidification on apoptosis and the relationship with hyperthermia-induced upregulation of hsp70 in DB-1 xenografts grown up from cell stably transfected with the gene for enhanced green fluorescent protein (egfp) under control of the hsp70 promoter. Aim 5 with Project 3 supports Project 4 to confirm whether nucleolin translocation is a determinant of heat response in vivo by measuring nucleolin movement from the nucleolus into the nucleo-plasm in DB-1 xenografts as a function of acidification during hyperthermia. Acute tumor acidification will have the clinical effect of increased tumor temperature with additional benefit from increased tumor oxygenation. These results will help direct a Phase I/II trial conducted by Dr. Douglas Fraker, Univ. of Penn. To demonstrate the effects of acidification of melanoma response to limb perfusion with melphalan at 42 degrees Centigrade.

Website: http://crisp.cit.nih.gov/crisp/Crisp_Query.Generate_Screen

- **Project Title: SIGNAL TRANSDUCTION AS THERAPY FOR MALIGNANT GLIOMAS**

Principal Investigator & Institution: Pollack, Ian F.; Walter Dandy Professor of Neurosurgery; University of Pittsburgh at Pittsburgh 350 Thackeray Hall Pittsburgh, Pa 15260

Timing: Fiscal Year 2002; Project Start 01-JUL-2002; Project End 31-MAY-2007

Summary: Malignant astrocytomas are the most common primary brain tumors, and are the group most poorly controlled with current treatments. Their limited response to conventional therapies in part reflects a resistance to undergoing apoptosis in response to DNA damage or mitogen depletion, which results from a combination of tumor suppressor gene mutations and aberrant activation of growth factor-stimulated pathways. However, our recent in vitro studies indicate that, despite the limitation of apoptotic triggering in these tumors, the effector pathways of apoptotic signaling remain intact and can be activated by inhibition of growth factor signaling or stimulation of death receptor pathways. Our preliminary studies also suggest a number of intriguing interactions between these strategies and other treatment approaches. We hypothesize that agents which block aberrantly activated growth signaling pathways, or directly activate apoptotic signaling, will have efficacy for inducing glioma apoptosis in vivo and will potential the efficacy of other therapeutic modalities. To test this hypothesis, we will examine the effects of glioma growth and viability in vitro and in vivo inhibitors of protein kinase C and ras, proteins that play critical roles in prolifer4ative signaling induced by aberrantly activated upstream receptors. These studies will incorporate a panel of established and low-passage cell lines with defined genetic alterations to assess whether genotypic features influence the response to these agents, and to establish reliable biological surrogates of tumor response. Second, we will examine whether apoptotic signaling can be directly induced by Apo2L/TRAIL, a ligand for the DR4 and DR5 members of the TNF4 family of death receptors, and evaluate TRAIL receptor expression patterns, genotypic features, and biological surrogates that may predict efficacy in vivo. Both studies will be integrated with Project 3, which will provide viral vectors for local delivery of TRAIL and for reversing selected tumor suppressor gene deletions. Third, we will determine whether signal transduction inhibition or activation of apoptotic signaling can enhance the efficacy of **radiotherapy** and conventional chemotherapy for promoting cytotoxicity in all, or a genotypically defined subset of, malignant gliomas. Fourth, because our preliminary studies indicate that induction of glioma cell apoptosis by signal transduction modulation may be an effective mechanism for "priming" dendritic cells to promote an anti-tumor immune response, we will build on longstanding interactions with Project 2 to determine whether signal transduction modulation can potentiate the efficacy of DC-based immunotherapy approaches. Taken together, these studies will provide a foundation for the clinical translation of signal transduction inhibition and death receptor activation as therapeutic approaches for malignant gliomas, and indicate ways in which these strategies can be used to enhance the efficacy of other therapies.

Website: http://crisp.cit.nih.gov/crisp/Crisp_Query.Generate_Screen

- **Project Title:** SIMULTANEOUS THERMORADIOTHERAPY FOR BREAST CARCINOMA

Principal Investigator & Institution: Moros, Eduardo G.; Associate Professor; Radiology; Washington University Lindell and Skinker Blvd St. Louis, Mo 63130

Timing: Fiscal Year 2003; Project Start 01-SEP-1996; Project End 31-DEC-2005

Summary: he overall objective of this proposal is to deliver true simultaneous radiation and hyperthermia treatments safely and with tumor thermal doses consistent with heat induced radiosensitization. There are three major components to this project: 1) Simultaneous superficial thermoradiotherapy clinical trials that seek to optimize thermal dose delivery and determine normal tissue tolerance; 2) Hyperthermia technology R&D; and 3) In vitro cell studies to define thermal dose objectives for the clinic. This proposal is for a new clinical trial that will evaluate the long-term normal tissue effects and local control of simultaneous thermal and **radiotherapy** vs. **radiotherapy** alone in curable but high risk patients with breast carcinoma. Hypotheses are: 1) It is possible to achieve minimum tumor thermal doses (equivalent times at 41C >60 minutes) in the clinic that are compatible with heat induced radiosensitization in vitro when radiation and hyperthermia are delivered simultaneously. Moreover, the overall minimum tumor thermal dose is improved with increasing number of hyperthermia sessions. 2) The thermal enhancement of subacute and late radiation injury from these thermal doses is tolerable and its thermal dose dependence can be characterized. 3) A minimum improvement of 10 to 15 percent in local control within the heated portion of the chest wall will be detected. Specific Aim: In a population of patients with no prior **radiotherapy** and minimal disease volume but high risk breast cancer, the aplicants will conduct a prospective clinical trial comparing skin and soft tissue changes between heated and non-heated portions of the chest wall (each patient is her own control) to determine the impact of superficial simultaneous hyperthermia and radiation on late radiation effects and local control. The **radiotherapy** will be conventionally fractionated and will include conventional boosts. The number of hyperthermia treatments will be four in the first arm of this study and will be escalated to eight in the second arm. The hyperthermia field size will be the maximum obtainable (12 cm x 12 cm) and will be directed to the medial or lateral portion of the chest wall (site selected by randomization). Skin/subcutaneous tissue changes will be graded according to the RTOG Late Effects of Normal Tissue (LENT) scale and contracture of skin will be measured by following reference tattoos in the heated and non-heated portions of the chest wall. The main potential benefit to patients is a greater likelihood of local control within the treated volume with tolerable long-term tissue effects. This benefit outweighs the potential risks from the therapy. This study may have a significant beneficial impact for patients with residual high-risk breast carcinoma.

Website: http://crisp.cit.nih.gov/crisp/Crisp_Query.Generate_Screen

- **Project Title: SMALL MOLECULAR INHIBITORS OF ARTEMIS AS RADIOSENSITIZER**

  Principal Investigator & Institution: Rundlett, Stephen E.; Athersys, Inc. 3201 Carnegie Ave Cleveland, Oh 441152634

  Timing: Fiscal Year 2004; Project Start 01-AUG-2004; Project End 31-JUL-2005

  Summary: (provided by applicant): Recent advances in our understanding of DNA repair mechanisms have led to the identification of the DNA repair specific nuclease, Artemis. Mutations in this enzyme do not affect viability, but enhance cellular sensitivity to ionizing radiation through the prevention of non-homologous-end-joining (NHEJ)-based DNA repair. Hence, small molecule drugs inhibiting the function of this enzyme are likely to be extremely useful as agents to enhance radiotherapeutic treatment of cancer while sparing normal tissue, thereby not adversely affecting patient quality of life. Importantly, administration of Artemis inhibitory compounds before, during, and after **radiotherapy** should sensitize tumor cells to radiation damage regardless of mitotic state at the time of treatment, effectively killing slow growing hypoxic tumor cells which are normally resistant to **radiotherapy.** This phase I application describe studies that will result in the screening of a small molecule library to identify inhibitors of Artemis activity. The subsequent Phase II application will be directed toward development and optimization of lead small molecule candidates that will be tested in-vitro and in-vivo to determine the extent to which these compounds sensitize tumor cells to radiation damage. There are three specific aims for this phase I application: 1) Purify Artemis in sufficient quantities for HTS and optimize screening methods. 2) Screen a approximately 100,000-member small molecule compound library for inhibitors of Artemis. 3) Determine compound specificity toward Artemis and obtain IC50 values for specific compounds.

  Website: http://crisp.cit.nih.gov/crisp/Crisp_Query.Generate_Screen

- **Project Title: SPORE IN PROSTATE CANCER**

  Principal Investigator & Institution: Coffey, Donald S.; Professor; Urology; Johns Hopkins University 3400 N Charles St Baltimore, Md 21218

  Timing: Fiscal Year 2002; Project Start 30-SEP-1992; Project End 31-MAY-2003

  Summary: Each year prostate cancer kills over 38,000 Americans, almost twice the number killed by handguns. Bone metastasis is devastating, and no effective therapy exists when the disease becomes hormone refractory. This Prostate SPORE renewal is a multidisciplinary approach to address methods to reduce the incidence, morbidity, and mortality of prostate cancer as follows. Prevention: DNA methylation changes in the human glutathione-S-transferase gene discovered in this grant are the most common genomic alterations reported in prostate cancer, and reversing this is a target of the proposed dietary and chemoprevention studies. Genetics: In families with pedigrees of prostate cancer, genetic linkage studies will identify candidate genes as the Hereditary

Prostate Cancer gene. Characterization of cancer genotypes and tumor suppressor gene sequencing will also be conducted. Early Detection and Diagnosis: The velocity of change in serum prostatic specific antigen and serum sex-steroid levels will be correlated with cancer risk in the Baltimore Longitudinal Study of Aging, the world's largest and longest longitudinal aging study. African-Americans have increased prostate cancer incidence and mortality, and this will be studied in the molecular epidemiology of the androgen receptor gene structure. Improved diagnosis and prognosis are studied by new algorithms using new SPORE discovered biomarkers and high resolution quantitative pathology techniques; study of the Kai-1 metastasis suppressor gene; and computational study of chromatin structure in human prostate cancer nuclei. Morbidity Reduction: To accelerate progress in improved prostate cancer patient quality of life, research is focused on the physiology of prostrate cancer bone metastases. Treatment: This SPORE developed the first human gene therapy for advanced prostate cancer which is now NIH RAC approved for clinical trials. New therapies using new vectors for gene therapy, topoisomerase-targeted drugs, immunotherapy, and **radiotherapy** are being designed. Pilot Projects are targeted on population studies of carcinogens and epidemiological factors; and new drug modalities to enhance cell death. A large core tissue bank has been established to accelerate translation of human prostate research to clinical medicine. New young investigators are being developed and established investigators in other fields are being attracted to study prostate cancer. This is a highly interactive clinical and basic research team dedicated to translate new discoveries to the control of prostrate cancer.

Website: http://crisp.cit.nih.gov/crisp/Crisp_Query.Generate_Screen

- **Project Title: SUPERHEATED DROP DETECTORS FOR DOSIMETRY IN RADIOTHERAPY**

Principal Investigator & Institution: Nath, Ravinder; Professor; Therapeutic Radiology; Yale University 47 College Street, Suite 203 New Haven, Ct 065208047

Timing: Fiscal Year 2003; Project Start 01-MAY-1995; Project End 31-JAN-2006

Summary: (provided by applicant): Microdroplets of halocarbons can serve as radiation dosimeters when maintained in a metastable superheated state suspended in a gel matrix. As ionizing radiation crosses the emulsion of droplets, it deposits energy along the tracks of released charged particles. This triggers the sudden vaporization of the superheated droplets, creating bubbles, which can be detected visually and/or electronically. A position sensitive reusable detector based on high resolution MR imaging of bubbles has been developed as a 3Dphoton dosimeter. The feasibility of using this superheated emulsion chamber (SEC) for dosimetry around a 1251brachytherapy source at distances larger than 1 cm has been demonstrated. The SEC offers the advantages of high spatial accuracy and resolution as well as good photon energy dependence. A unique advantage of the SEC is the possibility of including information about the linear energy transfer (LET) which may be of interest in characterizing the effects of low energy radiations that are present near the sources and near the interfaces of tissue with high atomic number materials, such as metallic stents, guide wires, calcifications, etc. The superheated droplets with diameters similar to cellular sizes (approximately 10 mum) provide the potential of developing a condensed-phase microdosimeter, which may lead to a new tool for better understanding the mechanisms of radiation effects. A mini SEC will be developed for high resolution dosimetry at millimeter distances using new emulsification and coating methods to achieve more uniform and smaller microdroplets An automated technique for rapid pressure cycling and high-speed image acquisition using 3D-echo planar imaging and optical tomography will be used to improve statistical accuracy and spatial resolution. The mini SEC will be used to determine reference dosimetry parameters at millimeter distances from typical gamma and beta sources used in ocular and intravascular brachytherapy. The ability of SEC for the determination of LET and interface effects for low energy photons will be investigated using a theoretical model of superheat and bubble formation. The SEC will be adapted to serve as an LET spectrometer for low energy photons using pressure steps. A Petri-dish-like micro SEC will be developed for the determination of doses at the interface of high Z materials and tissues with capability of measuring doses averaged over layers of about 10 pm thickness.

Website: http://crisp.cit.nih.gov/crisp/Crisp_Query.Generate_Screen

- **Project Title: TARGETED RADIOTHERAPY FOR EWING'S SARCOMA**

  Principal Investigator & Institution: Hawkins, Douglas S.; Children's Hospital and Reg Medical Ctr Box 5371, 4800 Sand Point Way Ne, Ms 6D-1 Seattle, Wa 98105

  Timing: Fiscal Year 2002; Project Start 04-AUG-2000; Project End 31-JUL-2005

  Summary: (Applicant's Description) Dr. Douglas Hawkins seeks to become a patient-oriented clinical investigator committed to improving the prognosis for pediatric sarcomas by developing a bone-seeking radiopharmaceutical. The prognosis for patients with recurrent or refractory Ewing's sarcoma family of tumors (ESFT) is quite poor, particularly for those with bone metastases. Although ESFT are radiosensitive, effective treatment with radiation therapy is limited by the toxicity of standard external beam radiation therapy to normal tissues, especially when bone metastases are widespread. A strategy that targets radiation to bone while sparing non-osseous tissue could allow the delivery of radiation to bone metastases with acceptable toxicity to normal organs. Holmium-166 (Ho)-DOTMP is a beta-particle emitting radiopharmaceutical that localizes to trabecular bone, with enhanced uptake in areas of active bone turnover. Studies in animals and in patients with multiple myeloma demonstrate that Ho-166-DOTMP delivers high doses of radiation to bone and bone marrow, with minimal non-hematopoietic toxicity. Dr. Hawkins will conduct a Phase I/II study of Ho-166-DOTMP in the treatment of recurrent or refractory ESFT with bone disease. The first specific aim of the project is to define the MTD and the range of toxicity for Ho-166-DOTMP using peripheral blood progenitor calls (PBPC) to support hematopoietic recovery. The second specific aim of the project is to determine the biodistribution and pharmacokinetics of Ho-166-DOTMP in ESFT, including estimation of the radiation dose to bone lesions. Because all patients will be required to have evaluable disease, the third specific aim of this project is to evaluate response to Ho-166-DOTMP. Once the MTD of Ho-166-DOTMP is defined, the fourth specific aim is to initiate a phase II study to estimate the response rate for recurrent or refractory ESFT with bone disease and to initiate a trial incorporating Ho-166-DOTMP into myeloablative therapy for poor risk ESFT. The clinical research environment at Children's Hospital and Regional Medical Center, the University of Washington, and the Fred Hutchinson Cancer Research Center are particularly well suited to the development of his clinical investigation. Dr. Irwin Bernstein, who has extensive clinical research and training experience, will serve as Dr. Hawkins' mentor. Dr. Hawkins also proposes to take courses in radiation biology, radiation pharmacology, biostatistics, and medical ethics at the University of Washington and Children's Hospital and Regional Medical Center. Upon completion of the five-year K23 award, he anticipates having acquired a strong foundation biostatistics and radiation biology, as well as considerable experience planning and conducting clinical trials enabling him to emerge as an independent clinical investigator.

  Website: http://crisp.cit.nih.gov/crisp/Crisp_Query.Generate_Screen

- **Project Title:** TARGETING CERAMIDE METABOLISM FOR CANCER TREATMENT

Principal Investigator & Institution: Cabot, Myles C.; Chief; John Wayne Cancer Institute 2200 Santa Monica Blvd Santa Monica, Ca 90404

Timing: Fiscal Year 2002; Project Start 01-APR-2002; Project End 31-MAR-2004

Summary: (provided by applicant): The long-term objective of this application is to evaluate a specific molecular target for discovery and clinical testing of new anticancer agents, based on molecular mechanisms that underlie chemotherapy resistance. Current research in anticancer drug mechanism of action and resistance biology has identified ceramide glycosylation as an event associated with progression of cancer. The focus of this application is to target glycosylation because it is essential for maintenance of the drug-resistant phenotype. It is believed that a new genre of agents can be brought forth for clinical assessment based on strong rationales. Drug-resistant human cancer cells which are known to demonstrate enhanced metabolism of ceramide through the glycosylation pathway catalyzed by glucosylceramide synthase (GCS), will be exposed to conventional chemotherapy, Adriamycin, Taxol, N-4(hydroxyphenyl)retinamide(4-HPR) in the absence or presence of agents that retard ceramide glycosylation, the latter being evaluated through screening of compounds in the Natural Products and Synthetic Repositories of the NCI. We will conduct analog searches of the repositories using lead compounds already shown to retard ceramide glycosylation and demonstrate synergistic cytotoxicity with classical chemotherapeutic agents. Other programs such as COMPARE and clustering algorithms will be employed to mine the NCI drug repositories. The impact of select agents on ceramide glycosylation will be evaluated in intact cancer cells and in in vitro cell-free assays, and based on results, regimens will be assessed for cytotoxicity either alone or in combination with chemotherapy, using standard cell proliferation and apoptosis assays. This study has two specific aims: 1) to screen compounds in the NCI Natural and Synthetic Products Repositories for ability to block ceramide metabolism by the glycosylation route; 2) to evaluate lead compounds alone and in combination with anticancer drugs for enhancement of chemotherapy-induced cytotoxicity in drug-resistant cancer cells. The limited efficacy of available drug therapies and the high incidence of chemotherapy resistance are strong reasons to pursue new approaches to treat patients with cancer. Dysfunctional ceramide metabolism is a significant contributor to chemo- and **radiotherapy** failure. Targeting ceramide metabolism is therefore an attractive strategy for anticancer drug development.

Website: http://crisp.cit.nih.gov/crisp/Crisp_Query.Generate_Screen

- **Project Title: THERAPEUTIC STUDIES OF PRIMARY CNS MALIGNANCIES-NABTT**

Principal Investigator & Institution: Barnett, Gene H.; Cleveland Clinic Foundation 9500 Euclid Ave Cleveland, Oh 44195

Timing: Fiscal Year 2004; Project Start 01-JAN-2004; Project End 31-DEC-2008

Summary: (provided by applicant): A major thrust of The Brain Tumor Institute (BTI) of the Cleveland Clinic Cancer Center is to advance knowledge of the mechanisms of brain tumor development and growth, through basic science, and to develop new treatment options, by way of engineering collaboration with industry and clinical research. We believe that an ongoing, long-term membership in the NABTT consortium will be our principal means of achieving this goal. The BTI performs more than 600 brain tumor operations per year, of which approximately 150 are on malignant glial neoplasms.

Through BTI's Center for Translational Therapeutics, we perform preclinical testing of new, promising brain tumor agents, determining their efficacy and optimum mode of delivery. Additional translational laboratory efforts include adoptive immunotherapy and immune system regulation for brain tumors, convection enhanced delivery of potential therapies, detection of serum tumor markers, and brain image post-processing or multimodality integration and longitudinal autosegmentation and fusion for assessment of treatment efficacy. It is our intention to contribute promising new agents and our expertise in these areas to the NABTT consortium. Since being accepted as a provisional member in NABTT 2 years ago, we have demonstrated our commitment to this organization by participating in or leading NABTT committees, protocol leadership, and having the highest second-year accrual of any active NABTT site, with a third-year projected accrual of about 28 patients. We believe that our yearly contribution of patients to the NABTT consortium will be in the range of 25 to 30 per year. Additional contributions to the Consortium will include 1) new agents with preclinical evidence of efficacy and optimal route of administration, 2) expertise in immunological strategies for brain tumor treatment, 3) new methods of integrating brain imaging and tracking changes over time, 4) expertise in advanced-agent delivery strategies such as convection enhanced delivery, 5) extensive expertise and state-of-art resources in **radiotherapy,** radiosurgery, surgical navigation, and neuro-imaging, 6) a broad, grant and endowment-supported basic science effort with capability to interface with other NABTT laboratories, 7) a large tumor bank with IRB-approved clinical/pathology/molecular/imaging database correlations, and 8) our expertise in generating and completing Phase I and II clinical trials.

Website: http://crisp.cit.nih.gov/crisp/Crisp_Query.Generate_Screen

- **Project Title: TNT IMAGING TO MONITOR THE EFFICACY OF CANCER THERAPY**

Principal Investigator & Institution: Epstein, Alan L.; Pathology; University of Southern California 2250 Alcazar Street, Csc-219 Los Angeles, Ca 90033

Timing: Fiscal Year 2002; Project Start 01-FEB-2000; Project End 31-JAN-2004

Summary: Cancer diagnosis as a discipline has been greatly improved with the advent of tumor imaging technologies which use radiolabeled monoclonal antibodies or their fragments to target primary and metastatic lesions in not detected by standard MRI or CAT scans. Serum markers, which generally use monoclonal antibodies to tumor cell products, have also helped the clinician to quantitate the size of the tumor burden and this information has helped to determine the effectiveness of treatment at the completion of each course of therapy. What is lacking is a method which can monitor the efficacy of cytoreductive therapy (chemotherapy, **radiotherapy,** or immunotherapy) during initial treatment to help the clinician know whether his/her chosen therapy is effective before a commitment to a given approach has been made. The ability to make this determination may enable clinicians to spare the patient undue toxicity if a given treatment approach appears unsuccessful and buy valuable time by enabling the therapist to switch to alternative treatment before actually completing each round of therapy. Imaging is an ideal tool for making this determination since it is non-invasive, rapid, and relatively inexpensive to perform. Our laboratory has developed a monoclonal antibody which targets necrotic regions in tumors and is especially effective in binding newly degenerating cells regardless of their cell of origin or disease status. In this proposal, we intend to construct a fast- clear derivative which after radiolabeling can be used to quantitative the amount of necrosis before and after therapy. Genetic engineering methods will be used to construct a single chain, diabody, and triabody derivative as well as F(ab) and F(ab')2 fragments of chimeric monoclonal antibody TNT-3. In vitro binding studies and in vivo biodistribution and imaging analyses will be used to determine which of the above constructs have the best imaging characteristics. At the completion of this phase of the work, in vivo tumor models consisting of chemotherapy resistant and sensitive tumor sublines will be used to demonstrate the potential of this approach to monitor the effectiveness of cytoreductive therapy. The results of these studies could provide the basis for future clinical trials by providing the nuclear medicine physician, oncologist, and radiation therapist with a new and valuable tool to assess the effectiveness of standard and experimental cancer therapy in a cost-effective and timely manner.

Website: http://crisp.cit.nih.gov/crisp/Crisp_Query.Generate_Screen

- **Project Title: TRANSLATIONAL MULTIMODALITY " ANTIBODY" THERAPY**

Principal Investigator & Institution: Denardo, Gerald L.; Professor Emeritus; Internal Medicine; University of California Davis Sponsored Programs, 118 Everson Hall Davis, Ca 956165200

Timing: Fiscal Year 2004; Project Start 09-MAY-1997; Project End 31-MAR-2007

Summary: (provided by applicant): The hypothesis for the competitive renewal of the grant, Translational Multimodality "Antibody" Therapy, is that the therapeutic index for radioisotopic molecular targeted **radiotherapy** (RMTR) can be dramatically improved using novel small molecules and delivery strategies. RMTR has expanded the usefulness of radiation to treat widespread cancer, and small radioisotope carrier molecules can achieve therapeutic indices 10-100X better than that currently achieved using macromolecular MAb carriers. This program has renewed its emphasis on translational research to apply novel science and resources for the development of drugs and strategies to be evaluated in preclinical studies (before transfer to patients). Although the proposals are potentially applicable to most cancers, the focus will be on lymphomas and prostate cancer because of the need for novel treatment and substantial progress achieved using conventional radioimmunotherapy. Using insights from our experience with Lym-1-MAb and HLA-DR targeting, and a combination of unusual capabilities, we have generated synthetic, high affinity (linked) ligands (SHALs) in Project 1 that selectively bind to unique sites on the beta subunit of HLA-DR, a protein shown to be relatively specific for the malignant lymphocytes of B-lymphomas and leukemias. These novel molecules have been shown to bind selectively to HLA-DR10 and human lymphoma cells and will be used as radioisotopic carriers for systemic **radiotherapy.** In Project 2, novel bispecific, multivalent single-chain MAbs, against the tandem repeat of the mucin protein characteristic of adenocarcinomas and against the DOTA chelator for radiometals, have been generated and placed on a PEGylated scaffold for use in a pretargeting RIT strategy for prostate cancer. Multivalent DOTA will be used as the radiometal carrier. PEGylated bivalent scFvs that bind selectively to prostate cancer have been synthesized. In Project 3, the inventor of the "one bead, one peptide" combinatorial libraries has generated serine protease (Activase(R), TNKase(R)) biodegradable linkers, stable in plasma, to reduce radiation doses to all normal tissues by eliminating radioisotope carriers from the blood "on demand". In the past, we showed that cathepsin-degradable peptides in radiometal-labeled MAbs reduced hepatic radiation dose. The proposed strategy decreases radiation dose to all normal tissues and is applicable to other radioisotopic targeting systems, both in development and approved, and as a clearance vehicle for pregargeting strategies. Four cores support the projects. Because of the focus on the development of novel molecules and strategies rather than trials, Core B has become a modeling core and biostatistics has been moved to Core A that supports all investigators. Substantial progress has been made and the likelihood of success is high.

Website: http://crisp.cit.nih.gov/crisp/Crisp_Query.Generate_Screen

- **Project Title: TUMOR ANTIGEN DISCOVERY IN ALL BY EXPRESSION PROFILING**

  Principal Investigator & Institution: Haining, W. Nicholas.; Dana-Farber Cancer Institute 44 Binney St Boston, Ma 02115

  Timing: Fiscal Year 2002; Project Start 15-JUL-2002; Project End 31-MAY-2007

  Summary: (provided by applicant): Many children and most adults with acute lymphoblastic leukemia (ALL) are not cured by conventional therapy. Moreover, the long-term effects of chemo-radiotherapy are now being manifest in survivors of childhood ALL. Immunotherapy may improve the therapeutic index of ALL treatment. We have shown that patients with B cell precursor ALL have tumor-specific T cells in their repertoire. This significant finding demonstrates that ALL cells express antigens which can be recognized by autologous T cells. Discovering the identity of these antigens is important because doing so will enable the characterization of host anti-tumor immunity in patients with ALL, and will offer new therapeutic targets. Tumor antigens can represent gene products overexpressed in tumor cells compared with non-malignant cells. We have developed a strategy that has identified successfully tumor antigens on the basis of their overexpression in cancer cells. However, in ALL, this approach has so far been limited by the small number of genes known to be overexpressed in leukemia cells. Gene expression profiling can identify genes that are overexpressed in B cell ALL relative to its normal counterpart, the B cell precursor, and relative to other normal tissues. These genes represent a pool of candidate tumor antigens that can be functionally validated. My hypothesis is therefore that GENOMIC APPROACHES TO TUMOR ANTIGEN DISCOVERY IN ACUTE LYMPHOBLASTIC LEUKEMIA WILL ADVANCE UNDERSTANDING OF HOST-TUMOR INTERACTIONS IN PATIENTS AND IDENTIFY NEW TARGETS FOR TREATMENT. To test this hypothesis I plan to: (1) define candidate tumor antigens bioinformatically using gene expression profiling; (2) validate candidate tumor antigens in vitro; and (3) credential tumor antigens in vivo. My career goal is to become an independent physician-scientist studying tumor immunology both in the laboratory and in the clinic. Specifically, I plan to study the biology of the host anti-tumor immune response in patients and determine how it contributes to disease outcome. Achieving this goal will require expertise in laboratory, translational and clinical research. To develop the necessary skills, I have the mentorship of co-sponsors with international reputations in laboratory research and translational medicine. I have also assembled a panel of advisors with great expertise in the field. My research environment is rich with opportunities for interaction and education, and I will enroll in didactic courses in biostatistics, study design and ethics to complement my research experience. This training will form the foundation of my career in translational research.

  Website: http://crisp.cit.nih.gov/crisp/Crisp_Query.Generate_Screen

- **Project Title: TUMOR OXYGENATION, VASCULARIZATION, AND RADIORESPONSE**

  Principal Investigator & Institution: Fenton, Bruce M.; Associate Professor; Radiation Oncology; University of Rochester 517 Hylan Bldg., Box 270140 Rochester, Ny 14627

  Timing: Fiscal Year 2002; Project Start 01-APR-1992; Project End 31-JUL-2004

Summary: Inhibition of tumor angiogenesis has emerged as a promising strategy to treat both primary and metastatic tumors. Although effective at shrinking tumors, antiangiogenic agents are not tumoricidal, and tumor regrowth frequently occurs after termination of treatment with the angiogenesis inhibitor. One strategy to overcome this limitation is to combine antiangiogenic agents with conventional therapies such as **radiotherapy,** although the underlying physiological rationale for such combinations remains unexplored. The primary focus of this proposal is to explore both physiological and molecular changes following both antiangiogenic and angiogenic stimuli. Although established, transplantable murine tumor models have long been the standard for radiobiological investigations, the dependence of physiological function on tumor derivation remains uncertain. Differences in vascular development, specifically in regards to relative proportions of host versus tumor vessels, could be vital in the evaluation of antiangiogenic and combined modality, preclinical strategies. The current application proposes to examine tumor microregional changes in vascular structure and hypoxia, in conjunction with alterations in angiogenic and antiangiogenic growth factor expression, among a panel of carefully chosen murine tumor models. First, spontaneous mammary carcinomas will be contrasted with slow and fast growing 1st generation transplants of these tumors. Second, nonmetastatic MCa-IV versus aggressive, metastatic MCa-35 established mammary carcinoma models will be studied. Our methods include: a) cryospectrophotometry to define intravascular oxygen levels, b) immunohistochemical staining to quantify total and perfused vessels, tumor cell proliferation, apoptosis, and percent necrosis, c) immunohistochemistry, in situ hybridization, and RNA protection assays to quantify growth factor and receptor levels, d) hypoxic marker uptake (EF5) to delineate regional changes in oxygenation, and e) growth delay assays to evaluate response to single and multi-fraction **radiotherapy,** as well as antiangiogenic agents. In view of an increasing interest in the use of multi-modality therapies that incorporate potentially angiogenic and antiangiogenic agents, this proposal will quantitate the effects of both angiogenic growth factors (VEGF and FGF2) and antiangiogenic agents (endostatin). Endostatin will also be combined with **radiotherapy** to determine whether the radiation is potentiated by the antiangiogenic agent. In summary, our primary goals are to determine the fundamental relationships between molecular and pathophysiological changes in disparate tumor models and whether observed differences can be therapeutically exploited.

Website: http://crisp.cit.nih.gov/crisp/Crisp_Query.Generate_Screen

- **Project Title: TUMOR RADIOSENSITIZATION BY PRENYLTRANSFERASE INHIBITORS**

  Principal Investigator & Institution: Bernhard, Eric J.; Associate Professor; Radiation Oncology; University of Pennsylvania 3451 Walnut Street Philadelphia, Pa 19104

  Timing: Fiscal Year 2003; Project Start 12-DEC-1997; Project End 31-JAN-2008

Summary: (provided by applicant): Our studies to date have demonstrated that inhibiting RAS reduces the radiation survival of tumor cells in which RAS is activated by mutation or epidermal growth factor receptor (EGFR) signaling. We have used a pharmacological approach to inhibit RAS post-translational processing. This processing is required for RAS membrane binding and activity. We have shown that farnesyltransferase inhibitor (FTI) treatment radiosensitizes tumor cells with H-ras mutations without altering the radiation sensitivity of normal cells. While the effect was significant in tissue culture, animal experiments led us to examine whether FTI treatment had additional effects in vivo. Subsequent studies revealed that FTI treatment led to increased oxygenation in tumors xenografts expressing oncogenic H-ras. We propose to further explore the ability of FTIs to alter the tumor microenvironment by determining whether mutant RAS is the target for this action of FTIs. We will investigate the mechanism through which FTIs alter the oxygenation of tumors and whether it involves changes in tumor vasculature. We have also shown, using a genetic approach, that oncogenic H-, K-, and N-RAS all contribute to radiation resistance. Signaling from the three RAS isoforms to down-stream effectors has been reported to differ. This raises the question of which pathways downstream of RAS contribute to the observed radiation resistance. We propose to explore the contribution of each RAS isoform to intrinsic radiation resistance and to investigate downstream pathways using both pharmacologic inhibitors as well as novel genetic reagents. Small interfering RNA (siRNA) will be used to specifically target expression of the different RAS isoforms as well as to specifically target oncogenic RAS expression. The results of these studies could be valuable in developing new molecular targets to improve the efficacy of **radiotherapy.** They may also provide a rationale for the application of FTIs in the treatment of tumors with RAS activation that is due to EGFR signaling.

Website: http://crisp.cit.nih.gov/crisp/Crisp_Query.Generate_Screen

- **Project Title: TUMOR UPTAKE OF GA-67 BY PHOTODEGRADED NIFEDIPINE**

Principal Investigator & Institution: Morton, Kathryn A.; Professor and Director; Div of Radiologic Sciences; Wake Forest University Health Sciences Winston-Salem, Nc 27157

Timing: Fiscal Year 2002; Project Start 12-FEB-1999; Project End 31-JUL-2005

Summary: (Provided by Applicant): This proposal is the first competing renewal of a 3-year RO1 grant to improve the uptake of gallium-67 for tumor imaging. Uptake of Ga-67 by tumors has traditionally thought to be mediated by transferrin (Tf) and Tf receptor-dependent mechanisms. We have found that uptake of Ga-67 by cells and tumors is also mediated by a Tf-independent process, which appears more important in tumors than normal tissues. More significantly, we have shown that the Tf-independent uptake of GA in cells and tumors can be regulated. It can be specifically induced in tumors by administration of compound, which we have named "nitrosipine," which is produced when nifedipine, a commonly used dihyropyridine calcium channel blocker, is exposed to fluorescent or UV light. We have generated evidence that nitrosipine may also enhance a variety of other metal cations as well. This may expand the utility of nitrosipine for gamma scintigraphy, PET imaging and **radiotherapy.** We propose to apply the knowledge gained during the last funding cycle to the following 6 specific aims: 1. To define the molecular features of nitrosipine that are necessary for promoting uptake of Ga-67. 2. To confirm and define the nature of the binding of nitrosipine (or other active derivatives) to metal cations. 3. To define the biological mechanism by which nitrosipine enhances the cellular Ga-67 uptake. 4. To define the in vivo kinetics and optimal method for dosing to maximize the visualization of tumors. 5. To test how broadly effective nitrosipine, and similar active derivatives, are in promoting uptake of GA-67 in tumors of a wide variety of histologic types in a murine tumor models. 6. To explore the potential for nitrosipine or active derivatives, to enhance the uptake of Cu-64.

Website: http://crisp.cit.nih.gov/crisp/Crisp_Query.Generate_Screen

- **Project Title: UNIVERSITY OF COLORADO SOUTHWEST ONCOLOGY GROUP**

Principal Investigator & Institution: Bearman, Scott I.; Medicine; University of Colorado Hlth Sciences Ctr P.O. Box 6508, Grants and Contracts Aurora, Co 800450508

Timing: Fiscal Year 2002; Project Start 21-JAN-1998; Project End 31-DEC-2003

Summary: Description (Adapted from the applicant s abstract): The University of Colorado Cancer Center is requesting continuing support for their participation in the Southwest Oncology Group (SWOG). The mission of the University of Colorado Cancer Center has, since it's founding, been the reduction of cancer mortality through basic laboratory research, moving scientific discoveries to the clinic through translational research, and the design, execution, and analysis of clinical trials. Their participation in SWOG has been an integral part of the mission of the University of Colorado Cancer Center. Institutional pilot studies conducted at the University of Colorado have been brought to the Group in the form of prospective randomized trials. SWOG members from the University of Colorado have and continue to contribute to the administrative, educational and scientific functions of SWOG. University of Colorado SWOG members are chairs or co-chairs of the following committees: Genitourinary (Dr. E. David Crawford), Blood and Marrow Transplantation (Dr. Elizabeth Shpall), GU Pathology (Dr. Gary Miller), and Lung Biology (Wilbur Franklin). Dr. Scott Bearman is Principal Investigator for SWOG and sits on the Board of Governors. In addition to these administrative contributions, University of Colorado Cancer Center members are coordinators or co-coordinators of 17 percent of the SWOG protocols activated during the previous grant period. Presently, University of Colorado members are important contributors to the Blood and Marrow Transplantation, Breast, Lung, and GU Committees. During the next five years they expect to continue to make important scientific and administrative contributions to those committees. In addition, they expect to contribute in other areas as well, including **radiotherapy** (Drs. Rachel Rabinovitch and Michael Weil), developmental therapeutics (Dr. Andrew Kraft), neuro-oncology (Dr. Bertrand Liang) and Cancer Control (Dr. Marie Wood). They are proud of our contributions to the Southwest Oncology Group and are committed to its mission. They expect their contributions to increase during the next 5 years.

Website: http://crisp.cit.nih.gov/crisp/Crisp_Query.Generate_Screen

E-Journals: PubMed Central[3]

PubMed Central (PMC) is a digital archive of life sciences journal literature developed and managed by the National Center for Biotechnology Information (NCBI) at the U.S. National Library of Medicine (NLM).[4] Access to this growing archive of e-journals is free and unrestricted.[5] To search, go to **http://www.ncbi.nlm.nih.gov/entrez/query.fcgi?db=Pmc**, and type "radiotherapy" (or synonyms) into the search box. This search gives you access to full-text articles. The following is a sample of items found for radiotherapy in the PubMed Central database:

- **Biological-effective versus conventional dose volume histograms correlated with late genitourinary and gastrointestinal toxicity after external beam radiotherapy for prostate cancer: a matched pair analysis.** by Jani AB, Hand CM, Pelizzari CA, Roeske JC, Krauz L, Vijayakumar S.; 2003;
  http://www.pubmedcentral.gov/articlerender.fcgi?tool=pmcentrez&artid=156635

---

[3] Adapted from the National Library of Medicine: **http://www.pubmedcentral.nih.gov/about/intro.html**.

[4] With PubMed Central, NCBI is taking the lead in preservation and maintenance of open access to electronic literature, just as NLM has done for decades with printed biomedical literature. PubMed Central aims to become a world-class library of the digital age.

[5] The value of PubMed Central, in addition to its role as an archive, lies in the availability of data from diverse sources stored in a common format in a single repository. Many journals already have online publishing operations, and there is a growing tendency to publish material online only, to the exclusion of print.

- **Breast cancer patients sue over radiotherapy wait times.** by Pengelley H.; 2004 May 25; http://www.pubmedcentral.gov/articlerender.fcgi?tool=pmcentrez&artid=408496

- **Clinical practice guidelines for the care and treatment of breast cancer: breast radiotherapy after breast-conserving surgery (summary of the 2003 update).** by Whelan T, Olivotto I, Levine M.; 2003 Feb 18; http://www.pubmedcentral.gov/articlerender.fcgi?tool=pmcentrez&artid=143551

- **Combined effects of radiotherapy and angiostatin gene therapy in glioma tumor model.** by Griscelli F, Li H, Cheong C, Opolon P, Bennaceur-Griscelli A, Vassal G, Soria J, Soria C, Lu H, Perricaudet M, Yeh P.; 2000 Jun 6; http://www.pubmedcentral.gov/articlerender.fcgi?tool=pmcentrez&artid=18707

- **Immediate versus delayed palliative thoracic radiotherapy in patients with unresectable locally advanced non-small cell lung cancer and minimal thoracic symptoms: randomised controlled trial.** by Falk SJ, Girling DJ, White RJ, Hopwood P, Harvey A, Qian W, Stephens RJ.; 2002 Aug 31; http://www.pubmedcentral.gov/articlerender.fcgi?tool=pmcentrez&artid=119441

- **Influence of local radiotherapy on penetration of fluconazole into human saliva.** by Oliary J, Tod M, Louchahi K, Petitjean O, Frachet B, Le Gros V, Brion N.; 1993 Dec; http://www.pubmedcentral.gov/picrender.fcgi?tool=pmcentrez&action=stream&blobtype=pdf&artid=192775

- **Mortality from cardiovascular disease more than 10 years after radiotherapy for breast cancer: nationwide cohort study of 90 000 Swedish women.** by Darby S, McGale P, Peto R, Granath F, Hall P, Ekbom A.; 2003 Feb 1; http://www.pubmedcentral.gov/articlerender.fcgi?tool=pmcentrez&artid=140764

- **Pretarget radiotherapy with an anti-CD25 antibody-streptavidin fusion protein was effective in therapy of leukemia /lymphoma xenografts.** by Zhang M, Zhang Z, Garmestani K, Schultz J, Axworthy DB, Goldman CK, Brechbiel MW, Carrasquillo JA, Waldmann TA.; 2003 Feb 18; http://www.pubmedcentral.gov/articlerender.fcgi?tool=pmcentrez&artid=149929

- **Radiation-resistant and repair-proficient human tumor cells may be associated with radiotherapy failure in head- and neck-cancer patients.** by Weichselbaum RR, Dahlberg W, Beckett M, Karrison T, Miller D, Clark J, Ervin TJ.; 1986 Apr; http://www.pubmedcentral.gov/picrender.fcgi?tool=pmcentrez&action=stream&blobtype=pdf&artid=323364

- **Solid tumor models for the assessment of different treatment modalities: systematics of response to radiotherapy and chemotherapy.** by Looney WB, Trefil JS, Schaffner JG, Kovacs CJ, Hopkins HA.; 1976 Mar; http://www.pubmedcentral.gov/picrender.fcgi?tool=pmcentrez&action=stream&blobtype=pdf&artid=336010

- **Spontaneous Enterocutaneous Fistula 27-years Following Radiotherapy in a Patient of Carcinoma Penis.** by Chintamani, Badran R, Rk D, Singhal V, Bhatnagar D.; 2003; http://www.pubmedcentral.gov/articlerender.fcgi?tool=pmcentrez&artid=269989

- **Targeting Radiotherapy to Cancer by Gene Transfer.** by Mairs RJ, Boyd M.; 2003; http://www.pubmedcentral.gov/articlerender.fcgi?tool=pmcentrez&artid=323955

- **The use of preoperative radiotherapy in the management of patients with clinically resectable rectal cancer: a practice guideline.** by Figueredo A, Zuraw L, Wong RK, Agboola O, Rumble RB, Tandan V.; 2003; http://www.pubmedcentral.gov/articlerender.fcgi?tool=pmcentrez&artid=281590

The National Library of Medicine: PubMed

One of the quickest and most comprehensive ways to find academic studies in both English and other languages is to use PubMed, maintained by the National Library of Medicine.[6] The advantage of PubMed over previously mentioned sources is that it covers a greater number of domestic and foreign references. It is also free to use. If the publisher has a Web site that offers full text of its journals, PubMed will provide links to that site, as well as to sites offering other related data. User registration, a subscription fee, or some other type of fee may be required to access the full text of articles in some journals.

To generate your own bibliography of studies dealing with radiotherapy, simply go to the PubMed Web site at **http://www.ncbi.nlm.nih.gov/pubmed**. Type "radiotherapy" (or synonyms) into the search box, and click "Go." The following is the type of output you can expect from PubMed for radiotherapy (hyperlinks lead to article summaries):

- **A prospective population-based management program including primary surgery and postoperative risk assessment by means of DNA ploidy and histopathology. Adjuvant radiotherapy is not necessary for the majority of patients with FIGO stage I-II endometrial cancer.**
  Author(s): Hogberg T, Fredstorp-Lidebring M, Alm P, Baldetorp B, Larsson G, Ottosen C, Svanberg L, Lindahl B; Southern Swedish Gynecologic Oncology Group.
  Source: International Journal of Gynecological Cancer : Official Journal of the International Gynecological Cancer Society. 2004 May-June; 14(3): 437-50.
  http://www.ncbi.nlm.nih.gov/entrez/query.fcgi?cmd=Retrieve&db=pubmed&dopt=Abstract&list_uids=15228416

- **A randomised trial of single-dose radiotherapy to prevent procedure tract metastasis by malignant mesothelioma.**
  Author(s): Bydder S, Phillips M, Joseph DJ, Cameron F, Spry NA, DeMelker Y, Musk AW.
  Source: British Journal of Cancer. 2004 July 5; 91(1): 9-10.
  http://www.ncbi.nlm.nih.gov/entrez/query.fcgi?cmd=Retrieve&db=pubmed&dopt=Abstract&list_uids=15199394

- **A randomized, controlled trial of aerobic exercise for treatment-related fatigue in men receiving radical external beam radiotherapy for localized prostate carcinoma.**
  Author(s): Windsor PM, Nicol KF, Potter J.
  Source: Cancer. 2004 August 1; 101(3): 550-7.
  http://www.ncbi.nlm.nih.gov/entrez/query.fcgi?cmd=Retrieve&db=pubmed&dopt=Abstract&list_uids=15274068

---

[6] PubMed was developed by the National Center for Biotechnology Information (NCBI) at the National Library of Medicine (NLM) at the National Institutes of Health (NIH). The PubMed database was developed in conjunction with publishers of biomedical literature as a search tool for accessing literature citations and linking to full-text journal articles at Web sites of participating publishers. Publishers that participate in PubMed supply NLM with their citations electronically prior to or at the time of publication.

- **A study of radiotherapy modalities combined with continuous 5-FU infusion for locally advanced gastrointestinal malignancies.**
  Author(s): Shibata SI, Pezner R, Chu D, Doroshow JH, Chow WA, Leong LA, Margolin KA, McNamara MV, Morgan RJ Jr, Raschko JW, Somlo G, Tetef ML, Yen Y, Synold TW, Wagman L, Vora N, Carroll M, Lin S, Longmate J.
  Source: European Journal of Surgical Oncology : the Journal of the European Society of Surgical Oncology and the British Association of Surgical Oncology. 2004 August; 30(6): 650-7.
  http://www.ncbi.nlm.nih.gov/entrez/query.fcgi?cmd=Retrieve&db=pubmed&dopt=Abstract&list_uids=15256240

- **A table top suited for CT and radiotherapy.**
  Author(s): Bratengeier K, Baur W, Baier K, Wulf J, Flentje M.
  Source: Z Med Phys. 2004; 14(2): 118-22.
  http://www.ncbi.nlm.nih.gov/entrez/query.fcgi?cmd=Retrieve&db=pubmed&dopt=Abstract&list_uids=15323290

- **A treatment planning study evaluating a 'simultaneous integrated boost' technique for accelerated radiotherapy of stage III non-small cell lung cancer.**
  Author(s): Dirkx ML, van Sornsen De Koste JR, Senan S.
  Source: Lung Cancer (Amsterdam, Netherlands). 2004 July; 45(1): 57-65.
  http://www.ncbi.nlm.nih.gov/entrez/query.fcgi?cmd=Retrieve&db=pubmed&dopt=Abstract&list_uids=15196735

- **Acute and chronic results of adjuvant radiotherapy after mastectomy and Transverse Rectus Abdominis Myocutaneous (TRAM) flap reconstruction for breast cancer.**
  Author(s): Halyard MY, McCombs KE, Wong WW, Buchel EW, Pockaj BA, Vora SA, Gray RJ, Schild SE.
  Source: American Journal of Clinical Oncology : the Official Publication of the American Radium Society. 2004 August; 27(4): 389-94.
  http://www.ncbi.nlm.nih.gov/entrez/query.fcgi?cmd=Retrieve&db=pubmed&dopt=Abstract&list_uids=15289733

- **Acute toxicity of chemo-radiotherapy for cervical cancer: the Addenbrooke's experience.**
  Author(s): Tan LT, Russell S, Burgess L.
  Source: Clin Oncol (R Coll Radiol). 2004 June; 16(4): 255-60.
  http://www.ncbi.nlm.nih.gov/entrez/query.fcgi?cmd=Retrieve&db=pubmed&dopt=Abstract&list_uids=15214649

- **Adding concurrent low dose continuous infusion of cisplatin to radiotherapy in locally advanced cervical carcinoma: a prospective randomized pilot study.**
  Author(s): Garipagaoglu M, Kayikcioglu F, Kose MF, Adli M, Gulkesen KH, Kocak Z, Tulunay G.
  Source: The British Journal of Radiology. 2004 July; 77(919): 581-7.
  http://www.ncbi.nlm.nih.gov/entrez/query.fcgi?cmd=Retrieve&db=pubmed&dopt=Abstract&list_uids=15238405

- **Adjuvant postoperative radiotherapy for colon carcinoma.**
  Author(s): Mendenhall WM, Amos EH, Rout WR, Zlotecki RA, Hochwald SN, Cance WG.
  Source: Cancer. 2004 September 15; 101(6): 1338-44. Review.
  http://www.ncbi.nlm.nih.gov/entrez/query.fcgi?cmd=Retrieve&db=pubmed&dopt=Abstract&list_uids=15316945

- **Adjuvant radiotherapy for breast cancer: effects of longer follow-up.**
  Author(s): Van de Steene J, Vinh-Hung V, Cutuli B, Storme G.
  Source: Radiotherapy and Oncology : Journal of the European Society for Therapeutic Radiology and Oncology. 2004 July; 72(1): 35-43.
  http://www.ncbi.nlm.nih.gov/entrez/query.fcgi?cmd=Retrieve&db=pubmed&dopt=Abstract&list_uids=15236872

- **An evaluation of radiation exposure from portal films taken during definitive course of pediatric radiotherapy.**
  Author(s): Kudchadker RJ, Chang EL, Bryan F, Maor MH, Famiglietti R.
  Source: International Journal of Radiation Oncology, Biology, Physics. 2004 July 15; 59(4): 1229-35. Erratum In: Int J Radiat Oncol Biol Phys. 2004 September 1; 60(1): 350.
  http://www.ncbi.nlm.nih.gov/entrez/query.fcgi?cmd=Retrieve&db=pubmed&dopt=Abstract&list_uids=15234060

- **Aneurysmal bone cyst of the sternum: a case report of successful treatment with radiotherapy.**
  Author(s): Yavuz AA, Sener M, Yavuz MN, Kosucu P, Cobanoglu U.
  Source: The British Journal of Radiology. 2004 July; 77(919): 610-4. Review.
  http://www.ncbi.nlm.nih.gov/entrez/query.fcgi?cmd=Retrieve&db=pubmed&dopt=Abstract&list_uids=15238410

- **Application of real-time tumor-tracking and gated radiotherapy system for unresectable pancreatic cancer.**
  Author(s): Ahn YC, Shimizu S, Shirato H, Hashimoto T, Osaka Y, Zhang XQ, Abe T, Hosokawa M, Miyasaka K.
  Source: Yonsei Medical Journal. 2004 August 31; 45(4): 584-90.
  http://www.ncbi.nlm.nih.gov/entrez/query.fcgi?cmd=Retrieve&db=pubmed&dopt=Abstract&list_uids=15344197

- **Are single fractions of radiotherapy suitable for plantar fasciitis?**
  Author(s): Schwarz F, Christie DR, Irving M.
  Source: Australasian Radiology. 2004 June; 48(2): 162-9.
  http://www.ncbi.nlm.nih.gov/entrez/query.fcgi?cmd=Retrieve&db=pubmed&dopt=Abstract&list_uids=15230750

- **Assessment of effective dose from concomitant exposures required in verification of the target volume in radiotherapy.**
  Author(s): Waddington SP, McKenzie AL.
  Source: The British Journal of Radiology. 2004 July; 77(919): 557-61.
  http://www.ncbi.nlm.nih.gov/entrez/query.fcgi?cmd=Retrieve&db=pubmed&dopt=Abstract&list_uids=15238401

- **Association of hemoglobin level with survival in cervical carcinoma patients treated with concurrent cisplatin and radiotherapy: a Gynecologic Oncology Group Study.**
  Author(s): Winter WE 3rd, Maxwell GL, Tian C, Sobel E, Rose GS, Thomas G, Carlson JW.
  Source: Gynecologic Oncology. 2004 August; 94(2): 495-501.
  http://www.ncbi.nlm.nih.gov/entrez/query.fcgi?cmd=Retrieve&db=pubmed&dopt=Abstract&list_uids=15297194

- **Association of percent positive prostate biopsies and perineural invasion with biochemical outcome after external beam radiotherapy for localized prostate cancer.**
  Author(s): Wong WW, Schild SE, Vora SA, Halyard MY.
  Source: International Journal of Radiation Oncology, Biology, Physics. 2004 September 1; 60(1): 24-9.
  http://www.ncbi.nlm.nih.gov/entrez/query.fcgi?cmd=Retrieve&db=pubmed&dopt=Abstract&list_uids=15337536

- **Atypical slipped capital femoral epiphysis after radiotherapy and chemotherapy.**
  Author(s): Liu SC, Tsai CC, Huang CH.
  Source: Clinical Orthopaedics and Related Research. 2004 Sep(426): 212-8. Review.
  http://www.ncbi.nlm.nih.gov/entrez/query.fcgi?cmd=Retrieve&db=pubmed&dopt=Abstract&list_uids=15346076

- **Bilateral renal artery stenosis after abdominal radiotherapy for Hodgkin's disease.**
  Author(s): Unsal D, Bora H.
  Source: Int J Clin Pract. 2003 December; 57(10): 923-4; Author Reply 924. No Abstract Available.
  http://www.ncbi.nlm.nih.gov/entrez/query.fcgi?cmd=Retrieve&db=pubmed&dopt=Abstract&list_uids=14712901

- **Bilateral renal artery stenosis after abdominal radiotherapy for Hodgkin's disease.**
  Author(s): Saka B, Bilge AK, Umman B, Yilmaz E, Nisanci Y, Erten N, Karan MA, Tascioglu C.
  Source: Int J Clin Pract. 2003 April; 57(3): 247-8.
  http://www.ncbi.nlm.nih.gov/entrez/query.fcgi?cmd=Retrieve&db=pubmed&dopt=Abstract&list_uids=12723735

- **Bilateral rhegmatogenous retinal detachment after external-beam radiotherapy: just a coincidence?**
  Author(s): Kodjikian L, Garweg JG, Fleury J, Rocher F, Burillon C, Grange JD.
  Source: Graefe's Archive for Clinical and Experimental Ophthalmology = Albrecht Von Graefes Archiv Fur Klinische Und Experimentelle Ophthalmologie. 2004 June; 242(6): 523-6. Epub 2004 March 24.
  http://www.ncbi.nlm.nih.gov/entrez/query.fcgi?cmd=Retrieve&db=pubmed&dopt=Abstract&list_uids=15042376

- **Biochemical failure as a determinant of distant metastasis and death in prostate cancer treated with radiotherapy.**
  Author(s): Pollack A, Hanlon AL, Movsas B, Hanks GE, Uzzo R, Horwitz EM.
  Source: International Journal of Radiation Oncology, Biology, Physics. 2003 September 1; 57(1): 19-23.
  http://www.ncbi.nlm.nih.gov/entrez/query.fcgi?cmd=Retrieve&db=pubmed&dopt=Abstract&list_uids=12909210

- **Biological factors and therapeutic modulation in brain tumor radiotherapy.**
  Author(s): De Santis M, Caiazza A, Simili A.
  Source: Rays. 2002 July-September; 27(3): 201-3.
  http://www.ncbi.nlm.nih.gov/entrez/query.fcgi?cmd=Retrieve&db=pubmed&dopt=Abstract&list_uids=12696250

- **Biological factors and therapeutic modulation in pancreatic carcinoma radiotherapy.**
  Author(s): Cellini N, Morganti AG, Macchia G, Smaniotto D, Luzi S, Mattiucci GC, Forni F, Valentini V.
  Source: Rays. 2002 July-September; 27(3): 215-7.
  http://www.ncbi.nlm.nih.gov/entrez/query.fcgi?cmd=Retrieve&db=pubmed&dopt=Abstract&list_uids=12696252

- **Biological factors and therapeutic modulation in prostate cancer radiotherapy.**
  Author(s): Cellini N, Luzi S, Morganit AG, Smaniotto D, Mattiucci GC, Digesu C, Mangiacotti MG, Cellini F, Valentini V.
  Source: Rays. 2002 July-September; 27(3): 205-14. Review.
  http://www.ncbi.nlm.nih.gov/entrez/query.fcgi?cmd=Retrieve&db=pubmed&dopt=Abstract&list_uids=12696251

- **Biological factors and therapeutic modulation in rectal cancer radiotherapy.**
  Author(s): Gambacorta MA, Micciche F, Corvari B, Mantini G, Valentini V.
  Source: Rays. 2002 July-September; 27(3): 219-22. Review.
  http://www.ncbi.nlm.nih.gov/entrez/query.fcgi?cmd=Retrieve&db=pubmed&dopt=Abstract&list_uids=12696253

- **Biological-effective versus conventional dose volume histograms correlated with late genitourinary and gastrointestinal toxicity after external beam radiotherapy for prostate cancer: a matched pair analysis.**
  Author(s): Jani AB, Hand CM, Pelizzari CA, Roeske JC, Krauz L, Vijayakumar S.
  Source: Bmc Cancer [electronic Resource]. 2003 May 13; 3(1): 16.
  http://www.ncbi.nlm.nih.gov/entrez/query.fcgi?cmd=Retrieve&db=pubmed&dopt=Abstract&list_uids=12744725

- **Biologically effective doses in radiotherapy of cervical carcinoma*.**
  Author(s): Urbanski K, Gasinska A, Pudelek J, Fowler JF, Lind B, Brahme A.
  Source: Neoplasma. 2004; 51(3): 228-38.
  http://www.ncbi.nlm.nih.gov/entrez/query.fcgi?cmd=Retrieve&db=pubmed&dopt=Abstract&list_uids=15254678

- **Black and white patients fare equally well when treated with postlumpectomy radiotherapy.**
  Author(s): Burri SH, Landry JC, Norton HJ, Davis LW.
  Source: Journal of the National Medical Association. 2004 July; 96(7): 961-7.
  http://www.ncbi.nlm.nih.gov/entrez/query.fcgi?cmd=Retrieve&db=pubmed&dopt=Abstract&list_uids=15253328

- **Brain metastases treated with radiosurgery alone: an alternative to whole brain radiotherapy?**
  Author(s): Hasegawa T, Kondziolka D, Flickinger JC, Germanwala A, Lunsford LD.
  Source: Neurosurgery. 2003 June; 52(6): 1318-26; Discussion 1326.
  http://www.ncbi.nlm.nih.gov/entrez/query.fcgi?cmd=Retrieve&db=pubmed&dopt=Abstract&list_uids=12762877

- **Breast cancer following radiotherapy and chemotherapy among young women with Hodgkin disease.**
  Author(s): Travis LB, Hill DA, Dores GM, Gospodarowicz M, van Leeuwen FE, Holowaty E, Glimelius B, Andersson M, Wiklund T, Lynch CF, Van't Veer MB, Glimelius I, Storm H, Pukkala E, Stovall M, Curtis R, Boice JD Jr, Gilbert E.
  Source: Jama : the Journal of the American Medical Association. 2003 July 23; 290(4): 465-75. Erratum In: Jama. 2003 September 10; 290(10): 1318.
  http://www.ncbi.nlm.nih.gov/entrez/query.fcgi?cmd=Retrieve&db=pubmed&dopt=Abstract&list_uids=12876089

- **Breast cancer patients sue over radiotherapy wait times.**
  Author(s): Pengelley H.
  Source: Cmaj : Canadian Medical Association Journal = Journal De L'association Medicale Canadienne. 2004 May 25; 170(11): 1655.
  http://www.ncbi.nlm.nih.gov/entrez/query.fcgi?cmd=Retrieve&db=pubmed&dopt=Abstract&list_uids=15159354

- **Breast conservation surgery, with and without radiotherapy, in women with lymph node-negative breast cancer: a randomised clinical trial in a population with access to public mammography screening.**
  Author(s): Malmstrom P, Holmberg L, Anderson H, Mattsson J, Jonsson PE, Tennvall-Nittby L, Balldin G, Loven L, Svensson JH, Ingvar C, Moller T, Holmberg E, Wallgren A; Swedisj Breast Cancer Group.
  Source: European Journal of Cancer (Oxford, England : 1990). 2003 August; 39(12): 1690-7.
  http://www.ncbi.nlm.nih.gov/entrez/query.fcgi?cmd=Retrieve&db=pubmed&dopt=Abstract&list_uids=12888363

- **Breast radiotherapy after lumpectomy--no longer always necessary.**
  Author(s): Smith IE, Ross GM.
  Source: The New England Journal of Medicine. 2004 September 2; 351(10): 1021-3.
  http://www.ncbi.nlm.nih.gov/entrez/query.fcgi?cmd=Retrieve&db=pubmed&dopt=Abstract&list_uids=15342811

- **Breast-conserving surgery has equivalent effect as mastectomy on stage I breast cancer prognosis only when followed by radiotherapy.**
  Author(s): Rapiti E, Fioretta G, Vlastos G, Kurtz J, Schafer P, Sappino AP, Spiliopoulos A, Renella R, Neyroud-Caspar I, Bouchardy C.
  Source: Radiotherapy and Oncology : Journal of the European Society for Therapeutic Radiology and Oncology. 2003 December; 69(3): 277-84.
  http://www.ncbi.nlm.nih.gov/entrez/query.fcgi?cmd=Retrieve&db=pubmed&dopt=Abstract&list_uids=14644487

- **Breast-conserving surgery with or without radiotherapy: pooled-analysis for risks of ipsilateral breast tumor recurrence and mortality.**
  Author(s): Vinh-Hung V, Verschraegen C.
  Source: Journal of the National Cancer Institute. 2004 January 21; 96(2): 115-21.
  http://www.ncbi.nlm.nih.gov/entrez/query.fcgi?cmd=Retrieve&db=pubmed&dopt=Abstract&list_uids=14734701

- **Breathing adapted radiotherapy of breast cancer: reduction of cardiac and pulmonary doses using voluntary inspiration breath-hold.**
  Author(s): Pedersen AN, Korreman S, Nystrom H, Specht L.
  Source: Radiotherapy and Oncology : Journal of the European Society for Therapeutic Radiology and Oncology. 2004 July; 72(1): 53-60.
  http://www.ncbi.nlm.nih.gov/entrez/query.fcgi?cmd=Retrieve&db=pubmed&dopt=Abstract&list_uids=15236874

- **Bulb of penis as a marker for prostatic apex in external beam radiotherapy of prostate cancer.**
  Author(s): Plants BA, Chen DT, Fiveash JB, Kim RY.
  Source: International Journal of Radiation Oncology, Biology, Physics. 2003 July 15; 56(4): 1079-84.
  http://www.ncbi.nlm.nih.gov/entrez/query.fcgi?cmd=Retrieve&db=pubmed&dopt=Abstract&list_uids=12829145

- **Cancer mortality after radiotherapy for a skin hemangioma during childhood.**
  Author(s): Dondon MG, de Vathaire F, Shamsaldin A, Doyon F, Diallo I, Ligot L, Paoletti C, Labbe M, Abbas M, Chavaudra J, Avril MF, Fragu P, Eschwege F.
  Source: Radiotherapy and Oncology : Journal of the European Society for Therapeutic Radiology and Oncology. 2004 July; 72(1): 87-93.
  http://www.ncbi.nlm.nih.gov/entrez/query.fcgi?cmd=Retrieve&db=pubmed&dopt=Abstract&list_uids=15236880

- **Cardiovascular status in long-term survivors of Hodgkin's disease treated with chest radiotherapy.**
  Author(s): Adams MJ, Lipsitz SR, Colan SD, Tarbell NJ, Treves ST, Diller L, Greenbaum N, Mauch P, Lipshultz SE.
  Source: Journal of Clinical Oncology : Official Journal of the American Society of Clinical Oncology. 2004 August 1; 22(15): 3139-48.
  http://www.ncbi.nlm.nih.gov/entrez/query.fcgi?cmd=Retrieve&db=pubmed&dopt=Abstract&list_uids=15284266

- Cerebral radionecrosis with cystic degeneration following radiotherapy for nasal cavity squamous cell carcinoma: a case report.
  Author(s): Hsu YC, Ho KY, Kuo WR, Wang LF, Lee KW, Huang SL.
  Source: Kaohsiung J Med Sci. 2004 June; 20(6): 308-12.
  http://www.ncbi.nlm.nih.gov/entrez/query.fcgi?cmd=Retrieve&db=pubmed&dopt=Abstract&list_uids=15253473

- Changing trends in national practice for external beam radiotherapy for clinically localized prostate cancer: 1999 Patterns of Care survey for prostate cancer.
  Author(s): Zelefsky MJ, Moughan J, Owen J, Zietman AL, Roach M 3rd, Hanks GE.
  Source: International Journal of Radiation Oncology, Biology, Physics. 2004 July 15; 59(4): 1053-61.
  http://www.ncbi.nlm.nih.gov/entrez/query.fcgi?cmd=Retrieve&db=pubmed&dopt=Abstract&list_uids=15234039

- Clinical evaluation of radiotherapy for advanced esophageal cancer after metallic stent placement.
  Author(s): Yu YT, Yang G, Liu Y, Shen BZ.
  Source: World Journal of Gastroenterology : Wjg. 2004 July 15; 10(14): 2145-6.
  http://www.ncbi.nlm.nih.gov/entrez/query.fcgi?cmd=Retrieve&db=pubmed&dopt=Abstract&list_uids=15237455

- Clinical nature and prognosis of locally recurrent rectal cancer after total mesorectal excision with or without preoperative radiotherapy.
  Author(s): van den Brink M, Stiggelbout AM, van den Hout WB, Kievit J, Klein Kranenbarg E, Marijnen CA, Nagtegaal ID, Rutten HJ, Wiggers T, van de Velde CJ.
  Source: Journal of Clinical Oncology : Official Journal of the American Society of Clinical Oncology. 2004 October 1; 22(19): 3958-64.
  http://www.ncbi.nlm.nih.gov/entrez/query.fcgi?cmd=Retrieve&db=pubmed&dopt=Abstract&list_uids=15459218

- Clinical outcomes of stereotactic radiotherapy for stage I non-small cell lung cancer using a novel irradiation technique: patient self-controlled breath-hold and beam switching using a combination of linear accelerator and CT scanner.
  Author(s): Onishi H, Kuriyama K, Komiyama T, Tanaka S, Sano N, Marino K, Ikenaga S, Araki T, Uematsu M.
  Source: Lung Cancer (Amsterdam, Netherlands). 2004 July; 45(1): 45-55.
  http://www.ncbi.nlm.nih.gov/entrez/query.fcgi?cmd=Retrieve&db=pubmed&dopt=Abstract&list_uids=15196734

- Clinical prioritisation for curative radiotherapy: a local waiting list initiative.
  Author(s): Martin JM, Ryan G, Duchesne G.
  Source: Clin Oncol (R Coll Radiol). 2004 June; 16(4): 299-306.
  http://www.ncbi.nlm.nih.gov/entrez/query.fcgi?cmd=Retrieve&db=pubmed&dopt=Abstract&list_uids=15214655

- **Clinical use of intensity-modulated radiotherapy: part I.**
  Author(s): Guerrero Urbano MT, Nutting CM.
  Source: The British Journal of Radiology. 2004 February; 77(914): 88-96. Review.
  http://www.ncbi.nlm.nih.gov/entrez/query.fcgi?cmd=Retrieve&db=pubmed&dopt=A
  bstract&list_uids=15010378

- **Clonogenic survival and cytokinesis-blocked binucleation of skin fibroblasts and normal tissue complications in soft tissue sarcoma patients treated with preoperative radiotherapy.**
  Author(s): Akudugu JM, Bell RS, Catton C, Davis AM, O'Sullivan B, Waldron J, Wunder JS, Hill RP.
  Source: Radiotherapy and Oncology : Journal of the European Society for Therapeutic Radiology and Oncology. 2004 July; 72(1): 103-12.
  http://www.ncbi.nlm.nih.gov/entrez/query.fcgi?cmd=Retrieve&db=pubmed&dopt=A
  bstract&list_uids=15236882

- **Combination epidermal growth factor receptor inhibition and radical radiotherapy for NSCLC.**
  Author(s): Rogers SJ, Harrington KJ, Eccles SA, Nutting CM.
  Source: Expert Review of Anticancer Therapy. 2004 August; 4(4): 569-83. Review.
  http://www.ncbi.nlm.nih.gov/entrez/query.fcgi?cmd=Retrieve&db=pubmed&dopt=A
  bstract&list_uids=15270661

- **Combined-modality therapy with gemcitabine and radiotherapy as a bladder preservation strategy: results of a phase I trial.**
  Author(s): Kent E, Sandler H, Montie J, Lee C, Herman J, Esper P, Fardig J, Smith DC.
  Source: Journal of Clinical Oncology : Official Journal of the American Society of Clinical Oncology. 2004 July 1; 22(13): 2540-5.
  http://www.ncbi.nlm.nih.gov/entrez/query.fcgi?cmd=Retrieve&db=pubmed&dopt=A
  bstract&list_uids=15226322

- Concomitant hydroxyurea plus radiotherapy versus radiotherapy for carcinoma of the uterine cervix: a systematic review.
  Author(s): Symonds RP, Collingwood M, Kirwan J, Humber CE, Tierney JF, Green JA, Williams C.
  Source: Cancer Treatment Reviews. 2004 August; 30(5): 405-14. Review.
  http://www.ncbi.nlm.nih.gov/entrez/query.fcgi?cmd=Retrieve&db=pubmed&dopt=A
  bstract&list_uids=15245773

- Concomitant radiochemotherapy vs radiotherapy alone in patients with head and neck cancer: a Hellenic Cooperative Oncology Group Phase III Study.
  Author(s): Fountzilas G, Ciuleanu E, Dafni U, Plataniotis G, Kalogera-Fountzila A, Samantas E, Athanassiou E, Tzitzikas J, Ciuleanu T, Nikolaou A, Pantelakos P, Zaraboukas T, Zamboglou N, Daniilidis J, Ghilezan N.
  Source: Medical Oncology (Northwood, London, England). 2004; 21(2): 95-107.
  http://www.ncbi.nlm.nih.gov/entrez/query.fcgi?cmd=Retrieve&db=pubmed&dopt=A
  bstract&list_uids=15299181

- **Considerations for post-operative radiotherapy to the hemithorax following extrapleural pneumonectomy in malignant pleural mesothelioma.**
  Author(s): Senan S, van de Pol M.
  Source: Lung Cancer (Amsterdam, Netherlands). 2004 August; 45 Suppl 1: S93-6. Review.
  http://www.ncbi.nlm.nih.gov/entrez/query.fcgi?cmd=Retrieve&db=pubmed&dopt=Abstract&list_uids=15261442

- **Continuous 28-day iododeoxyuridine infusion and hyperfractionated accelerated radiotherapy for malignant glioma: a phase I clinical study.**
  Author(s): Schulz CA, Mehta MP, Badie B, McGinn CJ, Robins HI, Hayes L, Chappell R, Volkman J, Binger K, Arzoomanian R, Simon K, Alberti D, Feierabend C, Tutsch KD, Kunugi KA, Wilding G, Kinsella TJ.
  Source: International Journal of Radiation Oncology, Biology, Physics. 2004 July 15; 59(4): 1107-15.
  http://www.ncbi.nlm.nih.gov/entrez/query.fcgi?cmd=Retrieve&db=pubmed&dopt=Abstract&list_uids=15234045

- **Daily electronic portal imaging for morbidly obese men undergoing radiotherapy for localized prostate cancer.**
  Author(s): Millender LE, Aubin M, Pouliot J, Shinohara K, Roach M 3rd.
  Source: International Journal of Radiation Oncology, Biology, Physics. 2004 May 1; 59(1): 6-10.
  http://www.ncbi.nlm.nih.gov/entrez/query.fcgi?cmd=Retrieve&db=pubmed&dopt=Abstract&list_uids=15093893

- **Daily ultrasound-based image-guided targeting for radiotherapy of upper abdominal malignancies.**
  Author(s): Fuss M, Salter BJ, Cavanaugh SX, Fuss C, Sadeghi A, Fuller CD, Ameduri A, Hevezi JM, Herman TS, Thomas CR Jr.
  Source: International Journal of Radiation Oncology, Biology, Physics. 2004 July 15; 59(4): 1245-56.
  http://www.ncbi.nlm.nih.gov/entrez/query.fcgi?cmd=Retrieve&db=pubmed&dopt=Abstract&list_uids=15234062

- **Decreased short- and long-term swallowing problems with altered radiotherapy dosing used in an organ-sparing protocol for advanced pharyngeal carcinoma.**
  Author(s): Smith RV, Goldman SY, Beitler JJ, Wadler SS.
  Source: Archives of Otolaryngology--Head & Neck Surgery. 2004 July; 130(7): 831-6.
  http://www.ncbi.nlm.nih.gov/entrez/query.fcgi?cmd=Retrieve&db=pubmed&dopt=Abstract&list_uids=15262759

- **Delay of postoperative radiotherapy in head and neck cancer patients.**
  Author(s): Blot E, Astruc E, Bastit L.
  Source: Journal of Clinical Oncology : Official Journal of the American Society of Clinical Oncology. 2004 April 1; 22(7): 1342; Author Reply 1343-4.
  http://www.ncbi.nlm.nih.gov/entrez/query.fcgi?cmd=Retrieve&db=pubmed&dopt=Abstract&list_uids=15051787

- **Delayed radiation toxicity after focal or whole brain radiotherapy for low-grade glioma.**
  Author(s): Swennen MH, Bromberg JE, Witkamp TD, Terhaard CH, Postma TJ, Taphoorn MJ.
  Source: Journal of Neuro-Oncology. 2004 February; 66(3): 333-9.
  http://www.ncbi.nlm.nih.gov/entrez/query.fcgi?cmd=Retrieve&db=pubmed&dopt=Abstract&list_uids=15015665

- **Dilated cardiomyopathy in a pregnant woman after doxorubicin and radiotherapy for Hodgkin's disease: a case report.**
  Author(s): Hadar A, Sheiner E, Press F, Katz A, Katz M.
  Source: J Reprod Med. 2004 May; 49(5): 401-3.
  http://www.ncbi.nlm.nih.gov/entrez/query.fcgi?cmd=Retrieve&db=pubmed&dopt=Abstract&list_uids=15214719

- **Do we need more trials of postoperative radiotherapy after esophagectomy?**
  Author(s): Pramesh CS, Mistry RC, Deshpande RK, Sharma S.
  Source: The Annals of Thoracic Surgery. 2004 May; 77(5): 1878-9.
  http://www.ncbi.nlm.nih.gov/entrez/query.fcgi?cmd=Retrieve&db=pubmed&dopt=Abstract&list_uids=15111224

- **Does radiotherapy around the time of pregnancy for Hodgkin's disease modify the risk of breast cancer?**
  Author(s): Chen J, Lee RJ, Tsodikov A, Smith L, Gaffney DK.
  Source: International Journal of Radiation Oncology, Biology, Physics. 2004 April 1; 58(5): 1474-9.
  http://www.ncbi.nlm.nih.gov/entrez/query.fcgi?cmd=Retrieve&db=pubmed&dopt=Abstract&list_uids=15050326

- **Dose and volume reduction for normal lung using intensity-modulated radiotherapy for advanced-stage non-small-cell lung cancer.**
  Author(s): Murshed H, Liu HH, Liao Z, Barker JL, Wang X, Tucker SL, Chandra A, Guerrero T, Stevens C, Chang JY, Jeter M, Cox JD, Komaki R, Mohan R, Change JY.
  Source: International Journal of Radiation Oncology, Biology, Physics. 2004 March 15; 58(4): 1258-67. Erratum In: Int J Radiat Oncol Biol Phys. 2004 July 1; 59(3): 921 Change Jt [corrected to Chang Jt].
  http://www.ncbi.nlm.nih.gov/entrez/query.fcgi?cmd=Retrieve&db=pubmed&dopt=Abstract&list_uids=15001271

- **Dose-escalated 3D conformal radiotherapy in prostate cancer.**
  Author(s): Malone S.
  Source: Expert Review of Anticancer Therapy. 2004 August; 4(4): 663-8. Review.
  http://www.ncbi.nlm.nih.gov/entrez/query.fcgi?cmd=Retrieve&db=pubmed&dopt=Abstract&list_uids=15270669

- **Dose-volume response analyses of late rectal bleeding after radiotherapy for prostate cancer.**
  Author(s): Tucker SL, Cheung R, Dong L, Liu HH, Thames HD, Huang EH, Kuban D, Mohan R.
  Source: International Journal of Radiation Oncology, Biology, Physics. 2004 June 1; 59(2): 353-65.
  http://www.ncbi.nlm.nih.gov/entrez/query.fcgi?cmd=Retrieve&db=pubmed&dopt=Abstract&list_uids=15145148

- **Dosimetric analysis of a simplified intensity modulation technique for prone breast radiotherapy.**
  Author(s): Goodman KA, Hong L, Wagman R, Hunt MA, McCormick B.
  Source: International Journal of Radiation Oncology, Biology, Physics. 2004 September 1; 60(1): 95-102.
  http://www.ncbi.nlm.nih.gov/entrez/query.fcgi?cmd=Retrieve&db=pubmed&dopt=Abstract&list_uids=15337544

- **Dosimetric correlates for acute esophagitis in patients treated with radiotherapy for lung carcinoma.**
  Author(s): Bradley J, Deasy JO, Bentzen S, El-Naqa I.
  Source: International Journal of Radiation Oncology, Biology, Physics. 2004 March 15; 58(4): 1106-13.
  http://www.ncbi.nlm.nih.gov/entrez/query.fcgi?cmd=Retrieve&db=pubmed&dopt=Abstract&list_uids=15001251

- **Dosimetric effect of respiratory motion in external beam radiotherapy of the lung.**
  Author(s): Mechalakos J, Yorke E, Mageras GS, Hertanto A, Jackson A, Obcemea C, Rosenzweig K, Clifton Ling C.
  Source: Radiotherapy and Oncology : Journal of the European Society for Therapeutic Radiology and Oncology. 2004 May; 71(2): 191-200.
  http://www.ncbi.nlm.nih.gov/entrez/query.fcgi?cmd=Retrieve&db=pubmed&dopt=Abstract&list_uids=15110453

- **Dosimetric effects within target and organs at risk of interfractional patient mispositioning in left breast cancer radiotherapy.**
  Author(s): Baroni G, Garibaldi C, Scabini M, Riboldi M, Catalano G, Tosi G, Orecchia R, Pedotti A.
  Source: International Journal of Radiation Oncology, Biology, Physics. 2004 July 1; 59(3): 861-71.
  http://www.ncbi.nlm.nih.gov/entrez/query.fcgi?cmd=Retrieve&db=pubmed&dopt=Abstract&list_uids=15183490

- **Dosimetry and radiobiologic model comparison of IMRT and 3D conformal radiotherapy in treatment of carcinoma of the prostate.**
  Author(s): Luxton G, Hancock SL, Boyer AL.
  Source: International Journal of Radiation Oncology, Biology, Physics. 2004 May 1; 59(1): 267-84.
  http://www.ncbi.nlm.nih.gov/entrez/query.fcgi?cmd=Retrieve&db=pubmed&dopt=Abstract&list_uids=15093924

- **Double-blind randomized, placebo-controlled study of pilocarpine to salvage salivary gland function during radiotherapy of patients with head and neck cancer.**
  Author(s): Gornitsky M, Shenouda G, Sultanem K, Katz H, Hier M, Black M, Velly AM.
  Source: Oral Surgery, Oral Medicine, Oral Pathology, Oral Radiology, and Endodontics. 2004 July; 98(1): 45-52.
  http://www.ncbi.nlm.nih.gov/entrez/query.fcgi?cmd=Retrieve&db=pubmed&dopt=Abstract&list_uids=15243470

- **Early prostate-specific antigen (PSA) kinetics following prostate carcinoma radiotherapy: prognostic value of a time-and-PSA threshold model.**
  Author(s): Cavanaugh SX, Kupelian PA, Fuller CD, Reddy C, Bradshaw P, Pollock BH, Fuss M.
  Source: Cancer. 2004 July 1; 101(1): 96-105.
  http://www.ncbi.nlm.nih.gov/entrez/query.fcgi?cmd=Retrieve&db=pubmed&dopt=Abstract&list_uids=15221994

- **Effect of intraoperative radiotherapy combined with external beam radiotherapy following internal drainage for advanced pancreatic carcinoma.**
  Author(s): Ma HB, Di ZL, Wang XJ, Kang HF, Deng HC, Bai MH.
  Source: World Journal of Gastroenterology : Wjg. 2004 June 1; 10(11): 1669-771.
  http://www.ncbi.nlm.nih.gov/entrez/query.fcgi?cmd=Retrieve&db=pubmed&dopt=Abstract&list_uids=15162548

- **Efficacy of radiotherapy for ovarian ablation: results of a breast intergroup study.**
  Author(s): Hughes LL, Gray RJ, Solin LJ, Robert NJ, Martino S, Tripathy D, Ingle JN, Wood WC; Eastern Cooperative Oncology Group; Southwest Oncology Group; Cancer and Leukemia Group B; North Central Cancer Treatment Group.
  Source: Cancer. 2004 September 1; 101(5): 969-72.
  http://www.ncbi.nlm.nih.gov/entrez/query.fcgi?cmd=Retrieve&db=pubmed&dopt=Abstract&list_uids=15329905

- **Efficacy of Sandostatin LAR (long-acting somatostatin analogue) is similar in patients with untreated acromegaly and in those previously treated with surgery and/or radiotherapy.**
  Author(s): Ayuk J, Stewart SE, Stewart PM, Sheppard MC; European Sandostatin LAR Group.
  Source: Clinical Endocrinology. 2004 March; 60(3): 375-81.
  http://www.ncbi.nlm.nih.gov/entrez/query.fcgi?cmd=Retrieve&db=pubmed&dopt=Abstract&list_uids=15009004

- **Enhanced systemic T-cell activation after in situ gene therapy with radiotherapy in prostate cancer patients.**
  Author(s): Satoh T, Teh BS, Timme TL, Mai WY, Gdor Y, Kusaka N, Fujita T, Pramudji CK, Vlachaki MT, Ayala G, Wheeler T, Amato R, Miles BJ, Kadmon D, Butler EB, Thompson TC.
  Source: International Journal of Radiation Oncology, Biology, Physics. 2004 June 1; 59(2): 562-71.
  http://www.ncbi.nlm.nih.gov/entrez/query.fcgi?cmd=Retrieve&db=pubmed&dopt=Abstract&list_uids=15145177

- **Enucleation versus preservation of blind eyes following plaque radiotherapy for choroidal melanoma.**
  Author(s): Augsburger JJ, Khouri L, Roumeliotis A, Kersten RC, Kulwin DR, Schneider S.
  Source: Can J Ophthalmol. 2004 June; 39(4): 372-9.
  http://www.ncbi.nlm.nih.gov/entrez/query.fcgi?cmd=Retrieve&db=pubmed&dopt=Abstract&list_uids=15327102

- **Erectile function following external beam radiotherapy for clinically organ-confined or locally advanced prostate cancer.**
  Author(s): Hisasue S, Kato R, Takahashi A, Masumori N, Itoh N, Miyao N, Takatsuka K, Yanase M, Oouchi A, Hareyama M, Tsukamoto T.
  Source: Japanese Journal of Clinical Oncology. 2004 May; 34(5): 269-73.
  http://www.ncbi.nlm.nih.gov/entrez/query.fcgi?cmd=Retrieve&db=pubmed&dopt=Abstract&list_uids=15231862

- **Estimation of an optimal radiotherapy utilization rate for gastrointestinal carcinoma: a review of the evidence.**
  Author(s): Delaney G, Barton M, Jacob S.
  Source: Cancer. 2004 August 15; 101(4): 657-70. Review.
  http://www.ncbi.nlm.nih.gov/entrez/query.fcgi?cmd=Retrieve&db=pubmed&dopt=Abstract&list_uids=15305395

- **Estimation of an optimal radiotherapy utilization rate for gynecologic carcinoma: part II--carcinoma of the endometrium.**
  Author(s): Delaney G, Jacob S, Barton M.
  Source: Cancer. 2004 August 15; 101(4): 682-92. Review.
  http://www.ncbi.nlm.nih.gov/entrez/query.fcgi?cmd=Retrieve&db=pubmed&dopt=Abstract&list_uids=15305397

- **Estimation of an optimal radiotherapy utilization rate for gynecologic carcinoma: part I--malignancies of the cervix, ovary, vagina and vulva.**
  Author(s): Delaney G, Jacob S, Barton M.
  Source: Cancer. 2004 August 15; 101(4): 671-81. Review.
  http://www.ncbi.nlm.nih.gov/entrez/query.fcgi?cmd=Retrieve&db=pubmed&dopt=Abstract&list_uids=15305396

- **Evaluation of a contour-alignment technique for CT-guided prostate radiotherapy: an intra- and interobserver study.**
  Author(s): Court LE, Dong L, Taylor N, Ballo M, Kitamura K, Lee AK, O'Daniel J, White RA, Cheung R, Kuban D.
  Source: International Journal of Radiation Oncology, Biology, Physics. 2004 June 1; 59(2): 412-8.
  http://www.ncbi.nlm.nih.gov/entrez/query.fcgi?cmd=Retrieve&db=pubmed&dopt=Abstract&list_uids=15145157

- **Evaluation of a radiotherapy protocol based on INT0116 for completely resected gastric adenocarcinoma.**
  Author(s): Chung HT, Shakespeare TP, Wynne CJ, Lu JJ, Mukherjee RK, Back MF.
  Source: International Journal of Radiation Oncology, Biology, Physics. 2004 August 1; 59(5): 1446-53.
  http://www.ncbi.nlm.nih.gov/entrez/query.fcgi?cmd=Retrieve&db=pubmed&dopt=Abstract&list_uids=15275731

- **Evaluation of arm and shoulder mobility and strength after modified radical mastectomy and radiotherapy.**
  Author(s): Blomqvist L, Stark B, Engler N, Malm M.
  Source: Acta Oncologica (Stockholm, Sweden). 2004; 43(3): 280-3.
  http://www.ncbi.nlm.nih.gov/entrez/query.fcgi?cmd=Retrieve&db=pubmed&dopt=Abstract&list_uids=15244252

- **Evaluation of the effect of radiotherapy for pituitary tumours on cognitive function and quality of life.**
  Author(s): Noad R, Narayanan KR, Howlett T, Lincoln NB, Page RC.
  Source: Clin Oncol (R Coll Radiol). 2004 June; 16(4): 233-7.
  http://www.ncbi.nlm.nih.gov/entrez/query.fcgi?cmd=Retrieve&db=pubmed&dopt=Abstract&list_uids=15214645

- **Ewing sarcoma: favourable results with combined modality therapy and conservative use of radiotherapy.**
  Author(s): Zogopoulos G, Teskey L, Sung L, Dix D, Grant R, Greenberg ML, Weitzman S.
  Source: Pediatric Blood & Cancer. 2004 July; 43(1): 35-9.
  http://www.ncbi.nlm.nih.gov/entrez/query.fcgi?cmd=Retrieve&db=pubmed&dopt=Abstract&list_uids=15170887

- **Extended prostate biopsy scheme improves reliability of Gleason grading: implications for radiotherapy patients.**
  Author(s): King CR, McNeal JE, Gill H, Presti JC Jr.
  Source: International Journal of Radiation Oncology, Biology, Physics. 2004 June 1; 59(2): 386-91.
  http://www.ncbi.nlm.nih.gov/entrez/query.fcgi?cmd=Retrieve&db=pubmed&dopt=Abstract&list_uids=15145152

- **External beam radiotherapy fails to prevent restenosis after iliac or femoropopliteal percutaneous transluminal angioplasty: results of a prospective randomized double-blind study.**
  Author(s): Fritz P, Stein U, Hasslacher C, Zierhut D, Wannenmacher M, Pritsch M.
  Source: International Journal of Radiation Oncology, Biology, Physics. 2004 July 1; 59(3): 815-21.
  http://www.ncbi.nlm.nih.gov/entrez/query.fcgi?cmd=Retrieve&db=pubmed&dopt=Abstract&list_uids=15183485

- **External beam radiotherapy for clinically node-negative, localized hormone-refractory prostate cancer: impact of pretreatment PSA value on radiotherapeutic outcomes.**
  Author(s): Akimoto T, Kitamoto Y, Saito J, Harashima K, Nakano T, Ito K, Yamamoto T, Kurokawa K, Yamanaka H, Takahashi M, Mitsuhashi N, Niibe H.
  Source: International Journal of Radiation Oncology, Biology, Physics. 2004 June 1; 59(2): 372-9.
  http://www.ncbi.nlm.nih.gov/entrez/query.fcgi?cmd=Retrieve&db=pubmed&dopt=Abstract&list_uids=15145150

- **Extranodal nonorbital indolent lymphomas of the head and neck: relationship between tumor control and radiotherapy.**
  Author(s): MacDermed D, Thurber L, George TI, Hoppe RT, Le QT.
  Source: International Journal of Radiation Oncology, Biology, Physics. 2004 July 1; 59(3): 788-95.
  http://www.ncbi.nlm.nih.gov/entrez/query.fcgi?cmd=Retrieve&db=pubmed&dopt=Abstract&list_uids=15183482

- **Failure of sentinel node identification following neo-adjuvant chemo-radiotherapy for locally advanced squamous cell carcinoma of the vulva.**
  Author(s): Levavi H, Sabah G, Hardoff R, Koren C, Gutman H.
  Source: Eur J Gynaecol Oncol. 2003; 24(5): 433-4.
  http://www.ncbi.nlm.nih.gov/entrez/query.fcgi?cmd=Retrieve&db=pubmed&dopt=Abstract&list_uids=14584664

- **Fanconi's anemia and clinical radiosensitivity report on two adult patients with locally advanced solid tumors treated by radiotherapy.**
  Author(s): Bremer M, Schindler D, Gross M, Dork T, Morlot S, Karstens JH.
  Source: Strahlentherapie Und Onkologie : Organ Der Deutschen Rontgengesellschaft. [et Al]. 2003 November; 179(11): 748-53.
  http://www.ncbi.nlm.nih.gov/entrez/query.fcgi?cmd=Retrieve&db=pubmed&dopt=Abstract&list_uids=14605744

- **Fatigue during breast radiotherapy and its relationship to biological factors.**
  Author(s): Wratten C, Kilmurray J, Nash S, Seldon M, Hamilton CS, O'Brien PC, Denham JW.
  Source: International Journal of Radiation Oncology, Biology, Physics. 2004 May 1; 59(1): 160-7.
  http://www.ncbi.nlm.nih.gov/entrez/query.fcgi?cmd=Retrieve&db=pubmed&dopt=Abstract&list_uids=15093912

- **FDG-PET in radiotherapy treatment planning: Pandora's box?**
  Author(s): Paulino AC, Johnstone PA.
  Source: International Journal of Radiation Oncology, Biology, Physics. 2004 May 1; 59(1): 4-5.
  http://www.ncbi.nlm.nih.gov/entrez/query.fcgi?cmd=Retrieve&db=pubmed&dopt=Abstract&list_uids=15093892

- **Feasibility of sparing lung and other thoracic structures with intensity-modulated radiotherapy for non-small-cell lung cancer.**
  Author(s): Liu HH, Wang X, Dong L, Wu Q, Liao Z, Stevens CW, Guerrero TM, Komaki R, Cox JD, Mohan R.
  Source: International Journal of Radiation Oncology, Biology, Physics. 2004 March 15; 58(4): 1268-79.
  http://www.ncbi.nlm.nih.gov/entrez/query.fcgi?cmd=Retrieve&db=pubmed&dopt=Abstract&list_uids=15001272

- **Feasibility of synchronization of real-time tumor-tracking radiotherapy and intensity-modulated radiotherapy from viewpoint of excessive dose from fluoroscopy.**
  Author(s): Shirato H, Oita M, Fujita K, Watanabe Y, Miyasaka K.
  Source: International Journal of Radiation Oncology, Biology, Physics. 2004 September 1; 60(1): 335-41.
  http://www.ncbi.nlm.nih.gov/entrez/query.fcgi?cmd=Retrieve&db=pubmed&dopt=Abstract&list_uids=15337573

- **Feasibility study of the simultaneous integrated boost (SIB) method for malignant gliomas using intensity-modulated radiotherapy (IMRT).**
  Author(s): Suzuki M, Nakamatsu K, Kanamori S, Okumra M, Uchiyama T, Akai F, Nishimura Y.
  Source: Japanese Journal of Clinical Oncology. 2003 June; 33(6): 271-7.
  http://www.ncbi.nlm.nih.gov/entrez/query.fcgi?cmd=Retrieve&db=pubmed&dopt=Abstract&list_uids=12913080

- **Fertility in women treated with cranial radiotherapy for childhood acute lymphoblastic leukemia.**
  Author(s): Byrne J, Fears TR, Mills JL, Zeltzer LK, Sklar C, Nicholson HS, Haupt R, Reaman GH, Meadows AT, Robison LL.
  Source: Pediatric Blood & Cancer. 2004 June; 42(7): 589-97.
  http://www.ncbi.nlm.nih.gov/entrez/query.fcgi?cmd=Retrieve&db=pubmed&dopt=Abstract&list_uids=15127413

- **Final results of the 94-01 French Head and Neck Oncology and Radiotherapy Group randomized trial comparing radiotherapy alone with concomitant radiochemotherapy in advanced-stage oropharynx carcinoma.**
  Author(s): Denis F, Garaud P, Bardet E, Alfonsi M, Sire C, Germain T, Bergerot P, Rhein B, Tortochaux J, Calais G.
  Source: Journal of Clinical Oncology : Official Journal of the American Society of Clinical Oncology. 2004 January 1; 22(1): 69-76. Epub 2003 December 02.
  http://www.ncbi.nlm.nih.gov/entrez/query.fcgi?cmd=Retrieve&db=pubmed&dopt=Abstract&list_uids=14657228

- **Finding dose-volume constraints to reduce late rectal toxicity following 3D-conformal radiotherapy (3D-CRT) of prostate cancer.**
  Author(s): Greco C, Mazzetta C, Cattani F, Tosi G, Castiglioni S, Fodor A, Orecchia R.
  Source: Radiotherapy and Oncology : Journal of the European Society for Therapeutic Radiology and Oncology. 2003 November; 69(2): 215-22.
  http://www.ncbi.nlm.nih.gov/entrez/query.fcgi?cmd=Retrieve&db=pubmed&dopt=Abstract&list_uids=14643961

- **First results of a phase I/II dose escalation trial in non-small cell lung cancer using three-dimensional conformal radiotherapy.**
  Author(s): Belderbos JS, De Jaeger K, Heemsbergen WD, Seppenwoolde Y, Baas P, Boersma LJ, Lebesque JV.
  Source: Radiotherapy and Oncology : Journal of the European Society for Therapeutic Radiology and Oncology. 2003 February; 66(2): 119-26.
  http://www.ncbi.nlm.nih.gov/entrez/query.fcgi?cmd=Retrieve&db=pubmed&dopt=Abstract&list_uids=12648783

- **Five compared with six fractions per week of conventional radiotherapy of squamous-cell carcinoma of head and neck: DAHANCA 6 and 7 randomised controlled trial.**
  Author(s): Overgaard J, Hansen HS, Specht L, Overgaard M, Grau C, Andersen E, Bentzen J, Bastholt L, Hansen O, Johansen J, Andersen L, Evensen JF.
  Source: Lancet. 2003 September 20; 362(9388): 933-40. Erratum In: Lancet. 2003 November 8; 362(9395): 1588.
  http://www.ncbi.nlm.nih.gov/entrez/query.fcgi?cmd=Retrieve&db=pubmed&dopt=Abstract&list_uids=14511925

- **Five-year outcomes after prostatectomy or radiotherapy for prostate cancer: the prostate cancer outcomes study.**
  Author(s): Potosky AL, Davis WW, Hoffman RM, Stanford JL, Stephenson RA, Penson DF, Harlan LC.
  Source: Journal of the National Cancer Institute. 2004 September 15; 96(18): 1358-67.
  http://www.ncbi.nlm.nih.gov/entrez/query.fcgi?cmd=Retrieve&db=pubmed&dopt=Abstract&list_uids=15367568

- **Fractionated low-dose radiotherapy after myeloablative stem cell transplantation for local control in patients with high-risk neuroblastoma.**
  Author(s): Bradfield SM, Douglas JG, Hawkins DS, Sanders JE, Park JR.
  Source: Cancer. 2004 March 15; 100(6): 1268-75.
  http://www.ncbi.nlm.nih.gov/entrez/query.fcgi?cmd=Retrieve&db=pubmed&dopt=Abstract&list_uids=15022296

- **Fractionated stereotactic conformal radiotherapy in the management of large chemodectomas of the skull base.**
  Author(s): Zabel A, Milker-Zabel S, Huber P, Schulz-Ertner D, Schlegel W, Wannenmacher M, Debus J.
  Source: International Journal of Radiation Oncology, Biology, Physics. 2004 April 1; 58(5): 1445-50.
  http://www.ncbi.nlm.nih.gov/entrez/query.fcgi?cmd=Retrieve&db=pubmed&dopt=Abstract&list_uids=15050322

- **Fractionated stereotactic radiotherapy in low-grade astrocytomas: long-term outcome and prognostic factors.**
  Author(s): Plathow C, Schulz-Ertner D, Thilman C, Zuna I, Lichy M, Weber MA, Schlemmer HP, Wannenmacher M, Debus J.
  Source: International Journal of Radiation Oncology, Biology, Physics. 2003 November 15; 57(4): 996-1003.
  http://www.ncbi.nlm.nih.gov/entrez/query.fcgi?cmd=Retrieve&db=pubmed&dopt=Abstract&list_uids=14575830

- **Fractionations in radiotherapy of brain metastases.**
  Author(s): Portaluri M, Bambace S, Giuliano G, Di Paola L, Gianicolo ME, Distante S, Casciaro S.
  Source: Tumori. 2004 January-February; 90(1): 80-5.
  http://www.ncbi.nlm.nih.gov/entrez/query.fcgi?cmd=Retrieve&db=pubmed&dopt=Abstract&list_uids=15143977

- **From physical dose constraints to equivalent uniform dose constraints in inverse radiotherapy planning.**
  Author(s): Thieke C, Bortfeld T, Niemierko A, Nill S.
  Source: Medical Physics. 2003 September; 30(9): 2332-9.
  http://www.ncbi.nlm.nih.gov/entrez/query.fcgi?cmd=Retrieve&db=pubmed&dopt=Abstract&list_uids=14528955

- **Full-dose intraoperative radiotherapy with electrons during breast-conserving surgery.**
  Author(s): Veronesi U, Gatti G, Luini A, Intra M, Ciocca M, Sanchez D, Zurrida S, Navarro S, Orecchia R.
  Source: Archives of Surgery (Chicago, Ill. : 1960). 2003 November; 138(11): 1253-6.
  http://www.ncbi.nlm.nih.gov/entrez/query.fcgi?cmd=Retrieve&db=pubmed&dopt=Abstract&list_uids=14609877

- **Fungal granuloma following ruthenium plaque radiotherapy of a choroidal melanoma.**
  Author(s): Okera S, Dodd T, Selva D, Muecke J.
  Source: Clinical & Experimental Ophthalmology. 2003 April; 31(2): 159-61.
  http://www.ncbi.nlm.nih.gov/entrez/query.fcgi?cmd=Retrieve&db=pubmed&dopt=Abstract&list_uids=12648052

- **Gamma knife radiosurgery for brain metastases: do patients benefit from adjuvant external-beam radiotherapy? An 18-month comparative analysis.**
  Author(s): Jawahar A, Willis BK, Smith DR, Ampil F, Datta R, Nanda A.
  Source: Stereotactic and Functional Neurosurgery. 2002; 79(3-4): 262-71.
  http://www.ncbi.nlm.nih.gov/entrez/query.fcgi?cmd=Retrieve&db=pubmed&dopt=Abstract&list_uids=12890985

- **Gamma knife stereotactic radiosurgical boost for patients treated primarily with neutron radiotherapy for salivary gland neoplasms.**
  Author(s): Douglas JG, Silbergeld DL, Laramore GE.
  Source: Stereotactic and Functional Neurosurgery. 2004; 82(2-3): 84-9. Epub 2004 March 25.
  http://www.ncbi.nlm.nih.gov/entrez/query.fcgi?cmd=Retrieve&db=pubmed&dopt=Abstract&list_uids=15305080

- **Gastric adenocarcinoma treated with R0-R1 surgical resection and intraoperative radiotherapy (IORT) plus external beam radiation therapy (EBRT).**
  Author(s): Glehen O, Beaujard AC, Romestaing P, Sentenac I, Francois Y, Peyrat P, Braillon G, Vignal J, Gerard JP, Gilly FN.
  Source: Suppl Tumori. 2003 September-October; 2(5): S51-3. No Abstract Available.
  http://www.ncbi.nlm.nih.gov/entrez/query.fcgi?cmd=Retrieve&db=pubmed&dopt=Abstract&list_uids=12914392

- **Genetic algorithm based deliverable segments optimization for static intensity-modulated radiotherapy.**
  Author(s): Li Y, Yao J, Yao D.
  Source: Physics in Medicine and Biology. 2003 October 21; 48(20): 3353-74.
  http://www.ncbi.nlm.nih.gov/entrez/query.fcgi?cmd=Retrieve&db=pubmed&dopt=Abstract&list_uids=14620063

- **Genetic effects of radiotherapy for childhood cancer.**
  Author(s): Boice JD Jr, Tawn EJ, Winther JF, Donaldson SS, Green DM, Mertens AC, Mulvihill JJ, Olsen JH, Robison LL, Stovall M.
  Source: Health Physics. 2003 July; 85(1): 65-80.
  http://www.ncbi.nlm.nih.gov/entrez/query.fcgi?cmd=Retrieve&db=pubmed&dopt=Abstract&list_uids=12852473

- **Genetically targeted radiotherapy for multiple myeloma.**
  Author(s): Dingli D, Diaz RM, Bergert ER, O'Connor MK, Morris JC, Russell SJ.
  Source: Blood. 2003 July 15; 102(2): 489-96. Epub 2003 March 20.
  http://www.ncbi.nlm.nih.gov/entrez/query.fcgi?cmd=Retrieve&db=pubmed&dopt=Abstract&list_uids=12649158

- **Geometric uncertainties in radiotherapy.**
  Author(s): Wilkinson JM.
  Source: The British Journal of Radiology. 2004 February; 77(914): 86-7.
  http://www.ncbi.nlm.nih.gov/entrez/query.fcgi?cmd=Retrieve&db=pubmed&dopt=Abstract&list_uids=15010377

- **Germ cell tumours of the central nervous system in children-controversies in radiotherapy.**
  Author(s): Borg M.
  Source: Medical and Pediatric Oncology. 2003 June; 40(6): 367-74. Review.
  http://www.ncbi.nlm.nih.gov/entrez/query.fcgi?cmd=Retrieve&db=pubmed&dopt=Abstract&list_uids=12692804

- **Germinoma with syncytiotrophoblastic giant cells recurring 13 years after radiotherapy for a pineal germinoma--case report.**
  Author(s): Fujikawa K, Kawahara Y, Hirano H, Yokoyama S, Niiro M, Kuratsu J.
  Source: Neurol Med Chir (Tokyo). 2003 March; 43(3): 146-9.
  http://www.ncbi.nlm.nih.gov/entrez/query.fcgi?cmd=Retrieve&db=pubmed&dopt=Abstract&list_uids=12699124

- **Gliomatosis cerebri: improved outcome with radiotherapy.**
  Author(s): Perkins GH, Schomer DF, Fuller GN, Allen PK, Maor MH.
  Source: International Journal of Radiation Oncology, Biology, Physics. 2003 July 15; 56(4): 1137-46.
  http://www.ncbi.nlm.nih.gov/entrez/query.fcgi?cmd=Retrieve&db=pubmed&dopt=Abstract&list_uids=12829152

- **GOG-99: ending the controversy regarding pelvic radiotherapy for endometrial carcinoma?**
  Author(s): Creutzberg CL.
  Source: Gynecologic Oncology. 2004 March; 92(3): 740-3.
  http://www.ncbi.nlm.nih.gov/entrez/query.fcgi?cmd=Retrieve&db=pubmed&dopt=Abstract&list_uids=14984935

- **Group II rhabdomyosarcoma and rhabdomyosarcomalike tumors: is radiotherapy necessary?**
  Author(s): Schuck A, Mattke AC, Schmidt B, Kunz DS, Harms D, Knietig R, Treuner J, Koscielniak E.
  Source: Journal of Clinical Oncology : Official Journal of the American Society of Clinical Oncology. 2004 January 1; 22(1): 143-9.
  http://www.ncbi.nlm.nih.gov/entrez/query.fcgi?cmd=Retrieve&db=pubmed&dopt=Abstract&list_uids=14701776

- **Growth hormone and pituitary radiotherapy, but not serum insulin-like growth factor-I concentrations, predict excess mortality in patients with acromegaly.**
  Author(s): Ayuk J, Clayton RN, Holder G, Sheppard MC, Stewart PM, Bates AS.
  Source: The Journal of Clinical Endocrinology and Metabolism. 2004 April; 89(4): 1613-7.
  http://www.ncbi.nlm.nih.gov/entrez/query.fcgi?cmd=Retrieve&db=pubmed&dopt=Abstract&list_uids=15070920

- **Guidelines for education and training of medical physicists in radiotherapy. Recommendations from an ESTRO/EFOMP working group.**
  Author(s): Eudaldo T, Huizenga H, Lamm IL, McKenzie A, Milano F, Schlegel W, Thwaites D, Heeren G; European Society of Therapeutic Radiology and Oncology; European Federation of Organisations for Medical Physics.
  Source: Radiotherapy and Oncology : Journal of the European Society for Therapeutic Radiology and Oncology. 2004 February; 70(2): 125-35.
  http://www.ncbi.nlm.nih.gov/entrez/query.fcgi?cmd=Retrieve&db=pubmed&dopt=Abstract&list_uids=15028400

- **Guidelines for the infrastructure of training institutes and teaching departments for radiotherapy in Europe.**
  Author(s): Rottinger E, Barrett A, Leer JW; European Board Of Radiotherapy.
  Source: Radiotherapy and Oncology : Journal of the European Society for Therapeutic Radiology and Oncology. 2004 February; 70(2): 123-4.
  http://www.ncbi.nlm.nih.gov/entrez/query.fcgi?cmd=Retrieve&db=pubmed&dopt=Abstract&list_uids=15028399

- **Hazards of dose escalation in prostate cancer radiotherapy.**
  Author(s): Kuban D, Pollack A, Huang E, Levy L, Dong L, Starkschall G, Rosen I.
  Source: International Journal of Radiation Oncology, Biology, Physics. 2003 December 1; 57(5): 1260-8.
  http://www.ncbi.nlm.nih.gov/entrez/query.fcgi?cmd=Retrieve&db=pubmed&dopt=Abstract&list_uids=14630260

- **Health-related quality of life in men after treatment of localized prostate cancer with external beam radiotherapy combined with (192)ir brachytherapy: a prospective study of 93 cases using the EORTC questionnaires QLQ-C30 and QLQ-PR25.**
  Author(s): Wahlgren T, Brandberg Y, Haggarth L, Hellstrom M, Nilsson S.
  Source: International Journal of Radiation Oncology, Biology, Physics. 2004 September 1; 60(1): 51-9.
  http://www.ncbi.nlm.nih.gov/entrez/query.fcgi?cmd=Retrieve&db=pubmed&dopt=Abstract&list_uids=15337539

- **Hepatic arterial infusion of 5-fluorouracil and extrabeam radiotherapy for liver metastases from pancreatic carcinoma.**
  Author(s): Ishii H, Furuse J, Nagase M, Yoshino M, Kawashima M, Satake M, Ogino T, Ikeda H.
  Source: Hepatogastroenterology. 2004 July-August; 51(58): 1175-8.
  http://www.ncbi.nlm.nih.gov/entrez/query.fcgi?cmd=Retrieve&db=pubmed&dopt=Abstract&list_uids=15239272

- **Her2/neu-positive disease does not increase risk of locoregional recurrence for patients treated with neoadjuvant doxorubicin-based chemotherapy, mastectomy, and radiotherapy.**
  Author(s): Buchholz TA, Huang EH, Berry D, Pusztai L, Strom EA, McNeese MD, Perkins GH, Schechter NR, Kuerer HM, Buzdar AU, Valero V, Hunt KK, Hortobagyi GN, Sahin AA.
  Source: International Journal of Radiation Oncology, Biology, Physics. 2004 August 1; 59(5): 1337-42.
  http://www.ncbi.nlm.nih.gov/entrez/query.fcgi?cmd=Retrieve&db=pubmed&dopt=Abstract&list_uids=15275718

- **High dose rate intraluminal brachytherapy in combination with external beam radiotherapy for palliative treatment of cancer rectum.**
  Author(s): Begum N, Asghar AH, N S, Khan SM, Khan A.
  Source: J Coll Physicians Surg Pak. 2003 November; 13(11): 633-6.
  http://www.ncbi.nlm.nih.gov/entrez/query.fcgi?cmd=Retrieve&db=pubmed&dopt=Abstract&list_uids=14700489

- **High-dose radiotherapy plus prolonged hormone therapy in CT2-3 prostatic carcinoma: is it useful?**
  Author(s): Cellini N, Pompei L, Fortuna G, Ammaturo MV, De Paula U, Luzi S, Mattiucci GC, Morganti AG, Digesu C, Rosetto ME, Palloni T, Petrongari MG, Gentile P, Deodato F, Valentini V.
  Source: Tumori. 2004 March-April; 90(2): 201-7.
  http://www.ncbi.nlm.nih.gov/entrez/query.fcgi?cmd=Retrieve&db=pubmed&dopt=Abstract&list_uids=15237583

- **High-dose-rate intraoperative radiotherapy for close or positive margins in patients with locally advanced or recurrent rectal cancer.**
  Author(s): Nuyttens JJ, Kolkman-Deurloo IK, Vermaas M, Ferenschild FT, Graveland WJ, De Wilt JH, Hanssens PE, Levendag PC.
  Source: International Journal of Radiation Oncology, Biology, Physics. 2004 January 1; 58(1): 106-12.
  http://www.ncbi.nlm.nih.gov/entrez/query.fcgi?cmd=Retrieve&db=pubmed&dopt=Abstract&list_uids=14697427

- **High-tech will improve radiotherapy of NSCLC: a hypothesis waiting to be validated.**
  Author(s): Ling CC, Yorke E, Amols H, Mechalakos J, Erdi Y, Leibel S, Rosenzweig K, Jackson A.
  Source: International Journal of Radiation Oncology, Biology, Physics. 2004 September 1; 60(1): 3-7.
  http://www.ncbi.nlm.nih.gov/entrez/query.fcgi?cmd=Retrieve&db=pubmed&dopt=Abstract&list_uids=15337533

- **Hormone therapy adjuvant to external beam radiotherapy for locally advanced prostate carcinoma: a complication-adjusted number-needed-to-treat analysis.**
  Author(s): Jani AB, Kao J, Hellman S.
  Source: Cancer. 2003 December 1; 98(11): 2351-61.
  http://www.ncbi.nlm.nih.gov/entrez/query.fcgi?cmd=Retrieve&db=pubmed&dopt=Abstract&list_uids=14635069

- **How safe is adjuvant chemotherapy and radiotherapy for rectal cancer?**
  Author(s): Chao MW, Tjandra JJ, Gibbs P, McLaughlin S.
  Source: Asian J Surg. 2004 April; 27(2): 147-61. Review.
  http://www.ncbi.nlm.nih.gov/entrez/query.fcgi?cmd=Retrieve&db=pubmed&dopt=Abstract&list_uids=15140670

- **How safe is Australian radiotherapy?**
  Author(s): Hamilton C, Oliver L, Coulter K.
  Source: Australasian Radiology. 2003 December; 47(4): 428-33.
  http://www.ncbi.nlm.nih.gov/entrez/query.fcgi?cmd=Retrieve&db=pubmed&dopt=Abstract&list_uids=14641197

- **How the implementation of an in-vivo dosimetry protocol improved the dose delivery accuracy in head and neck radiotherapy.**
  Author(s): Malicki J, Litoborski M, Kierzkowski J, Kosicka G.
  Source: Neoplasma. 2004; 51(2): 155-8.
  http://www.ncbi.nlm.nih.gov/entrez/query.fcgi?cmd=Retrieve&db=pubmed&dopt=Abstract&list_uids=15190426

- **Hyperfractionated accelerated radiotherapy alone and with concomitant chemotherapy to the head and neck: treated within and outside of randomized clinical trials.**
  Author(s): Hehr T, Classen J, Schreck U, Glocker S, Bamberg M, Budach W.
  Source: International Journal of Radiation Oncology, Biology, Physics. 2004 April 1; 58(5): 1424-30.
  http://www.ncbi.nlm.nih.gov/entrez/query.fcgi?cmd=Retrieve&db=pubmed&dopt=A bstract&list_uids=15050319

- **Hyperfractionated radiotherapy and concomitant cisplatin for locally advanced laryngeal and hypopharyngeal carcinomas: final results of a single institutional program.**
  Author(s): de la Vega FA, Garcia RV, Dominguez D, Iturre EV, Lopez EM, Alonso SM, Romero P, Sola JM.
  Source: American Journal of Clinical Oncology : the Official Publication of the American Radium Society. 2003 December; 26(6): 550-7.
  http://www.ncbi.nlm.nih.gov/entrez/query.fcgi?cmd=Retrieve&db=pubmed&dopt=A bstract&list_uids=14663370

- **Hyperfractionated radiotherapy for T2N0 glottic carcinoma: a retrospective analysis at 10 years follow-up in a series of 60 consecutive patients.**
  Author(s): Bignardi M, Antognoni P, Sanguineti G, Magli A, Molteni M, Merlotti A, Richetti A, Tordiglione M, Conte L, Magno L.
  Source: Tumori. 2004 May-June; 90(3): 317-23.
  http://www.ncbi.nlm.nih.gov/entrez/query.fcgi?cmd=Retrieve&db=pubmed&dopt=A bstract&list_uids=15315312

- **Hypofractionated conformal radiotherapy in carcinoma of the prostate: five-year outcome analysis.**
  Author(s): Livsey JE, Cowan RA, Wylie JP, Swindell R, Read G, Khoo VS, Logue JP.
  Source: International Journal of Radiation Oncology, Biology, Physics. 2003 December 1; 57(5): 1254-9.
  http://www.ncbi.nlm.nih.gov/entrez/query.fcgi?cmd=Retrieve&db=pubmed&dopt=A bstract&list_uids=14630259

- **Hypofractionated external beam radiotherapy as retreatment for symptomatic non-small-cell lung carcinoma: an effective treatment?**
  Author(s): Kramer GW, Gans S, Ullmann E, van Meerbeeck JP, Legrand CC, Leer JW.
  Source: International Journal of Radiation Oncology, Biology, Physics. 2004 April 1; 58(5): 1388-93.
  http://www.ncbi.nlm.nih.gov/entrez/query.fcgi?cmd=Retrieve&db=pubmed&dopt=A bstract&list_uids=15050314

- **Hypofractionated palliative radiotherapy (17 Gy per two fractions) in advanced non-small-cell lung carcinoma is comparable to standard fractionation for symptom control and survival: a national phase III trial.**
  Author(s): Sundstrom S, Bremnes R, Aasebo U, Aamdal S, Hatlevoll R, Brunsvig P, Johannessen DC, Klepp O, Fayers PM, Kaasa S.
  Source: Journal of Clinical Oncology : Official Journal of the American Society of Clinical Oncology. 2004 March 1; 22(5): 801-10.
  http://www.ncbi.nlm.nih.gov/entrez/query.fcgi?cmd=Retrieve&db=pubmed&dopt=Abstract&list_uids=14990635

- **Hypofractionated radiotherapy for advanced non-small-cell lung cancer: is the LINAC half full?**
  Author(s): Bogart JA.
  Source: Journal of Clinical Oncology : Official Journal of the American Society of Clinical Oncology. 2004 March 1; 22(5): 765-8.
  http://www.ncbi.nlm.nih.gov/entrez/query.fcgi?cmd=Retrieve&db=pubmed&dopt=Abstract&list_uids=14990629

- **Imaging perfusion and hypoxia with PET to predict radiotherapy response in head-and-neck cancer.**
  Author(s): Lehtio K, Eskola O, Viljanen T, Oikonen V, Gronroos T, Sillanmaki L, Grenman R, Minn H.
  Source: International Journal of Radiation Oncology, Biology, Physics. 2004 July 15; 59(4): 971-82.
  http://www.ncbi.nlm.nih.gov/entrez/query.fcgi?cmd=Retrieve&db=pubmed&dopt=Abstract&list_uids=15234030

- **Immunohistochemical study of cell cycle-associated proteins in adenocarcinoma of the uterine cervix treated with radiotherapy alone: P53 status has a strong impact on prognosis.**
  Author(s): Suzuki Y, Nakano T, Kato S, Ohno T, Tsujii H, Oka K.
  Source: International Journal of Radiation Oncology, Biology, Physics. 2004 September 1; 60(1): 231-6.
  http://www.ncbi.nlm.nih.gov/entrez/query.fcgi?cmd=Retrieve&db=pubmed&dopt=Abstract&list_uids=15337561

- **Impact of margin for target volume in low-dose involved field radiotherapy after induction chemotherapy for intracranial germinoma.**
  Author(s): Shirato H, Aoyama H, Ikeda J, Fujieda K, Kato N, Ishi N, Miyasaka K, Iwasaki Y, Sawamura Y.
  Source: International Journal of Radiation Oncology, Biology, Physics. 2004 September 1; 60(1): 214-7.
  http://www.ncbi.nlm.nih.gov/entrez/query.fcgi?cmd=Retrieve&db=pubmed&dopt=Abstract&list_uids=15337558

- **Impact of mean rectal dose on late rectal bleeding after conformal radiotherapy for prostate cancer: dose-volume effect.**
  Author(s): Zapatero A, Garcia-Vicente F, Modolell I, Alcantara P, Floriano A, Cruz-Conde A, Torres JJ, Perez-Torrubia A.
  Source: International Journal of Radiation Oncology, Biology, Physics. 2004 August 1; 59(5): 1343-51.
  http://www.ncbi.nlm.nih.gov/entrez/query.fcgi?cmd=Retrieve&db=pubmed&dopt=Abstract&list_uids=15275719

- **Impact on cytoprotective efficacy of intermediate interval between amifostine administration and radiotherapy: a retrospective analysis.**
  Author(s): Kouloulias VE, Kouvaris JR, Kokakis JD, Kostakopoulos A, Mallas E, Metafa A, Vlahos LJ.
  Source: International Journal of Radiation Oncology, Biology, Physics. 2004 July 15; 59(4): 1148-56.
  http://www.ncbi.nlm.nih.gov/entrez/query.fcgi?cmd=Retrieve&db=pubmed&dopt=Abstract&list_uids=15234050

- **Improved sphincter preservation in low rectal cancer with high-dose preoperative radiotherapy: the lyon R96-02 randomized trial.**
  Author(s): Gerard JP, Chapet O, Nemoz C, Hartweig J, Romestaing P, Coquard R, Barbet N, Maingon P, Mahe M, Baulieux J, Partensky C, Papillon M, Glehen O, Crozet B, Grandjean JP, Adeleine P.
  Source: Journal of Clinical Oncology : Official Journal of the American Society of Clinical Oncology. 2004 June 15; 22(12): 2404-9.
  http://www.ncbi.nlm.nih.gov/entrez/query.fcgi?cmd=Retrieve&db=pubmed&dopt=Abstract&list_uids=15197202

- **In regard to Fiorino et al.: Rectal dose-volume constraints in high-dose radiotherapy of localized prostate cancer (Int J Radiat Oncol Biol Phys 2003;57:953-962).**
  Author(s): Bauman G, Rodrigues G.
  Source: International Journal of Radiation Oncology, Biology, Physics. 2004 July 1; 59(3): 912-4; Author Reply 914-5. Review.
  http://www.ncbi.nlm.nih.gov/entrez/query.fcgi?cmd=Retrieve&db=pubmed&dopt=Abstract&list_uids=15183497

- **Increased cure rate of glioblastoma using concurrent therapy with radiotherapy and arsenic trioxide.**
  Author(s): Ning S, Knox SJ.
  Source: International Journal of Radiation Oncology, Biology, Physics. 2004 September 1; 60(1): 197-203.
  http://www.ncbi.nlm.nih.gov/entrez/query.fcgi?cmd=Retrieve&db=pubmed&dopt=Abstract&list_uids=15337556

- **Induction chemotherapy and radiotherapy in locally advanced non-small cell lung cancer.**
  Author(s): Cohen EE, Vokes EE.
  Source: Hematology/Oncology Clinics of North America. 2004 February; 18(1): 81-90. Review.
  http://www.ncbi.nlm.nih.gov/entrez/query.fcgi?cmd=Retrieve&db=pubmed&dopt=Abstract&list_uids=15005282

- **Intensity-modulated radiotherapy and the Internet.**
  Author(s): Schomas DA, Milano MT, Roeske JC, Mell LK, Mundt AJ.
  Source: Cancer. 2004 July 15; 101(2): 412-20.
  http://www.ncbi.nlm.nih.gov/entrez/query.fcgi?cmd=Retrieve&db=pubmed&dopt=Abstract&list_uids=15241841

- **Intensity-modulated radiotherapy for early-stage nasopharyngeal carcinoma: a prospective study on disease control and preservation of salivary function.**
  Author(s): Kwong DL, Pow EH, Sham JS, McMillan AS, Leung LH, Leung WK, Chua DT, Cheng AC, Wu PM, Au GK.
  Source: Cancer. 2004 October 1; 101(7): 1584-93.
  http://www.ncbi.nlm.nih.gov/entrez/query.fcgi?cmd=Retrieve&db=pubmed&dopt=Abstract&list_uids=15378492

- **Intensive cisplatin and cyclophosphamide-based chemotherapy without radiotherapy for intracranial germinomas: failure of a primary chemotherapy approach.**
  Author(s): Kellie SJ, Boyce H, Dunkel IJ, Diez B, Rosenblum M, Brualdi L, Finlay JL.
  Source: Pediatric Blood & Cancer. 2004 August; 43(2): 126-33.
  http://www.ncbi.nlm.nih.gov/entrez/query.fcgi?cmd=Retrieve&db=pubmed&dopt=Abstract&list_uids=15236278

- **Intracranial subfrontal schwannoma treated with surgery and 3D conformal radiotherapy.**
  Author(s): Prasad D, Jalali R, Shet T.
  Source: Neurology India. 2004 June; 52(2): 248-50.
  http://www.ncbi.nlm.nih.gov/entrez/query.fcgi?cmd=Retrieve&db=pubmed&dopt=Abstract&list_uids=15269484

- **Inverse planning in three-dimensional conformal and intensity-modulated radiotherapy of mid-thoracic oesophageal cancer.**
  Author(s): Wu VW, Sham JS, Kwong DL.
  Source: The British Journal of Radiology. 2004 July; 77(919): 568-72.
  http://www.ncbi.nlm.nih.gov/entrez/query.fcgi?cmd=Retrieve&db=pubmed&dopt=Abstract&list_uids=15238403

- **Involution of retinochoroidal shunt vessel after radiotherapy for optic nerve sheath meningioma.**
  Author(s): Mashayekhi A, Shields JA, Shields CL.
  Source: Eur J Ophthalmol. 2004 January-February; 14(1): 61-4.
  http://www.ncbi.nlm.nih.gov/entrez/query.fcgi?cmd=Retrieve&db=pubmed&dopt=Abstract&list_uids=15005588

- **Is "no treatment" better than radiotherapy and chemotherapy?**
  Author(s): Debevec L.
  Source: Lung Cancer (Amsterdam, Netherlands). 2004 July; 45(1): 125; Author Reply 127.
  http://www.ncbi.nlm.nih.gov/entrez/query.fcgi?cmd=Retrieve&db=pubmed&dopt=Abstract&list_uids=15196743

- **Isolated plexiform neurofibroma: treatment with three-dimensional conformal radiotherapy.**
  Author(s): Robertson TC, Buck DA, Schmidt-Ullrich R, Powers CN, Reiter ER.
  Source: The Laryngoscope. 2004 July; 114(7): 1139-42.
  http://www.ncbi.nlm.nih.gov/entrez/query.fcgi?cmd=Retrieve&db=pubmed&dopt=Abstract&list_uids=15235336

- **Ki-67 staining is a strong predictor of distant metastasis and mortality for men with prostate cancer treated with radiotherapy plus androgen deprivation: Radiation Therapy Oncology Group Trial 92-02.**
  Author(s): Pollack A, DeSilvio M, Khor LY, Li R, Al-Saleem TI, Hammond ME, Venkatesan V, Lawton CA, Roach M 3rd, Shipley WU, Hanks GE, Sandler HM.
  Source: Journal of Clinical Oncology : Official Journal of the American Society of Clinical Oncology. 2004 June 1; 22(11): 2133-40.
  http://www.ncbi.nlm.nih.gov/entrez/query.fcgi?cmd=Retrieve&db=pubmed&dopt=Abstract&list_uids=15169799

- **Late effects of radiotherapy for pediatric extremity sarcomas.**
  Author(s): Paulino AC.
  Source: International Journal of Radiation Oncology, Biology, Physics. 2004 September 1; 60(1): 265-74.
  http://www.ncbi.nlm.nih.gov/entrez/query.fcgi?cmd=Retrieve&db=pubmed&dopt=Abstract&list_uids=15337565

- **Late toxicity following conventional radiotherapy for prostate cancer: analysis of the EORTC trial 22863.**
  Author(s): Ataman F, Zurlo A, Artignan X, van Tienhoven G, Blank LE, Warde P, Dubois JB, Jeanneret W, Keuppens F, Bernier J, Kuten A, Collette L, Pierart M, Bolla M.
  Source: European Journal of Cancer (Oxford, England : 1990). 2004 July; 40(11): 1674-81.
  http://www.ncbi.nlm.nih.gov/entrez/query.fcgi?cmd=Retrieve&db=pubmed&dopt=Abstract&list_uids=15251156

- **Late-course accelerated hyperfractionated radiotherapy for localized esophageal carcinoma.**
  Author(s): Zhao KL, Shi XH, Jiang GL, Wang Y.
  Source: International Journal of Radiation Oncology, Biology, Physics. 2004 September 1; 60(1): 123-9.
  http://www.ncbi.nlm.nih.gov/entrez/query.fcgi?cmd=Retrieve&db=pubmed&dopt=Abstract&list_uids=15337547

- **Limitations of adjuvant radiotherapy for uterine sarcomas spread beyond the uterus.**
  Author(s): Dusenbery KE, Potish RA, Judson P.
  Source: Gynecologic Oncology. 2004 July; 94(1): 191-6.
  http://www.ncbi.nlm.nih.gov/entrez/query.fcgi?cmd=Retrieve&db=pubmed&dopt=Abstract&list_uids=15262141

- **Linac radiosurgery versus whole brain radiotherapy for brain metastases. A survival comparison based on the RTOG recursive partitioning analysis.**
  Author(s): Kocher M, Maarouf M, Bendel M, Voges J, Muller RP, Sturm V.
  Source: Strahlentherapie Und Onkologie : Organ Der Deutschen Rontgengesellschaft. [et Al]. 2004 May; 180(5): 263-7.
  http://www.ncbi.nlm.nih.gov/entrez/query.fcgi?cmd=Retrieve&db=pubmed&dopt=Abstract&list_uids=15127155

- **Literature-based recommendations for treatment planning and execution in high-dose radiotherapy for lung cancer.**
  Author(s): Senan S, De Ruysscher D, Giraud P, Mirimanoff R, Budach V; Radiotherapy Group of European Organization for Research and Treatment of Cancer.
  Source: Radiotherapy and Oncology : Journal of the European Society for Therapeutic Radiology and Oncology. 2004 May; 71(2): 139-46. Review.
  http://www.ncbi.nlm.nih.gov/entrez/query.fcgi?cmd=Retrieve&db=pubmed&dopt=Abstract&list_uids=15110446

- **Local control and recurrence of stage I non-small cell lung cancer after carbon ion radiotherapy.**
  Author(s): Koto M, Miyamoto T, Yamamoto N, Nishimura H, Yamada S, Tsujii H.
  Source: Radiotherapy and Oncology : Journal of the European Society for Therapeutic Radiology and Oncology. 2004 May; 71(2): 147-56.
  http://www.ncbi.nlm.nih.gov/entrez/query.fcgi?cmd=Retrieve&db=pubmed&dopt=Abstract&list_uids=15110447

- **Local recurrence in breast cancer after conservative surgery: timing of radiotherapy and sequencing of chemotherapy.**
  Author(s): Donato V, Monaco A, Messina F, De Sanctis V, Messineo D, Banelli E, Maurizi Enrici R.
  Source: Anticancer Res. 2004 March-April; 24(2C): 1303-6.
  http://www.ncbi.nlm.nih.gov/entrez/query.fcgi?cmd=Retrieve&db=pubmed&dopt=Abstract&list_uids=15154664

- **Local recurrence of prostate cancer after external beam radiotherapy: early experience of salvage therapy using high-intensity focused ultrasonography.**
  Author(s): Gelet A, Chapelon JY, Poissonnier L, Bouvier R, Rouviere O, Curiel L, Janier M, Vallancien G.
  Source: Urology. 2004 April; 63(4): 625-9.
  http://www.ncbi.nlm.nih.gov/entrez/query.fcgi?cmd=Retrieve&db=pubmed&dopt=Abstract&list_uids=15072864

- **Loco-regional conformal radiotherapy of the breast: delineation of the regional lymph node clinical target volumes in treatment position.**
  Author(s): Dijkema IM, Hofman P, Raaijmakers CP, Lagendijk JJ, Battermann JJ, Hillen B.
  Source: Radiotherapy and Oncology : Journal of the European Society for Therapeutic Radiology and Oncology. 2004 June; 71(3): 287-95.
  http://www.ncbi.nlm.nih.gov/entrez/query.fcgi?cmd=Retrieve&db=pubmed&dopt=Abstract&list_uids=15172144

- **Long-term clinical outcomes of postoperative pelvic radiotherapy with or without prophylactic paraaortic irradiation for stage I-II cervical carcinoma with positive lymph nodes: retrospective analysis of predictive variables regarding survival and failure patterns.**
  Author(s): Kodaira T, Fuwa N, Nakanishi T, Kuzuya K, Sasaoka M, Tachibana H, Furutani K.
  Source: American Journal of Clinical Oncology : the Official Publication of the American Radium Society. 2004 April; 27(2): 140-8.
  http://www.ncbi.nlm.nih.gov/entrez/query.fcgi?cmd=Retrieve&db=pubmed&dopt=Abstract&list_uids=15057153

- **Long-term follow-up of patients treated with radiotherapy alone for early-stage histologically aggressive non-Hodgkin's lymphoma.**
  Author(s): Spicer J, Smith P, Maclennan K, Hoskin P, Hancock B, Linch D, Pettengell R.
  Source: British Journal of Cancer. 2004 March 22; 90(6): 1151-5.
  http://www.ncbi.nlm.nih.gov/entrez/query.fcgi?cmd=Retrieve&db=pubmed&dopt=Abstract&list_uids=15026794

- **Long-term follow-up of radiotherapy for prostate cancer.**
  Author(s): Swanson GP, Riggs MW, Earle JD.
  Source: International Journal of Radiation Oncology, Biology, Physics. 2004 June 1; 59(2): 406-11.
  http://www.ncbi.nlm.nih.gov/entrez/query.fcgi?cmd=Retrieve&db=pubmed&dopt=Abstract&list_uids=15145156

- **Long-term treatment results of invasive cervical cancer patients undergoing inadvertent hysterectomy followed by salvage radiotherapy.**
  Author(s): Hsu WL, Shueng PW, Jen YM, Wu CJ, Hwang JM, Chang LP, Chen CM, Lin LC, Teh BS.
  Source: International Journal of Radiation Oncology, Biology, Physics. 2004 June 1; 59(2): 521-7.
  http://www.ncbi.nlm.nih.gov/entrez/query.fcgi?cmd=Retrieve&db=pubmed&dopt=Abstract&list_uids=15145172

- **Malignant pheochromocytoma of the urinary bladder: effectiveness of radiotherapy in conjunction with chemotherapy.**
  Author(s): Yoshida S, Nakagomi K, Goto S, Kobayashi S.
  Source: International Journal of Urology : Official Journal of the Japanese Urological Association. 2004 March; 11(3): 175-7.
  http://www.ncbi.nlm.nih.gov/entrez/query.fcgi?cmd=Retrieve&db=pubmed&dopt=Abstract&list_uids=15009367

- **Management of radiotherapy-induced cataracts in eyes with retinoblastoma.**
  Author(s): Sinha R, Titiyal JS, Sharma N, Vajpayee RB.
  Source: Journal of Cataract and Refractive Surgery. 2004 May; 30(5): 1145-6.
  http://www.ncbi.nlm.nih.gov/entrez/query.fcgi?cmd=Retrieve&db=pubmed&dopt=A
  bstract&list_uids=15130661

- **Mesenteric vein thrombosis after surgery and radiotherapy for pancreatic carcinoma. A case report.**
  Author(s): Macchia G, Morganti AG, Valentini V, Trodella L, Brizi MG, Cina G, Alfieri S, Doglietto G, Cellini N.
  Source: Tumori. 2004 March-April; 90(2): 262-4.
  http://www.ncbi.nlm.nih.gov/entrez/query.fcgi?cmd=Retrieve&db=pubmed&dopt=A
  bstract&list_uids=15237596

- **Modeling and computer simulations of tumor growth and tumor response to radiotherapy.**
  Author(s): Borkenstein K, Levegrun S, Peschke P.
  Source: Radiation Research. 2004 July; 162(1): 71-83.
  http://www.ncbi.nlm.nih.gov/entrez/query.fcgi?cmd=Retrieve&db=pubmed&dopt=A
  bstract&list_uids=15222799

- **Molecular prognostic factors in locally irresectable rectal cancer treated preoperatively by chemo-radiotherapy.**
  Author(s): Reerink O, Karrenbeld A, Plukker JT, Verschueren RC, Szabo BG, Sluiter WJ, Hospers GA, Mulder NH.
  Source: Anticancer Res. 2004 March-April; 24(2C): 1217-21.
  http://www.ncbi.nlm.nih.gov/entrez/query.fcgi?cmd=Retrieve&db=pubmed&dopt=A
  bstract&list_uids=15154650

- **Monotherapy for stage T1-T2 prostate cancer: radical prostatectomy, external beam radiotherapy, or permanent seed implantation.**
  Author(s): Potters L, Klein EA, Kattan MW, Reddy CA, Ciezki JP, Reuther AM, Kupelian PA.
  Source: Radiotherapy and Oncology : Journal of the European Society for Therapeutic Radiology and Oncology. 2004 April; 71(1): 29-33.
  http://www.ncbi.nlm.nih.gov/entrez/query.fcgi?cmd=Retrieve&db=pubmed&dopt=A
  bstract&list_uids=15066293

- **Monte Carlo dose calculations for radiotherapy machines: Theratron 780-C teletherapy case study.**
  Author(s): Sichani BT, Sohrabpour M.
  Source: Physics in Medicine and Biology. 2004 March 7; 49(5): 807-18.
  http://www.ncbi.nlm.nih.gov/entrez/query.fcgi?cmd=Retrieve&db=pubmed&dopt=A
  bstract&list_uids=15070204

- **Monte Carlo simulation of the photoneutron field in linac radiotherapy treatments with different collimation systems.**
  Author(s): Zanini A, Durisi E, Fasolo F, Ongaro C, Visca L, Nastasi U, Burn KW, Scielzo G, Adler JO, Annand JR, Rosner G.
  Source: Physics in Medicine and Biology. 2004 February 21; 49(4): 571-82.
  http://www.ncbi.nlm.nih.gov/entrez/query.fcgi?cmd=Retrieve&db=pubmed&dopt=Abstract&list_uids=15005166

- **Motes and beams: some observations on an IR(ME)R inspection in radiotherapy.**
  Author(s): Munro AJ.
  Source: The British Journal of Radiology. 2004 April; 77(916): 273-5.
  http://www.ncbi.nlm.nih.gov/entrez/query.fcgi?cmd=Retrieve&db=pubmed&dopt=Abstract&list_uids=15107315

- **Multifocal basal cell carcinoma developing in a facial port wine stain treated with argon and pulsed dye laser: a possible role for previous radiotherapy.**
  Author(s): Jasim ZF, Woo WK, Walsh MY, Handley JM.
  Source: Dermatologic Surgery : Official Publication for American Society for Dermatologic Surgery [et Al.]. 2004 August; 30(8): 1155-7.
  http://www.ncbi.nlm.nih.gov/entrez/query.fcgi?cmd=Retrieve&db=pubmed&dopt=Abstract&list_uids=15274710

- **Nasal and paranasal sinus changes after radiotherapy for nasopharyngeal carcinoma.**
  Author(s): Kamel R, Al-Badawy S, Khairy A, Kandil T, Sabry A.
  Source: Acta Oto-Laryngologica. 2004 May; 124(4): 532-5.
  http://www.ncbi.nlm.nih.gov/entrez/query.fcgi?cmd=Retrieve&db=pubmed&dopt=Abstract&list_uids=15224889

- **Nemaline myopathy in neck muscle after radiotherapy.**
  Author(s): Zamecnik M, Mukensnabl P, Kracik M.
  Source: Human Pathology. 2004 May; 35(5): 642-3.
  http://www.ncbi.nlm.nih.gov/entrez/query.fcgi?cmd=Retrieve&db=pubmed&dopt=Abstract&list_uids=15138944

- **Neoadjuvant chemotherapy followed by radiotherapy in epidermoid carcinoma of anus.**
  Author(s): Chie EK, Wu HG, Heo DS, Bang YJ, Kim NK, Ha SW.
  Source: Tumori. 2004 May-June; 90(3): 299-302.
  http://www.ncbi.nlm.nih.gov/entrez/query.fcgi?cmd=Retrieve&db=pubmed&dopt=Abstract&list_uids=15315309

- **Neoadjuvant hormonal therapy impairs sexual outcome among younger men who undergo external beam radiotherapy for localized prostate cancer.**
  Author(s): Hollenbeck BK, Wei JT, Sanda MG, Dunn RL, Sandler HM.
  Source: Urology. 2004 May; 63(5): 946-50.
  http://www.ncbi.nlm.nih.gov/entrez/query.fcgi?cmd=Retrieve&db=pubmed&dopt=Abstract&list_uids=15134986

- **New radiotherapy technologies for meningiomas: 3D conformal radiotherapy? Radiosurgery? Stereotactic radiotherapy? Intensity-modulated radiotherapy? Proton beam radiotherapy? Spot scanning proton radiation therapy. or nothing at all?**
  Author(s): Mirimanoff RO.
  Source: Radiotherapy and Oncology : Journal of the European Society for Therapeutic Radiology and Oncology. 2004 June; 71(3): 247-9. Review.
  http://www.ncbi.nlm.nih.gov/entrez/query.fcgi?cmd=Retrieve&db=pubmed&dopt=Abstract&list_uids=15172138

- **Next generation of targeted radiotherapy drugs emerging from the clinical pipeline.**
  Author(s): Goldman B.
  Source: Journal of the National Cancer Institute. 2004 June 16; 96(12): 903-4.
  http://www.ncbi.nlm.nih.gov/entrez/query.fcgi?cmd=Retrieve&db=pubmed&dopt=Abstract&list_uids=15199108

- **Nodal control and surgical salvage after primary radiotherapy in 1782 patients with laryngeal and pharyngeal carcinoma.**
  Author(s): Johansen LV, Grau C, Overgaard J.
  Source: Acta Oncologica (Stockholm, Sweden). 2004; 43(5): 486-94.
  http://www.ncbi.nlm.nih.gov/entrez/query.fcgi?cmd=Retrieve&db=pubmed&dopt=Abstract&list_uids=15360054

- **Nonocular second primary tumors after retinoblastoma: retrospective study of 111 patients treated by electron beam radiotherapy with or without TEM.**
  Author(s): Schlienger P, Campana F, Vilcoq JR, Asselain B, Dendale R, Desjardins L, Dorval T, Quintana E, Rodriguez J.
  Source: American Journal of Clinical Oncology : the Official Publication of the American Radium Society. 2004 August; 27(4): 411-9.
  http://www.ncbi.nlm.nih.gov/entrez/query.fcgi?cmd=Retrieve&db=pubmed&dopt=Abstract&list_uids=15289737

- **Non-randomised phase II trial of hyperbaric oxygen therapy in patients with chronic arm lymphoedema and tissue fibrosis after radiotherapy for early breast cancer.**
  Author(s): Gothard L, Stanton A, MacLaren J, Lawrence D, Hall E, Mortimer P, Parkin E, Pritchard J, Risdall J, Sawyer R, Woods M, Yarnold J.
  Source: Radiotherapy and Oncology : Journal of the European Society for Therapeutic Radiology and Oncology. 2004 March; 70(3): 217-24.
  http://www.ncbi.nlm.nih.gov/entrez/query.fcgi?cmd=Retrieve&db=pubmed&dopt=Abstract&list_uids=15064005

- **Nutrition intervention is beneficial in oncology outpatients receiving radiotherapy to the gastrointestinal or head and neck area.**
  Author(s): Isenring EA, Capra S, Bauer JD.
  Source: British Journal of Cancer. 2004 August 2; 91(3): 447-52.
  http://www.ncbi.nlm.nih.gov/entrez/query.fcgi?cmd=Retrieve&db=pubmed&dopt=Abstract&list_uids=15226773

- **On the use of margins for geometrical uncertainties around the rectum in radiotherapy planning.**
  Author(s): Muren LP, Ekerold R, Kvinnsland Y, Karlsdottir A, Dahl O.
  Source: Radiotherapy and Oncology : Journal of the European Society for Therapeutic Radiology and Oncology. 2004 January; 70(1): 11-9.
  http://www.ncbi.nlm.nih.gov/entrez/query.fcgi?cmd=Retrieve&db=pubmed&dopt=Abstract&list_uids=15036847

- **On-line aSi portal imaging of implanted fiducial markers for the reduction of interfraction error during conformal radiotherapy of prostate carcinoma.**
  Author(s): Chung PW, Haycocks T, Brown T, Cambridge Z, Kelly V, Alasti H, Jaffray DA, Catton CN.
  Source: International Journal of Radiation Oncology, Biology, Physics. 2004 September 1; 60(1): 329-34.
  http://www.ncbi.nlm.nih.gov/entrez/query.fcgi?cmd=Retrieve&db=pubmed&dopt=Abstract&list_uids=15337572

- **Online ultrasound image guidance for radiotherapy of prostate cancer: impact of image acquisition on prostate displacement.**
  Author(s): Artignan X, Smitsmans MH, Lebesque JV, Jaffray DA, van Her M, Bartelink H.
  Source: International Journal of Radiation Oncology, Biology, Physics. 2004 June 1; 59(2): 595-601.
  http://www.ncbi.nlm.nih.gov/entrez/query.fcgi?cmd=Retrieve&db=pubmed&dopt=Abstract&list_uids=15145181

- **Optic neuropathy secondary to radiotherapy for nasal melanoma.**
  Author(s): Garrott H, O'Day J.
  Source: Clinical & Experimental Ophthalmology. 2004 June; 32(3): 330-3.
  http://www.ncbi.nlm.nih.gov/entrez/query.fcgi?cmd=Retrieve&db=pubmed&dopt=Abstract&list_uids=15180849

- **Optimization of the primary collimator settings for fractionated IMRT stereotactic radiotherapy.**
  Author(s): Tobler M, Leavitt DD, Watson G.
  Source: Medical Dosimetry : Official Journal of the American Association of Medical Dosimetrists. 2004 Summer; 29(2): 72-9.
  http://www.ncbi.nlm.nih.gov/entrez/query.fcgi?cmd=Retrieve&db=pubmed&dopt=Abstract&list_uids=15191751

- **Optimization of tumour control probability for heterogeneous tumours in fractionated radiotherapy treatment protocols.**
  Author(s): Levin-Plotnik D, Hamilton RJ.
  Source: Physics in Medicine and Biology. 2004 February 7; 49(3): 407-24.
  http://www.ncbi.nlm.nih.gov/entrez/query.fcgi?cmd=Retrieve&db=pubmed&dopt=Abstract&list_uids=15012010

- Oral health-related quality of life in southern Chinese following radiotherapy for nasopharyngeal carcinoma.
  Author(s): McMillan AS, Pow EH, Leung WK, Wong MC, Kwong DL.
  Source: Journal of Oral Rehabilitation. 2004 June; 31(6): 600-8.
  http://www.ncbi.nlm.nih.gov/entrez/query.fcgi?cmd=Retrieve&db=pubmed&dopt=Abstract&list_uids=15189320

- Outcome following initial external beam radiotherapy in patients with Reese-Ellsworth group Vb retinoblastoma.
  Author(s): Abramson DH, Beaverson KL, Chang ST, Dunkel IJ, McCormick B.
  Source: Archives of Ophthalmology. 2004 September; 122(9): 1316-23.
  http://www.ncbi.nlm.nih.gov/entrez/query.fcgi?cmd=Retrieve&db=pubmed&dopt=Abstract&list_uids=15364710

- Outcome of split-thickness skin grafts after external beam radiotherapy.
  Author(s): Bui DT, Chunilal A, Mehrara BJ, Disa JJ, Alektiar KM, Cordeiro PG.
  Source: Annals of Plastic Surgery. 2004 June; 52(6): 551-6; Discussion 557.
  http://www.ncbi.nlm.nih.gov/entrez/query.fcgi?cmd=Retrieve&db=pubmed&dopt=Abstract&list_uids=15166977

- Overexpression of Bcl2 abrogates chemo- and radiotherapy-induced sensitisation of NCI-H460 non-small-cell lung cancer cells to adenovirus-mediated expression of full-length TRAIL.
  Author(s): Abou El Hassan MA, Mastenbroek DC, Gerritsen WR, Giaccone G, Kruyt FA.
  Source: British Journal of Cancer. 2004 July 5; 91(1): 171-7.
  http://www.ncbi.nlm.nih.gov/entrez/query.fcgi?cmd=Retrieve&db=pubmed&dopt=Abstract&list_uids=15173860

- Pathological changes of advanced lower-rectal cancer by preoperative radiotherapy.
  Author(s): Kinoshita H, Watanabe T, Yanagisawa A, Nagawa H, Kato Y, Muto T.
  Source: Hepatogastroenterology. 2004 September-October; 51(59): 1362-6.
  http://www.ncbi.nlm.nih.gov/entrez/query.fcgi?cmd=Retrieve&db=pubmed&dopt=Abstract&list_uids=15362753

- Phenomenologic model describing flow reduction for parotid gland irradiation with intensity-modulated radiotherapy: evidence of significant recovery effect.
  Author(s): Scrimger RA, Stavrev P, Parliament MB, Field C, Thompson H, Stavreva N, Fallone BG.
  Source: International Journal of Radiation Oncology, Biology, Physics. 2004 September 1; 60(1): 178-85.
  http://www.ncbi.nlm.nih.gov/entrez/query.fcgi?cmd=Retrieve&db=pubmed&dopt=Abstract&list_uids=15337554

- Plaque radiotherapy for choroidal and ciliochoroidal melanomas with limited nodular extrascleral extension.
  Author(s): Augsburger JJ, Schneider S, Narayana A, Breneman JC, Aron BS, Barrett WL, Trichopoulos N.
  Source: Can J Ophthalmol. 2004 June; 39(4): 380-7.
  http://www.ncbi.nlm.nih.gov/entrez/query.fcgi?cmd=Retrieve&db=pubmed&dopt=Abstract&list_uids=15327103

- **Postoperative radiotherapy in stage II or IIIA completely resected non-small cell lung cancer: a systematic review and practice guideline.**
  Author(s): Okawara G, Ung YC, Markman BR, Mackay JA, Evans WK; Lung Cancer Disease Site Group of Cancer Care Ontario's Program in Evidence-Based Care.
  Source: Lung Cancer (Amsterdam, Netherlands). 2004 April; 44(1): 1-11. Review.
  http://www.ncbi.nlm.nih.gov/entrez/query.fcgi?cmd=Retrieve&db=pubmed&dopt=Abstract&list_uids=15013578

- **Post-operative sequential chemo-radiotherapy in high-grade cerebral gliomas with fotemustine.**
  Author(s): Ozkan M, Altinbas M, Er O, Kaplan B, Coskun HS, Karahacioglu E, Menku A, Cihan Y, Kontas O, Akdemir H.
  Source: J Chemother. 2004 June; 16(3): 298-302.
  http://www.ncbi.nlm.nih.gov/entrez/query.fcgi?cmd=Retrieve&db=pubmed&dopt=Abstract&list_uids=15330329

- **Prediction of respiratory tumour motion for real-time image-guided radiotherapy.**
  Author(s): Sharp GC, Jiang SB, Shimizu S, Shirato H.
  Source: Physics in Medicine and Biology. 2004 February 7; 49(3): 425-40.
  http://www.ncbi.nlm.nih.gov/entrez/query.fcgi?cmd=Retrieve&db=pubmed&dopt=Abstract&list_uids=15012011

- **Prognostic significance of Bax, Bcl-2, and p53 expressions in cervical squamous cell carcinoma treated by radiotherapy.**
  Author(s): Wootipoom V, Lekhyananda N, Phungrassami T, Boonyaphiphat P, Thongsuksai P.
  Source: Gynecologic Oncology. 2004 September; 94(3): 636-42.
  http://www.ncbi.nlm.nih.gov/entrez/query.fcgi?cmd=Retrieve&db=pubmed&dopt=Abstract&list_uids=15350352

- **Prospective validation of serum CYFRA 21-1, beta-2-microglobulin, and ferritin levels as prognostic markers in patients with nonmetastatic nasopharyngeal carcinoma undergoing radiotherapy.**
  Author(s): Ma BB, Leungm SF, Hui EP, Mo F, Kwan WH, Zee B, Yuen J, Chan AT.
  Source: Cancer. 2004 August 15; 101(4): 776-81.
  http://www.ncbi.nlm.nih.gov/entrez/query.fcgi?cmd=Retrieve&db=pubmed&dopt=Abstract&list_uids=15305409

- **Quality assurance of axillary radiotherapy in the EORTC AMAROS trial 10981/22023: the dummy run.**
  Author(s): Hurkmans CW, Borger JH, Rutgers EJ, van Tienhoven G; EORTC Breast Cancer Cooperative Group; Radiotherapy Cooperative Group.
  Source: Radiotherapy and Oncology : Journal of the European Society for Therapeutic Radiology and Oncology. 2003 September; 68(3): 233-40.
  http://www.ncbi.nlm.nih.gov/entrez/query.fcgi?cmd=Retrieve&db=pubmed&dopt=Abstract&list_uids=13129630

- **Quality assurance of the EORTC 26981/22981; NCIC CE3 intergroup trial on radiotherapy with or without temozolomide for newly-diagnosed glioblastoma multiforme: the individual case review.**
  Author(s): Ataman F, Poortmans P, Stupp R, Fisher B, Mirimanoff RO.
  Source: European Journal of Cancer (Oxford, England : 1990). 2004 July; 40(11): 1724-30.
  http://www.ncbi.nlm.nih.gov/entrez/query.fcgi?cmd=Retrieve&db=pubmed&dopt=Abstract&list_uids=15251162

- **Quality of life after treatment for prostate cancer: no difference between surgery and radiotherapy?**
  Author(s): Vordermark D, Koelbl O.
  Source: Journal of Clinical Oncology : Official Journal of the American Society of Clinical Oncology. 2003 December 15; 21(24): 4655; Author Reply 4655-6.
  http://www.ncbi.nlm.nih.gov/entrez/query.fcgi?cmd=Retrieve&db=pubmed&dopt=Abstract&list_uids=14673059

- **Quality of life as a survival predictor for esophageal squamous cell carcinoma treated with radiotherapy.**
  Author(s): Fang FM, Tsai WL, Chiu HC, Kuo WR, Hsiung CY.
  Source: International Journal of Radiation Oncology, Biology, Physics. 2004 April 1; 58(5): 1394-404.
  http://www.ncbi.nlm.nih.gov/entrez/query.fcgi?cmd=Retrieve&db=pubmed&dopt=Abstract&list_uids=15050315

- **Quality of life as a survival predictor for patients with advanced head and neck carcinoma treated with radiotherapy.**
  Author(s): Fang FM, Liu YT, Tang Y, Wang CJ, Ko SF.
  Source: Cancer. 2004 January 15; 100(2): 425-32.
  http://www.ncbi.nlm.nih.gov/entrez/query.fcgi?cmd=Retrieve&db=pubmed&dopt=Abstract&list_uids=14716781

- **Quality of life following resection, free flap reconstruction and postoperative external beam radiotherapy for squamous cell carcinoma of the base of tongue.**
  Author(s): Winter SC, Cassell O, Corbridge RJ, Goodacre T, Cox GJ.
  Source: Clinical Otolaryngology and Allied Sciences. 2004 June; 29(3): 274-8.
  http://www.ncbi.nlm.nih.gov/entrez/query.fcgi?cmd=Retrieve&db=pubmed&dopt=Abstract&list_uids=15142075

- **Quality-of-life questionnaire results 2 and 3 years after radiotherapy for prostate cancer in a randomized dose-escalation study.**
  Author(s): Little DJ, Kuban DA, Levy LB, Zagars GK, Pollack A.
  Source: Urology. 2003 October; 62(4): 707-13.
  http://www.ncbi.nlm.nih.gov/entrez/query.fcgi?cmd=Retrieve&db=pubmed&dopt=Abstract&list_uids=14550448

- **Quantification of tumour response to radiotherapy.**
  Author(s): Gong QY, Eldridge PR, Brodbelt AR, Garcia-Finana M, Zaman A, Jones B, Roberts N.
  Source: The British Journal of Radiology. 2004 May; 77(917): 405-13.
  http://www.ncbi.nlm.nih.gov/entrez/query.fcgi?cmd=Retrieve&db=pubmed&dopt=Abstract&list_uids=15121704

- **Quantification of volumetric and geometric changes occurring during fractionated radiotherapy for head-and-neck cancer using an integrated CT/linear accelerator system.**
  Author(s): Barker JL Jr, Garden AS, Ang KK, O'Daniel JC, Wang H, Court LE, Morrison WH, Rosenthal DI, Chao KS, Tucker SL, Mohan R, Dong L.
  Source: International Journal of Radiation Oncology, Biology, Physics. 2004 July 15; 59(4): 960-70.
  http://www.ncbi.nlm.nih.gov/entrez/query.fcgi?cmd=Retrieve&db=pubmed&dopt=Abstract&list_uids=15234029

- **Quantitative analysis of three-dimensional conformal radiotherapy techniques for posterior fossa treatment in children.**
  Author(s): Timmerman RD, Ewing M, Donges M, Wilson J, Jakacki R, Randall ME.
  Source: Technology in Cancer Research & Treatment. 2003 December; 2(6): 587-93.
  http://www.ncbi.nlm.nih.gov/entrez/query.fcgi?cmd=Retrieve&db=pubmed&dopt=Abstract&list_uids=14640770

- **Radioimmunoscintigraphy for postprostatectomy radiotherapy: analysis of toxicity and biochemical control.**
  Author(s): Jani AB, Blend MJ, Hamilton R, Brendler C, Pelizzari C, Krauz L, Sapra B, Vijayakumar S, Awan A, Weichselbaum RR.
  Source: Journal of Nuclear Medicine : Official Publication, Society of Nuclear Medicine. 2004 August; 45(8): 1315-22.
  http://www.ncbi.nlm.nih.gov/entrez/query.fcgi?cmd=Retrieve&db=pubmed&dopt=Abstract&list_uids=15299055

- **Radiotherapy and chemotherapy in locally advanced non-small cell lung cancer: preclinical and early clinical data.**
  Author(s): Reboul FL.
  Source: Hematology/Oncology Clinics of North America. 2004 February; 18(1): 41-53. Review.
  http://www.ncbi.nlm.nih.gov/entrez/query.fcgi?cmd=Retrieve&db=pubmed&dopt=Abstract&list_uids=15005280

- **Radiotherapy for hypersplenism from congestive splenomegaly.**
  Author(s): Liu MT, Hsieh CY, Chang TH, Lin JP, Huang CC.
  Source: Ann Saudi Med. 2004 May-June; 24(3): 198-200. No Abstract Available.
  http://www.ncbi.nlm.nih.gov/entrez/query.fcgi?cmd=Retrieve&db=pubmed&dopt=Abstract&list_uids=15307459

- **Radiotherapy for pediatric central nervous system tumors: a regional cancer centre experience.**
  Author(s): Bauman G, Fisher B, Cairney E, Ranger A, Dar AR, Ross J, Stitt L, MacDonald D.
  Source: Journal of Neuro-Oncology. 2004 July; 68(3): 285-94. Review.
  http://www.ncbi.nlm.nih.gov/entrez/query.fcgi?cmd=Retrieve&db=pubmed&dopt=Abstract&list_uids=15332333

- **Radiotherapy in the treatment of stage III-IV hypopharyngeal carcinoma.**
  Author(s): Tombolini V, Santarelli M, Raffetto N, Donato V, Valeriani M, Ferretti A, Enrici RM.
  Source: Anticancer Res. 2004 January-February; 24(1): 349-54.
  http://www.ncbi.nlm.nih.gov/entrez/query.fcgi?cmd=Retrieve&db=pubmed&dopt=Abstract&list_uids=15015620

- **Radiotherapy plus either transdermal fentanyl or paracetamol and codeine for painful bone metastases: a randomised study of pain relief and quality of life.**
  Author(s): Pistevou-Gompaki K, Kouloulias VE, Varveris C, Mystakidou K, Georgakopoulos G, Eleftheriadis N, Gompakis N, Kouvaris J.
  Source: Current Medical Research and Opinion. 2004; 20(2): 159-63.
  http://www.ncbi.nlm.nih.gov/entrez/query.fcgi?cmd=Retrieve&db=pubmed&dopt=Abstract&list_uids=15006009

- **Re: Breast-conserving surgery with or without radiotherapy: pooled-analysis for risks of ipsilateral breast tumor recurrence and mortality.**
  Author(s): Kunkler I, Williams L, Prescott R, King C.
  Source: Journal of the National Cancer Institute. 2004 August 18; 96(16): 1255; Author Reply 1255-7.
  http://www.ncbi.nlm.nih.gov/entrez/query.fcgi?cmd=Retrieve&db=pubmed&dopt=Abstract&list_uids=15316061

- **Recurrent squamous cell carcinoma of cervix after definitive radiotherapy.**
  Author(s): Hong JH, Tsai CS, Lai CH, Chang TC, Wang CC, Chou HH, Lee SP, Hsueh S.
  Source: International Journal of Radiation Oncology, Biology, Physics. 2004 September 1; 60(1): 249-57.
  http://www.ncbi.nlm.nih.gov/entrez/query.fcgi?cmd=Retrieve&db=pubmed&dopt=Abstract&list_uids=15337563

- **Regional radiotherapy to axilla and supraclavicular fossa for adjuvant breast treatment: a comparison of four techniques.**
  Author(s): Jephcott CR, Tyldesley S, Swift CL.
  Source: International Journal of Radiation Oncology, Biology, Physics. 2004 September 1; 60(1): 103-10.
  http://www.ncbi.nlm.nih.gov/entrez/query.fcgi?cmd=Retrieve&db=pubmed&dopt=Abstract&list_uids=15337545

- **Report of a multicenter Canadian phase III randomized trial of 3 months vs. 8 months neoadjuvant androgen deprivation before standard-dose radiotherapy for clinically localized prostate cancer.**
  Author(s): Crook J, Ludgate C, Malone S, Lim J, Perry G, Eapen L, Bowen J, Robertson S, Lockwood G.
  Source: International Journal of Radiation Oncology, Biology, Physics. 2004 September 1; 60(1): 15-23.
  http://www.ncbi.nlm.nih.gov/entrez/query.fcgi?cmd=Retrieve&db=pubmed&dopt=Abstract&list_uids=15337535

- **Salvage esophagectomy after definitive chemotherapy and radiotherapy for advanced esophageal cancer.**
  Author(s): Nakamura T, Hayashi K, Ota M, Eguchi R, Ide H, Takasaki K, Mitsuhashi N.
  Source: American Journal of Surgery. 2004 September; 188(3): 261-6.
  http://www.ncbi.nlm.nih.gov/entrez/query.fcgi?cmd=Retrieve&db=pubmed&dopt=Abstract&list_uids=15450831

- **Sphincter preservation following preoperative radiotherapy for rectal cancer: report of a randomised trial comparing short-term radiotherapy vs. conventionally fractionated radiochemotherapy.**
  Author(s): Bujko K, Nowacki MP, Nasierowska-Guttmejer A, Michalski W, Bebenek M, Pudelko M, Kryj M, Oledzki J, Szmeja J, Sluszniak J, Serkies K, Kladny J, Pamucka M, Kukolowicz P.
  Source: Radiotherapy and Oncology : Journal of the European Society for Therapeutic Radiology and Oncology. 2004 July; 72(1): 15-24.
  http://www.ncbi.nlm.nih.gov/entrez/query.fcgi?cmd=Retrieve&db=pubmed&dopt=Abstract&list_uids=15236870

- **Squamous cell carcinoma of the scalp after radiotherapy for tinea capitis.**
  Author(s): Ronel DN, Schwager RG, Avram MR.
  Source: Dermatologic Surgery : Official Publication for American Society for Dermatologic Surgery [et Al.]. 2004 March; 30(3): 446-9.
  http://www.ncbi.nlm.nih.gov/entrez/query.fcgi?cmd=Retrieve&db=pubmed&dopt=Abstract&list_uids=15008881

- **Status of postmastectomy radiotherapy in the United States: a patterns of care study.**
  Author(s): White J, Moughan J, Pierce LJ, Morrow M, Owen J, Wilson JF.
  Source: International Journal of Radiation Oncology, Biology, Physics. 2004 September 1; 60(1): 77-85.
  http://www.ncbi.nlm.nih.gov/entrez/query.fcgi?cmd=Retrieve&db=pubmed&dopt=Abstract&list_uids=15337542

- **Stereotactic conformal radiotherapy in patients with growth hormone-secreting pituitary adenoma.**
  Author(s): Milker-Zabel S, Zabel A, Huber P, Schlegel W, Wannenmacher M, Debus J.
  Source: International Journal of Radiation Oncology, Biology, Physics. 2004 July 15; 59(4): 1088-96.
  http://www.ncbi.nlm.nih.gov/entrez/query.fcgi?cmd=Retrieve&db=pubmed&dopt=Abstract&list_uids=15234043

- **Stereotactic radiotherapy for primary lung cancer and pulmonary metastases: a noninvasive treatment approach in medically inoperable patients.**
  Author(s): Wulf J, Haedinger U, Oppitz U, Thiele W, Mueller G, Flentje M.
  Source: International Journal of Radiation Oncology, Biology, Physics. 2004 September 1; 60(1): 186-96.
  http://www.ncbi.nlm.nih.gov/entrez/query.fcgi?cmd=Retrieve&db=pubmed&dopt=Abstract&list_uids=15337555

- **Successful removal after radiotherapy and vascular embolization in a huge tentorial epithelioid hemangioendothelioma: a case report.**
  Author(s): Kubota T, Sato K, Takeuchi H, Handa Y.
  Source: Journal of Neuro-Oncology. 2004 June; 68(2): 177-83. Review.
  http://www.ncbi.nlm.nih.gov/entrez/query.fcgi?cmd=Retrieve&db=pubmed&dopt=Abstract&list_uids=15218955

- **Survey on use of palliative radiotherapy in hospice care.**
  Author(s): Lutz S, Spence C, Chow E, Janjan N, Connor S.
  Source: Journal of Clinical Oncology : Official Journal of the American Society of Clinical Oncology. 2004 September 1; 22(17): 3581-6.
  http://www.ncbi.nlm.nih.gov/entrez/query.fcgi?cmd=Retrieve&db=pubmed&dopt=Abstract&list_uids=15337808

- **Survivin expression is an independent prognostic factor in rectal cancer patients with and without preoperative radiotherapy.**
  Author(s): Knutsen A, Adell G, Sun XF.
  Source: International Journal of Radiation Oncology, Biology, Physics. 2004 September 1; 60(1): 149-55.
  http://www.ncbi.nlm.nih.gov/entrez/query.fcgi?cmd=Retrieve&db=pubmed&dopt=Abstract&list_uids=15337550

- **The application of number needed to treat (NNT) to clinical problems in radiotherapy.**
  Author(s): Jani AB, Myrianthopoulos L, Vijayakumar S.
  Source: Cancer Investigation. 2004; 22(2): 262-70.
  http://www.ncbi.nlm.nih.gov/entrez/query.fcgi?cmd=Retrieve&db=pubmed&dopt=Abstract&list_uids=15199609

- **The comparison of radiotherapy techniques for treatment of the prostate cancer: the three-field vs. the four-field.**
  Author(s): Milecki P, Piotrowski T, Dymnicka M.
  Source: Neoplasma. 2004; 51(1): 64-9.
  http://www.ncbi.nlm.nih.gov/entrez/query.fcgi?cmd=Retrieve&db=pubmed&dopt=Abstract&list_uids=15004663

- **The experience of radiotherapy for localized prostate cancer: the men's perspective.**
  Author(s): Kelsey SG, Owens J, White A.
  Source: European Journal of Cancer Care. 2004 July; 13(3): 272-8.
  http://www.ncbi.nlm.nih.gov/entrez/query.fcgi?cmd=Retrieve&db=pubmed&dopt=Abstract&list_uids=15196231

- **The role of abdominal-pelvic radiotherapy in the management of uterine papillary serous carcinoma.**
  Author(s): Kwon J, Ackerman I, Franssen E.
  Source: International Journal of Radiation Oncology, Biology, Physics. 2004 August 1; 59(5): 1439-45.
  http://www.ncbi.nlm.nih.gov/entrez/query.fcgi?cmd=Retrieve&db=pubmed&dopt=Abstract&list_uids=15275730

- **The role of external radiotherapy in patients treated with permanent prostate brachytherapy.**
  Author(s): Potters L, Fearn P, Kattan M.
  Source: Prostate Cancer and Prostatic Diseases. 2002; 5(1): 47-53. Review.
  http://www.ncbi.nlm.nih.gov/entrez/query.fcgi?cmd=Retrieve&db=pubmed&dopt=Abstract&list_uids=15195130

- **Therapeutic effects and prognostic factors in three-dimensional conformal radiotherapy combined with transcatheter arterial chemoembolization for hepatocellular carcinoma.**
  Author(s): Wu DH, Liu L, Chen LH.
  Source: World Journal of Gastroenterology : Wjg. 2004 August 1; 10(15): 2184-9.
  http://www.ncbi.nlm.nih.gov/entrez/query.fcgi?cmd=Retrieve&db=pubmed&dopt=Abstract&list_uids=15259062

- **Three-dimensional conformal radiotherapy versus intracavitary brachytherapy for salvage treatment of locally persistent nasopharyngeal carcinoma.**
  Author(s): Zheng XK, Chen LH, Chen YQ, Deng XG.
  Source: International Journal of Radiation Oncology, Biology, Physics. 2004 September 1; 60(1): 165-70.
  http://www.ncbi.nlm.nih.gov/entrez/query.fcgi?cmd=Retrieve&db=pubmed&dopt=Abstract&list_uids=15337552

- **Treatment of patients with cardiac pacemakers and implantable cardioverter-defibrillators during radiotherapy.**
  Author(s): Solan AN, Solan MJ, Bednarz G, Goodkin MB.
  Source: International Journal of Radiation Oncology, Biology, Physics. 2004 July 1; 59(3): 897-904. Review.
  http://www.ncbi.nlm.nih.gov/entrez/query.fcgi?cmd=Retrieve&db=pubmed&dopt=Abstract&list_uids=15183493

- **Tumor hypoxia is independent of hemoglobin and prognostic for loco-regional tumor control after primary radiotherapy in advanced head and neck cancer.**
  Author(s): Nordsmark M, Overgaard J.
  Source: Acta Oncologica (Stockholm, Sweden). 2004; 43(4): 396-403.
  http://www.ncbi.nlm.nih.gov/entrez/query.fcgi?cmd=Retrieve&db=pubmed&dopt=Abstract&list_uids=15303502

- **Uncertainties regarding pelvic radiotherapy for prostate cancer.**
  Author(s): Ennis RD.
  Source: Journal of Clinical Oncology : Official Journal of the American Society of Clinical Oncology. 2004 June 1; 22(11): 2254-5; Author Reply 2255-7.
  http://www.ncbi.nlm.nih.gov/entrez/query.fcgi?cmd=Retrieve&db=pubmed&dopt=Abstract&list_uids=15169820

- **Univariate analysis of factors correlated with tumor control probability of three-dimensional conformal hypofractionated high-dose radiotherapy for small pulmonary or hepatic tumors.**
  Author(s): Wada H, Takai Y, Nemoto K, Yamada S.
  Source: International Journal of Radiation Oncology, Biology, Physics. 2004 March 15; 58(4): 1114-20.
  http://www.ncbi.nlm.nih.gov/entrez/query.fcgi?cmd=Retrieve&db=pubmed&dopt=Abstract&list_uids=15001252

- **Unusual chromaffin cell differentiation of a neuroblastoma after chemotherapy and radiotherapy: report of an autopsy case with immunohistochemical evaluations.**
  Author(s): Miyauchi J, Kiyotani C, Shioda Y, Kumagai M, Honna T, Matsuoka K, Masaki H, Aiba M, Hata J, Tsunematsu Y.
  Source: The American Journal of Surgical Pathology. 2004 April; 28(4): 548-53.
  http://www.ncbi.nlm.nih.gov/entrez/query.fcgi?cmd=Retrieve&db=pubmed&dopt=Abstract&list_uids=15087676

- **Updated European core curriculum for radiotherapists (radiation oncologists). Recommended curriculum for the specialist training of medical practitioners in radiotherapy (radiation oncology) within Europe.**
  Author(s): Baumann M, Leer JW, Dahl O, De Neve W, Hunter R, Rampling R, Verfaillie C; European Core Curriculum for Radiotherapists Working Party, The European Society for Therapeutic Radiology and Oncology; European Core Curriculum for Radiotherapists Working Party, European Board of Radiotherapy.
  Source: Radiotherapy and Oncology : Journal of the European Society for Therapeutic Radiology and Oncology. 2004 February; 70(2): 107-13.
  http://www.ncbi.nlm.nih.gov/entrez/query.fcgi?cmd=Retrieve&db=pubmed&dopt=Abstract&list_uids=15028397

- **Use and timing of radiotherapy in high-risk prostate cancer.**
  Author(s): Ward JF, Blute ML.
  Source: Jama : the Journal of the American Medical Association. 2004 June 16; 291(23): 2817; Author Reply 2817-8.
  http://www.ncbi.nlm.nih.gov/entrez/query.fcgi?cmd=Retrieve&db=pubmed&dopt=Abstract&list_uids=15199027

- **Use of artificial neural networks to predict biological outcomes for patients receiving radical radiotherapy of the prostate.**
  Author(s): Gulliford SL, Webb S, Rowbottom CG, Corne DW, Dearnaley DP.
  Source: Radiotherapy and Oncology : Journal of the European Society for Therapeutic Radiology and Oncology. 2004 April; 71(1): 3-12.
  http://www.ncbi.nlm.nih.gov/entrez/query.fcgi?cmd=Retrieve&db=pubmed&dopt=Abstract&list_uids=15066290

- Use of pathologic factors to assist in establishing adequacy of excision before radiotherapy in patients treated with breast-conserving therapy.
  Author(s): Vicini FA, Goldstein NS, Pass H, Kestin LL.
  Source: International Journal of Radiation Oncology, Biology, Physics. 2004 September 1; 60(1): 86-94.
  http://www.ncbi.nlm.nih.gov/entrez/query.fcgi?cmd=Retrieve&db=pubmed&dopt=Abstract&list_uids=15337543

- Use of the humanized anti-epidermal growth factor receptor monoclonal antibody h-R3 in combination with radiotherapy in the treatment of locally advanced head and neck cancer patients.
  Author(s): Crombet T, Osorio M, Cruz T, Roca C, del Castillo R, Mon R, Iznaga-Escobar N, Figueredo R, Koropatnick J, Renginfo E, Fernandez E, Alvarez D, Torres O, Ramos M, Leonard I, Perez R, Lage A.
  Source: Journal of Clinical Oncology : Official Journal of the American Society of Clinical Oncology. 2004 May 1; 22(9): 1646-54.
  http://www.ncbi.nlm.nih.gov/entrez/query.fcgi?cmd=Retrieve&db=pubmed&dopt=Abstract&list_uids=15117987

- Use of the small pelvic field instead of the classic whole pelvic field in postoperative radiotherapy for cervical cancer: reduction of adverse events.
  Author(s): Ohara K, Tsunoda H, Satoh T, Oki A, Sugahara S, Yoshikawa H.
  Source: International Journal of Radiation Oncology, Biology, Physics. 2004 September 1; 60(1): 258-64.
  http://www.ncbi.nlm.nih.gov/entrez/query.fcgi?cmd=Retrieve&db=pubmed&dopt=Abstract&list_uids=15337564

- Utilization of custom electron bolus in head and neck radiotherapy.
  Author(s): Kudchadker RJ, Antolak JA, Morrison WH, Wong PF, Hogstrom KR.
  Source: Journal of Applied Clinical Medical Physics [electronic Resource] / American College of Medical Physics. 2003 Autumn; 4(4): 321-33.
  http://www.ncbi.nlm.nih.gov/entrez/query.fcgi?cmd=Retrieve&db=pubmed&dopt=Abstract&list_uids=14604422

- Validation of a method for automatic image fusion (BrainLAB System) of CT data and 11C-methionine-PET data for stereotactic radiotherapy using a LINAC: first clinical experience.
  Author(s): Grosu AL, Lachner R, Wiedenmann N, Stark S, Thamm R, Kneschaurek P, Schwaiger M, Molls M, Weber WA.
  Source: International Journal of Radiation Oncology, Biology, Physics. 2003 August 1; 56(5): 1450-63.
  http://www.ncbi.nlm.nih.gov/entrez/query.fcgi?cmd=Retrieve&db=pubmed&dopt=Abstract&list_uids=12873691

- Variations in 6MV x-ray radiotherapy build-up dose with treatment distance.
  Author(s): Butson MJ, Cheung T, Yu PK.
  Source: Australas Phys Eng Sci Med. 2003 June; 26(2): 88-90.
  http://www.ncbi.nlm.nih.gov/entrez/query.fcgi?cmd=Retrieve&db=pubmed&dopt=Abstract&list_uids=12956192

- **Vascular endothelial growth factor independently predicts the efficacy of postoperative radiotherapy in node-negative breast cancer patients.**
Author(s): Manders P, Sweep FC, Tjan-Heijnen VC, Geurts-Moespot A, van Tienoven DT, Foekens JA, Span PN, Bussink J, Beex LV.
Source: Clinical Cancer Research : an Official Journal of the American Association for Cancer Research. 2003 December 15; 9(17): 6363-70.
http://www.ncbi.nlm.nih.gov/entrez/query.fcgi?cmd=Retrieve&db=pubmed&dopt=Abstract&list_uids=14695136

- **Vitamin D3 and vitamin D3 analogues as an adjunct to cancer chemo-therapy and radiotherapy.**
Author(s): Gewirtz DA, Gupta MS, Sundaram S.
Source: Current Medicinal Chemistry. Anti-Cancer Agents. 2002 November; 2(6): 683-90. Review.
http://www.ncbi.nlm.nih.gov/entrez/query.fcgi?cmd=Retrieve&db=pubmed&dopt=Abstract&list_uids=12678720

- **Vocal fold paralysis following radiotherapy for nasopharyngeal carcinoma: laryngeal electromyography findings.**
Author(s): Lau DP, Lo YL, Wee J, Tan NG, Low WK.
Source: Journal of Voice : Official Journal of the Voice Foundation. 2003 March; 17(1): 82-7.
http://www.ncbi.nlm.nih.gov/entrez/query.fcgi?cmd=Retrieve&db=pubmed&dopt=Abstract&list_uids=12705821

- **Voice quality after laser surgery or radiotherapy for T1a glottic carcinoma.**
Author(s): Tamura E, Kitahara S, Ogura M, Kohno N.
Source: The Laryngoscope. 2003 May; 113(5): 910-4.
http://www.ncbi.nlm.nih.gov/entrez/query.fcgi?cmd=Retrieve&db=pubmed&dopt=Abstract&list_uids=12792332

- **Voice quality after treatment for T1a glottic carcinoma--radiotherapy versus laser cordectomy.**
Author(s): Krengli M, Policarpo M, Manfredda I, Aluffi P, Gambaro G, Panella M, Pia F.
Source: Acta Oncologica (Stockholm, Sweden). 2004; 43(3): 284-9.
http://www.ncbi.nlm.nih.gov/entrez/query.fcgi?cmd=Retrieve&db=pubmed&dopt=Abstract&list_uids=15244253

- **Volume-based radiotherapy targeting in soft tissue sarcoma.**
Author(s): Ward I, Haycocks T, Sharpe M, Griffin A, Catton C, Jaffray D, O'Sullivan B.
Source: Cancer Treat Res. 2004; 120: 17-42. Review. No Abstract Available.
http://www.ncbi.nlm.nih.gov/entrez/query.fcgi?cmd=Retrieve&db=pubmed&dopt=Abstract&list_uids=15217216

- **Volumetric and histologic responses to radiotherapy or radiochemotherapy of metastatic cervical lymph nodes of oral squamous cell carcinoma.**
  Author(s): Yusa H, Yoshida H, Noguchi M, Ohara K.
  Source: Journal of Oral and Maxillofacial Surgery : Official Journal of the American Association of Oral and Maxillofacial Surgeons. 2003 August; 61(8): 904-8.
  http://www.ncbi.nlm.nih.gov/entrez/query.fcgi?cmd=Retrieve&db=pubmed&dopt=Abstract&list_uids=12905442

- **Vulvar cancer in a patient with Fanconi's anemia, treated with 3D conformal radiotherapy.**
  Author(s): Harper JL, Jenrette JM, Goddu SM, Lal A, Smith T.
  Source: American Journal of Hematology. 2004 June; 76(2): 148-51.
  http://www.ncbi.nlm.nih.gov/entrez/query.fcgi?cmd=Retrieve&db=pubmed&dopt=Abstract&list_uids=15164381

- **Waiting times for radiotherapy: consequences of volume increase for the TCP in oropharyngeal carcinoma.**
  Author(s): Waaijer A, Terhaard CH, Dehnad H, Hordijk GJ, van Leeuwen MS, Raaymakers CP, Lagendijk JJ.
  Source: Radiotherapy and Oncology : Journal of the European Society for Therapeutic Radiology and Oncology. 2003 March; 66(3): 271-6.
  http://www.ncbi.nlm.nih.gov/entrez/query.fcgi?cmd=Retrieve&db=pubmed&dopt=Abstract&list_uids=12742266

- **Waiting times for radiotherapy--a survey of patients' attitudes.**
  Author(s): Lehman M, Jacob S, Delaney G, Papadatos G, Jalaludin B, Cail S, McCourt J, Wright S, O'Brien C, Barton M.
  Source: Radiotherapy and Oncology : Journal of the European Society for Therapeutic Radiology and Oncology. 2004 March; 70(3): 283-9.
  http://www.ncbi.nlm.nih.gov/entrez/query.fcgi?cmd=Retrieve&db=pubmed&dopt=Abstract&list_uids=15064014

- **Web-based submission, archive, and review of radiotherapy data for clinical quality assurance: a new paradigm.**
  Author(s): Palta JR, Frouhar VA, Dempsey JF.
  Source: International Journal of Radiation Oncology, Biology, Physics. 2003 December 1; 57(5): 1427-36.
  http://www.ncbi.nlm.nih.gov/entrez/query.fcgi?cmd=Retrieve&db=pubmed&dopt=Abstract&list_uids=14630282

- **What can the Cancer Services Collaborative do for your radiotherapy department?**
  Author(s): Kirkbride P, Roberts T, Craig A.
  Source: Clin Oncol (R Coll Radiol). 2003 June; 15(4): 172-3. No Abstract Available.
  http://www.ncbi.nlm.nih.gov/entrez/query.fcgi?cmd=Retrieve&db=pubmed&dopt=Abstract&list_uids=12846493

- **Whole abdomen radiotherapy for patients with peritoneal dissemination of endometrial adenocarcinoma.**
  Author(s): Lee SW, Russell AH, Kinney WK.
  Source: International Journal of Radiation Oncology, Biology, Physics. 2003 July 1; 56(3): 788-92.
  http://www.ncbi.nlm.nih.gov/entrez/query.fcgi?cmd=Retrieve&db=pubmed&dopt=Abstract&list_uids=12788186

- **Whole abdominopelvic radiotherapy (WAPRT) using intensity-modulated arc therapy (IMAT): first clinical experience.**
  Author(s): Duthoy W, De Gersem W, Vergote K, Coghe M, Boterberg T, De Deene Y, De Wagter C, Van Belle S, De Neve W.
  Source: International Journal of Radiation Oncology, Biology, Physics. 2003 November 15; 57(4): 1019-32.
  http://www.ncbi.nlm.nih.gov/entrez/query.fcgi?cmd=Retrieve&db=pubmed&dopt=Abstract&list_uids=14575833

- **Widespread morphoea following radiotherapy for carcinoma of the breast.**
  Author(s): Ardern-Jones MR, Black MM.
  Source: Clinical and Experimental Dermatology. 2003 March; 28(2): 160-2.
  http://www.ncbi.nlm.nih.gov/entrez/query.fcgi?cmd=Retrieve&db=pubmed&dopt=Abstract&list_uids=12653704

- **XRCC1 and glutathione-S-transferase gene polymorphisms and susceptibility to radiotherapy-related malignancies in survivors of Hodgkin disease.**
  Author(s): Mertens AC, Mitby PA, Radloff G, Jones IM, Perentesis J, Kiffmeyer WR, Neglia JP, Meadows A, Potter JD, Friedman D, Yasui Y, Robison LL, Davies SM.
  Source: Cancer. 2004 September 15; 101(6): 1463-72.
  http://www.ncbi.nlm.nih.gov/entrez/query.fcgi?cmd=Retrieve&db=pubmed&dopt=Abstract&list_uids=15368334

CHAPTER 2. NUTRITION AND RADIOTHERAPY

Overview

In this chapter, we will show you how to find studies dedicated specifically to nutrition and radiotherapy.

Finding Nutrition Studies on Radiotherapy

The National Institutes of Health's Office of Dietary Supplements (ODS) offers a searchable bibliographic database called the IBIDS (International Bibliographic Information on Dietary Supplements; National Institutes of Health, Building 31, Room 1B29, 31 Center Drive, MSC 2086, Bethesda, Maryland 20892-2086, Tel: 301-435-2920, Fax: 301-480-1845, E-mail: ods@nih.gov). The IBIDS contains over 460,000 scientific citations and summaries about dietary supplements and nutrition as well as references to published international, scientific literature on dietary supplements such as vitamins, minerals, and botanicals.[7] The IBIDS includes references and citations to both human and animal research studies.

As a service of the ODS, access to the IBIDS database is available free of charge at the following Web address: **http://ods.od.nih.gov/databases/ibids.html**. After entering the search area, you have three choices: (1) IBIDS Consumer Database, (2) Full IBIDS Database, or (3) Peer Reviewed Citations Only.

Now that you have selected a database, click on the "Advanced" tab. An advanced search allows you to retrieve up to 100 fully explained references in a comprehensive format. Type "radiotherapy" (or synonyms) into the search box, and click "Go." To narrow the search, you can also select the "Title" field.

---

[7] Adapted from **http://ods.od.nih.gov**. IBIDS is produced by the Office of Dietary Supplements (ODS) at the National Institutes of Health to assist the public, healthcare providers, educators, and researchers in locating credible, scientific information on dietary supplements. IBIDS was developed and will be maintained through an interagency partnership with the Food and Nutrition Information Center of the National Agricultural Library, U.S. Department of Agriculture.

The following information is typical of that found when using the "Full IBIDS Database" to search for "radiotherapy" (or a synonym):

- **Changing role and decreasing size: current trends in radiotherapy for Hodgkin's disease.**
  Author(s): Department of Radiation Oncology, Memorial Sloan-Kettering Cancer Center, Weill Medical College of Cornell University, 1275 York Avenue, New York, NY 10021, USA. yahalomj@mskcc.org
  Source: Yahalom, J Curr-Oncol-Repage 2002 September; 4(5): 415-23 1523-3790

- **Combination chemotherapy and radiotherapy for primary central nervous system lymphoma: Radiation Therapy Oncology Group Study 93-10.**
  Author(s): Memorial Sloan-Kettering Cancer Center, New York, NY 10021, USA. deangell@mskcc.org
  Source: DeAngelis, L M Seiferheld, W Schold, S C Fisher, B Schultz, C J J-Clin-Oncol. 2002 December 15; 20(24): 4643-8 0732-183X

- **Concurrent administration of Docetaxel and Stealth liposomal doxorubicin with radiotherapy in non-small cell lung cancer : excellent tolerance using subcutaneous amifostine for cytoprotection.**
  Author(s): Tumour and Angiogenesis Research Group, PO Box 12, Democritus University of Thrace, Alexandroupolis 68100, Greece. targ@her.forthnet.gr
  Source: Koukourakis, M I Romanidis, K Froudarakis, M Kyrgias, G Koukourakis, G V Retalis, G Bahlitzanakis, N Br-J-Cancer. 2002 August 12; 87(4): 385-92 0007-0920

- **Dose-escalation study of weekly irinotecan and daily carboplatin with concurrent thoracic radiotherapy for unresectable stage III non-small cell lung cancer.**
  Author(s): First Department of Internal Medicine, Osaka City University Medical School, 1-4-3 Asahi-machi, Abeno-ku, Osaka 545-8585, Japan. yamachan-pe@msic.med.osaka-cu.ac.jp
  Source: Yamada, M Kudoh, S Fukuda, H Nakagawa, K Yamamoto, N Nishimura, Y Negoro, S Takeda, K Tanaka, M Fukuoka, M Br-J-Cancer. 2002 July 29; 87(3): 258-63 0007-0920

- **Is postoperative radiotherapy useful for the rectal carcinoma in the era of total mesorectal excision?**
  Author(s): Department of Surgery, Ajou University School of Medicine, San-5 Paldal ku, Wonchon dong, Suwon 442-749, Korea. kwsuh@madang.ajou.ac.kr
  Source: Suh, K W Kim, B W Chun, M Lim, H Y Hepatogastroenterology. 2002 Mar-April; 49(44): 399-403 0172-6390

- **Neoadjuvant androgen withdrawal prior to external radiotherapy for locally advanced adenocarcinoma of the prostate.**
  Author(s): Department of Urology, Kobe University School of Medicine, Japan. hara@med.kobe-u.ac.jp
  Source: Hara, I Miyake, H Yamada, Y Takechi, Y Hara, S Gotoh, A Fujisawa, M Okada, H Arakawa, S Soejima, T Sugimura, K Kamidono, S Int-J-Urol. 2002 June; 9(6): 322-8; discussion 328 0919-8172

- **Outpatient weekly neoadjuvant chemotherapy followed by radiotherapy for advanced nasopharyngeal carcinoma: high complete response and low toxicity rates.**
  Author(s): Department of Radiation Oncology, Taichung Veterans General Hospital, Taiwan. jclin@mail.vghtc.gov.tw
  Source: Lin, J C January, J S Hsu, C Y Jiang, R S Wang, W Y Br-J-Cancer. 2003 Jan 27; 88(2): 187-94 0007-0920

- **Randomized comparison of low-dose involved-field radiotherapy and no radiotherapy for children with Hodgkin's disease who achieve a complete response to chemotherapy.**
  Author(s): Section of Pediatric Hematology-Oncology, University of Chicago, Chicago, IL, USA. jnachman@peds.bsd.uchicago.edu
  Source: Nachman, J B Sposto, R Herzog, P Gilchrist, G S Wolden, S L Thomson, J Kadin, M E Pattengale, P Davis, P C Hutchinson, R J White, K J-Clin-Oncol. 2002 September 15; 20(18): 3765-71 0732-183X

- **Stanford V and radiotherapy for Hodgkin's disease.**
  Author(s): Department of Medicine, Memorial Sloan-Kettering Cancer Center, 1275 York Avenue, New York, NY 10021, USA.
  Source: Portlock, C S Curr-Oncol-Repage 2002 September; 4(5): 413 1523-3790

Federal Resources on Nutrition

In addition to the IBIDS, the United States Department of Health and Human Services (HHS) and the United States Department of Agriculture (USDA) provide many sources of information on general nutrition and health. Recommended resources include:

- healthfinder®, HHS's gateway to health information, including diet and nutrition: **http://www.healthfinder.gov/scripts/SearchContext.asp?topic=238&page=0**

- The United States Department of Agriculture's Web site dedicated to nutrition information: **www.nutrition.gov**

- The Food and Drug Administration's Web site for federal food safety information: **www.foodsafety.gov**

- The National Action Plan on Overweight and Obesity sponsored by the United States Surgeon General: **http://www.surgeongeneral.gov/topics/obesity/**

- The Center for Food Safety and Applied Nutrition has an Internet site sponsored by the Food and Drug Administration and the Department of Health and Human Services: **http://vm.cfsan.fda.gov/**

- Center for Nutrition Policy and Promotion sponsored by the United States Department of Agriculture: **http://www.usda.gov/cnpp/**

- Food and Nutrition Information Center, National Agricultural Library sponsored by the United States Department of Agriculture: **http://www.nal.usda.gov/fnic/**

- Food and Nutrition Service sponsored by the United States Department of Agriculture: **http://www.fns.usda.gov/fns/**

Additional Web Resources

A number of additional Web sites offer encyclopedic information covering food and nutrition. The following is a representative sample:

- AOL: **http://search.aol.com/cat.adp?id=174&layer=&from=subcats**

- Family Village: **http://www.familyvillage.wisc.edu/med_nutrition.html**

- Google: **http://directory.google.com/Top/Health/Nutrition/**

- Healthnotes: **http://www.healthnotes.com/**
- Open Directory Project: **http://dmoz.org/Health/Nutrition/**
- Yahoo.com: **http://dir.yahoo.com/Health/Nutrition/**
- WebMD®Health: **http://my.webmd.com/nutrition**
- WholeHealthMD.com: **http://www.wholehealthmd.com/reflib/0,1529,00.html**

The following is a specific Web list relating to radiotherapy; please note that any particular subject below may indicate either a therapeutic use, or a contraindication (potential danger), and does not reflect an official recommendation:

- **Minerals**

   Cisplatin
   Source: Healthnotes, Inc.; www.healthnotes.com

CHAPTER 3. ALTERNATIVE MEDICINE AND RADIOTHERAPY

Overview

In this chapter, we will begin by introducing you to official information sources on complementary and alternative medicine (CAM) relating to radiotherapy. At the conclusion of this chapter, we will provide additional sources.

National Center for Complementary and Alternative Medicine

The National Center for Complementary and Alternative Medicine (NCCAM) of the National Institutes of Health (http://nccam.nih.gov/) has created a link to the National Library of Medicine's databases to facilitate research for articles that specifically relate to radiotherapy and complementary medicine. To search the database, go to the following Web site: http://www.nlm.nih.gov/nccam/camonpubmed.html. Select "CAM on PubMed." Enter "radiotherapy" (or synonyms) into the search box. Click "Go." The following references provide information on particular aspects of complementary and alternative medicine that are related to radiotherapy:

- **70 Gy thoracic radiotherapy is feasible concurrent with chemotherapy for limited-stage small-cell lung cancer: analysis of Cancer and Leukemia Group B study 39808.**
  Author(s): Bogart JA, Herndon JE 2nd, Lyss AP, Watson D, Miller AA, Lee ME, Turrisi AT, Green MR; Cancer and Leukemia Group B study 39808.
  Source: International Journal of Radiation Oncology, Biology, Physics. 2004 June 1; 59(2): 460-8.
  http://www.ncbi.nlm.nih.gov/entrez/query.fcgi?cmd=Retrieve&db=pubmed&dopt=Abstract&list_uids=15145163

- **A little to a lot or a lot to a little? An analysis of pneumonitis risk from dose-volume histogram parameters of the lung in patients with lung cancer treated with 3-D conformal radiotherapy.**
  Author(s): Willner J, Jost A, Baier K, Flentje M.

Source: Strahlentherapie Und Onkologie : Organ Der Deutschen Rontgengesellschaft. [et Al]. 2003 August; 179(8): 548-56.
http://www.ncbi.nlm.nih.gov/entrez/query.fcgi?cmd=Retrieve&db=pubmed&dopt=Abstract&list_uids=14509954

- **A Phase I-II study in the use of acupuncture-like transcutaneous nerve stimulation in the treatment of radiation-induced xerostomia in head-and-neck cancer patients treated with radical radiotherapy.**
  Author(s): Wong RK, Jones GW, Sagar SM, Babjak AF, Whelan T.
  Source: International Journal of Radiation Oncology, Biology, Physics. 2003 October 1; 57(2): 472-80.
  http://www.ncbi.nlm.nih.gov/entrez/query.fcgi?cmd=Retrieve&db=pubmed&dopt=Abstract&list_uids=12957259

- **A randomized study of primary bleomycin, vincristine, mitomycin and cisplatin (BOMP) chemotherapy followed by radiotherapy versus radiotherapy alone in stage IIIB and IVA squamous cell carcinoma of the cervix.**
  Author(s): Tabata T, Takeshima N, Nishida H, Hirai Y, Hasumi K.
  Source: Anticancer Res. 2003 May-June; 23(3C): 2885-90.
  http://www.ncbi.nlm.nih.gov/entrez/query.fcgi?cmd=Retrieve&db=pubmed&dopt=Abstract&list_uids=12926129

- **ABVD plus subtotal nodal versus involved-field radiotherapy in early-stage Hodgkin's disease: long-term results.**
  Author(s): Bonadonna G, Bonfante V, Viviani S, Di Russo A, Villani F, Valagussa P.
  Source: Journal of Clinical Oncology : Official Journal of the American Society of Clinical Oncology. 2004 July 15; 22(14): 2835-41. Epub 2004 June 15.
  http://www.ncbi.nlm.nih.gov/entrez/query.fcgi?cmd=Retrieve&db=pubmed&dopt=Abstract&list_uids=15199092

- **Acute toxicity of adjuvant radiotherapy in locally advanced differentiated thyroid carcinoma. First results of the multicenter study differentiated thyroid carcinoma (MSDS).**
  Author(s): Schuck A, Biermann M, Pixberg MK, Muller SB, Heinecke A, Schober O, Willich N.
  Source: Strahlentherapie Und Onkologie : Organ Der Deutschen Rontgengesellschaft. [et Al]. 2003 December; 179(12): 832-9.
  http://www.ncbi.nlm.nih.gov/entrez/query.fcgi?cmd=Retrieve&db=pubmed&dopt=Abstract&list_uids=14652672

- **Aggressive simultaneous radiochemotherapy with cisplatin and paclitaxel in combination with accelerated hyperfractionated radiotherapy in locally advanced head and neck tumors. Results of a phase I-II trial.**
  Author(s): Kuhnt T, Becker A, Pigorsch S, Pelz T, Bloching M, Passmann M, Lotterer E, Hansgen G, Dunst J.
  Source: Strahlentherapie Und Onkologie : Organ Der Deutschen Rontgengesellschaft. [et Al]. 2003 October; 179(10): 673-81.
  http://www.ncbi.nlm.nih.gov/entrez/query.fcgi?cmd=Retrieve&db=pubmed&dopt=Abstract&list_uids=14566475

- **C225 antiepidermal growth factor receptor antibody enhances the efficacy of docetaxel chemoradiotherapy.**
  Author(s): Nakata E, Hunter N, Mason K, Fan Z, Ang KK, Milas L.
  Source: International Journal of Radiation Oncology, Biology, Physics. 2004 July 15; 59(4): 1163-73.
  http://www.ncbi.nlm.nih.gov/entrez/query.fcgi?cmd=Retrieve&db=pubmed&dopt=Abstract&list_uids=15234052

- **Can chemotherapy replace radiotherapy in low-grade gliomas? Time for randomized studies.**
  Author(s): van den Bent MJ.
  Source: Seminars in Oncology. 2003 December; 30(6 Suppl 19): 39-44. Review.
  http://www.ncbi.nlm.nih.gov/entrez/query.fcgi?cmd=Retrieve&db=pubmed&dopt=Abstract&list_uids=14765384

- **Causes of chemoreduction failure in retinoblastoma and analysis of associated factors leading to eventual treatment with external beam radiotherapy and enucleation.**
  Author(s): Gunduz K, Gunalp I, Yalcindag N, Unal E, Tacyildiz N, Erden E, Geyik PO.
  Source: Ophthalmology. 2004 October; 111(10): 1917-24.
  http://www.ncbi.nlm.nih.gov/entrez/query.fcgi?cmd=Retrieve&db=pubmed&dopt=Abstract&list_uids=15465557

- **Chemotherapy with or without radiotherapy in limited-stage diffuse aggressive non-Hodgkin's lymphoma: Eastern Cooperative Oncology Group study 1484.**
  Author(s): Horning SJ, Weller E, Kim K, Earle JD, O'Connell MJ, Habermann TM, Glick JH.
  Source: Journal of Clinical Oncology : Official Journal of the American Society of Clinical Oncology. 2004 August 1; 22(15): 3032-8. Epub 2004 June 21.
  http://www.ncbi.nlm.nih.gov/entrez/query.fcgi?cmd=Retrieve&db=pubmed&dopt=Abstract&list_uids=15210738

- **Chronomics: circadian and circaseptan timing of radiotherapy, drugs, calories, perhaps nutriceuticals and beyond.**
  Author(s): Halberg F, Cornelissen G, Wang Z, Wan C, Ulmer W, Katinas G, Singh R, Singh RK, Singh RK, Gupta BD, Singh RB, Kumar A, Kanabrocki E, Sothern RB, Rao G, Bhatt ML, Srivastava M, Rai G, Singh S, Pati AK, Nath P, Halberg F, Halberg J, Schwartzkopff O, Bakken E, Governor Shri Vishnu Kant Shastri.
  Source: Journal of Experimental Therapeutics & Oncology. 2003 September-October; 3(5): 223-60. Review.
  http://www.ncbi.nlm.nih.gov/entrez/query.fcgi?cmd=Retrieve&db=pubmed&dopt=Abstract&list_uids=14641812

- **Combination chemotherapy (cyclophosphamide, doxorubicin, and vincristine with continuous-infusion cisplatin and etoposide) and radiotherapy with stem cell support can be beneficial for adolescents and adults with estheisoneuroblastoma.**
  Author(s): Mishima Y, Nagasaki E, Terui Y, Irie T, Takahashi S, Ito Y, Oguchi M, Kawabata K, Kamata S, Hatake K.
  Source: Cancer. 2004 September 15; 101(6): 1437-44.
  http://www.ncbi.nlm.nih.gov/entrez/query.fcgi?cmd=Retrieve&db=pubmed&dopt=Abstract&list_uids=15368332

- **Combination chemotherapy plus low-dose involved-field radiotherapy for early clinical stage Hodgkin's lymphoma.**
  Author(s): Vassilakopoulos TP, Angelopoulou MK, Siakantaris MP, Kontopidou FN, Dimopoulou MN, Kokoris SI, Kyrtsonis MC, Tsaftaridis P, Karkantaris C, Anargyrou K, Boutsis DE, Variamis E, Michalopoulos T, Boussiotis VA, Panayiotidis P, Papavassiliou C, Pangalis GA.
  Source: International Journal of Radiation Oncology, Biology, Physics. 2004 July 1; 59(3): 765-81.
  http://www.ncbi.nlm.nih.gov/entrez/query.fcgi?cmd=Retrieve&db=pubmed&dopt=Abstract&list_uids=15183480

- **Comparison of retinoblastoma reduction for chemotherapy vs external beam radiotherapy.**
  Author(s): Sussman DA, Escalona-Benz E, Benz MS, Hayden BC, Feuer W, Cicciarelli N, Toledano S, Markoe A, Murray TG.
  Source: Archives of Ophthalmology. 2003 July; 121(7): 979-84.
  http://www.ncbi.nlm.nih.gov/entrez/query.fcgi?cmd=Retrieve&db=pubmed&dopt=Abstract&list_uids=12860801

- **Complementary and alternative medicine in radiotherapy patients--more harm than expected? In regard to D'Amico et al.: self-administration of untested medical therapy for treatment of prostate cancer can lead to clinically significant adverse events. IJROBP 2002;54:1311-1313.**
  Author(s): Micke O, Mucke R, Schonekaes K, Buntzel J.
  Source: International Journal of Radiation Oncology, Biology, Physics. 2003 November 15; 57(4): 1197-8; Author Reply 1198.
  http://www.ncbi.nlm.nih.gov/entrez/query.fcgi?cmd=Retrieve&db=pubmed&dopt=Abstract&list_uids=14575856

- **Concurrent cisplatin, paclitaxel, and radiotherapy as preoperative treatment for patients with locoregional esophageal carcinoma.**
  Author(s): Urba SG, Orringer MB, Ianettonni M, Hayman JA, Satoru H.
  Source: Cancer. 2003 November 15; 98(10): 2177-83.
  http://www.ncbi.nlm.nih.gov/entrez/query.fcgi?cmd=Retrieve&db=pubmed&dopt=Abstract&list_uids=14601087

- **Consolidation radiotherapy following brief chemotherapy for localized diffuse large B-cell lymphoma: a prospective study.**
  Author(s): Isobe K, Kawakami H, Tamaru J, Yasuda S, Uno T, Aruga T, Kawata T, Shigematsu N, Hatano K, Takagi T, Mikata A, Ito H.
  Source: Leukemia & Lymphoma. 2003 September; 44(9): 1535-9.
  http://www.ncbi.nlm.nih.gov/entrez/query.fcgi?cmd=Retrieve&db=pubmed&dopt=Abstract&list_uids=14565656

- **Consolidation radiotherapy may improve outcomes in people with Hodgkin's disease achieving complete remission after combination chemotherapy.**
  Author(s): Specht L.
  Source: Cancer Treatment Reviews. 2004 August; 30(5): 479-82.
  http://www.ncbi.nlm.nih.gov/entrez/query.fcgi?cmd=Retrieve&db=pubmed&dopt=Abstract&list_uids=15245780

- **Coping of cancer patients during and after radiotherapy--a follow-up of 2 years.**
  Author(s): Sehlen S, Song R, Fahmuller H, Herschbach P, Lenk M, Hollenhorst H, Schymura B, Aydemir U, Duhmke E.
  Source: Onkologie. 2003 December; 26(6): 557-63.
  http://www.ncbi.nlm.nih.gov/entrez/query.fcgi?cmd=Retrieve&db=pubmed&dopt=Abstract&list_uids=14709930

- **Current and potential role of thermoradiotherapy for solid tumours.**
  Author(s): Hehr T, Wust P, Bamberg M, Budach W.
  Source: Onkologie. 2003 June; 26(3): 295-302. Review.
  http://www.ncbi.nlm.nih.gov/entrez/query.fcgi?cmd=Retrieve&db=pubmed&dopt=Abstract&list_uids=12845217

- **Differential attenuation of clavicle growth after asymmetric mantle radiotherapy.**
  Author(s): Merchant TE, Nguyen L, Nguyen D, Wu S, Hudson MM, Kaste SC.
  Source: International Journal of Radiation Oncology, Biology, Physics. 2004 June 1; 59(2): 556-61.
  http://www.ncbi.nlm.nih.gov/entrez/query.fcgi?cmd=Retrieve&db=pubmed&dopt=Abstract&list_uids=15145176

- **Docetaxel and radiotherapy and pancreatic cancer.**
  Author(s): Viret F, Ychou M, Goncalves A, Moutardier V, Magnin V, Braud AC, Dubois JB, Bories E, Gravis G, Camerlo J, Genre D, Maraninchi D, Viens P, Giovannini M.
  Source: Pancreas. 2003 October; 27(3): 214-9.
  http://www.ncbi.nlm.nih.gov/entrez/query.fcgi?cmd=Retrieve&db=pubmed&dopt=Abstract&list_uids=14508124

- **Docetaxel with concurrent radiotherapy in head and neck cancer.**
  Author(s): Nabell L, Spencer S.
  Source: Seminars in Oncology. 2003 December; 30(6 Suppl 18): 89-93. Review.
  http://www.ncbi.nlm.nih.gov/entrez/query.fcgi?cmd=Retrieve&db=pubmed&dopt=Abstract&list_uids=14727247

- **Docetaxel, carboplatin and concomitant radiotherapy for unresectable squamous cell carcinoma of the head and neck: pharmacokinetic and clinical data of a phase I-II study.**
  Author(s): Airoldi M, Cattel L, Cortesina G, Giordano C, Pedani F, Recalenda V, Danova M, Gabriele AM, Tagini V, Porta C, Bumma C.
  Source: American Journal of Clinical Oncology : the Official Publication of the American Radium Society. 2004 April; 27(2): 155-63.
  http://www.ncbi.nlm.nih.gov/entrez/query.fcgi?cmd=Retrieve&db=pubmed&dopt=Abstract&list_uids=15057155

- **Docetaxel-based combined-modality chemoradiotherapy for locally advanced non-small cell lung cancer.**
  Author(s): Scagliotti GV, Turrisi AT 3rd.
  Source: The Oncologist. 2003; 8(4): 361-74. Review.
  http://www.ncbi.nlm.nih.gov/entrez/query.fcgi?cmd=Retrieve&db=pubmed&dopt=Abstract&list_uids=12897333

- **Dose escalation of docetaxel concomitant with hypofractionated, once weekly chest radiotherapy for non-small-cell lung cancer: a phase I study.**
  Author(s): Schwarzenberger P, Theodossiou C, Barron S, Diethelm L, Boyle M, Harrison L, Wynn RB, Salazar OM, Fariss A.
  Source: American Journal of Clinical Oncology : the Official Publication of the American Radium Society. 2004 August; 27(4): 395-9.
  http://www.ncbi.nlm.nih.gov/entrez/query.fcgi?cmd=Retrieve&db=pubmed&dopt=Abstract&list_uids=15289734

- **Early concurrent chemoradiotherapy with prolonged oral etoposide and cisplatin for limited-stage small-cell lung cancer.**
  Author(s): Lee SH, Ahn YC, Kim HJ, Lim do H, Lee SI, Nam E, Park SH, Park J, Lee KE, Park JO, Kim K, Kim WS, Jung CW, Im YH, Kang WK, Lee MH, Park K.
  Source: Japanese Journal of Clinical Oncology. 2003 December; 33(12): 620-5.
  http://www.ncbi.nlm.nih.gov/entrez/query.fcgi?cmd=Retrieve&db=pubmed&dopt=Abstract&list_uids=14769839

- **Effect of oral zinc supplementation on agents of oropharyngeal infection in patients receiving radiotherapy for head and neck cancer.**
  Author(s): Ertekin MV, Uslu H, Karslioglu I, Ozbek E, Ozbek A.
  Source: J Int Med Res. 2003 July-August; 31(4): 253-66.
  http://www.ncbi.nlm.nih.gov/entrez/query.fcgi?cmd=Retrieve&db=pubmed&dopt=Abstract&list_uids=12964500

- **Effects of amifostine on acute toxicity from concurrent chemotherapy and radiotherapy for inoperable non-small-cell lung cancer: report of a randomized comparative trial.**
  Author(s): Komaki R, Lee JS, Milas L, Lee HK, Fossella FV, Herbst RS, Allen PK, Liao Z, Stevens CW, Lu C, Zinner RG, Papadimitrakopoulou VA, Kies MS, Blumenschein GR Jr, Pisters KM, Glisson BS, Kurie J, Kaplan B, Garza VP, Mooring D, Tucker SL, Cox JD.
  Source: International Journal of Radiation Oncology, Biology, Physics. 2004 April 1; 58(5): 1369-77.
  http://www.ncbi.nlm.nih.gov/entrez/query.fcgi?cmd=Retrieve&db=pubmed&dopt=Abstract&list_uids=15050312

- **Effects of oral Ginkgo biloba supplementation on cataract formation and oxidative stress occurring in lenses of rats exposed to total cranium radiotherapy.**
  Author(s): Ertekin MV, Kocer I, Karslioglu I, Taysi S, Gepdiremen A, Sezen O, Balci E, Bakan N.
  Source: Japanese Journal of Ophthalmology. 2004 September-October; 48(5): 499-502.
  http://www.ncbi.nlm.nih.gov/entrez/query.fcgi?cmd=Retrieve&db=pubmed&dopt=Abstract&list_uids=15486777

- **Efficacy of vinblastine, bleomycin, methotrexate (VBM) combination chemotherapy with involved field radiotherapy in early stage (I-IIA) Hodgkin disease patients.**
  Author(s): Martinelli G, Cocorocchio E, Saletti PC, Orecchia R, Bernier J, Tradati N, Santoro P, Robertson C, Peccatori FA, Zucca E, Cavalli F.
  Source: Leukemia & Lymphoma. 2003 November; 44(11): 1919-23. Review.
  http://www.ncbi.nlm.nih.gov/entrez/query.fcgi?cmd=Retrieve&db=pubmed&dopt=Abstract&list_uids=14738143

- **Esophageal cancer: outcomes of surgery, neoadjuvant chemotherapy, and three-dimension conformal radiotherapy.**
  Author(s): Frechette E, Buck DA, Kaplan BJ, Chung TD, Shaw JE, Kachnic LA, Neifeld JP.
  Source: Journal of Surgical Oncology. 2004 August 1; 87(2): 68-74.
  http://www.ncbi.nlm.nih.gov/entrez/query.fcgi?cmd=Retrieve&db=pubmed&dopt=Abstract&list_uids=15282698

- **Flavopiridol increases therapeutic ratio of radiotherapy by preferentially enhancing tumor radioresponse.**
  Author(s): Mason KA, Hunter NR, Raju U, Ariga H, Husain A, Valdecanas D, Neal R, Ang KK, Milas L.
  Source: International Journal of Radiation Oncology, Biology, Physics. 2004 July 15; 59(4): 1181-9.
  http://www.ncbi.nlm.nih.gov/entrez/query.fcgi?cmd=Retrieve&db=pubmed&dopt=Abstract&list_uids=15234054

- **Grade III dermatitis in a patient treated with paclitaxel and radiotherapy.**
  Author(s): de Freitas R, Freitas NM, de Abreu WC, Falcao MF, Bezerril CF, de Oliveira AM, Goulart FB.
  Source: The Breast Journal. 2003 November-December; 9(6): 503-4.
  http://www.ncbi.nlm.nih.gov/entrez/query.fcgi?cmd=Retrieve&db=pubmed&dopt=Abstract&list_uids=14616948

- **How patients manage gastrointestinal symptoms after pelvic radiotherapy.**
  Author(s): Gami B, Harrington K, Blake P, Dearnaley D, Tait D, Davies J, Norman AR, Andreyev HJ.
  Source: Alimentary Pharmacology & Therapeutics. 2003 November 15; 18(10): 987-94.
  http://www.ncbi.nlm.nih.gov/entrez/query.fcgi?cmd=Retrieve&db=pubmed&dopt=Abstract&list_uids=14616164

- **Hyperfractionated radiotherapy and chemotherapy for childhood ependymoma: final results of the first prospective AIEOP (Associazione Italiana di Ematologia-Oncologia Pediatrica) study.**
  Author(s): Massimino M, Gandola L, Giangaspero F, Sandri A, Valagussa P, Perilongo G, Garre ML, Ricardi U, Forni M, Genitori L, Scarzello G, Spreafico F, Barra S, Mascarin M, Pollo B, Gardiman M, Cama A, Navarria P, Brisigotti M, Collini P, Balter R, Fidani P, Stefanelli M, Burnelli R, Potepan P, Podda M, Sotti G, Madon E; AIEOP Pediatric Neuro-Oncology Group.
  Source: International Journal of Radiation Oncology, Biology, Physics. 2004 April 1; 58(5): 1336-45.
  http://www.ncbi.nlm.nih.gov/entrez/query.fcgi?cmd=Retrieve&db=pubmed&dopt=Abstract&list_uids=15050308

- **Impact of radiotherapy parameters on outcome in the International Society of Paediatric Oncology/United Kingdom Children's Cancer Study Group PNET-3 study of preradiotherapy chemotherapy for M0-M1 medulloblastoma.**
  Author(s): Taylor RE, Bailey CC, Robinson KJ, Weston CL, Ellison D, Ironside J, Lucraft H, Gilbertson R, Tait DM, Saran F, Walker DA, Pizer BL, Lashford LS; United Kingdom

Children's Cancer Study Group Brain Tumour Committee; International Society of Paediatric Oncology.
Source: International Journal of Radiation Oncology, Biology, Physics. 2004 March 15; 58(4): 1184-93.
http://www.ncbi.nlm.nih.gov/entrez/query.fcgi?cmd=Retrieve&db=pubmed&dopt=Abstract&list_uids=15001263

- **Improvement in efficacy of chemoradiotherapy by addition of an antiangiogenic agent in a murine tumor model.**
Author(s): McDonnell CO, Holden G, Sheridan ME, Foley D, Moriarty M, Walsh TN, Bouchier-Hayes DJ.
Source: The Journal of Surgical Research. 2004 January; 116(1): 19-23.
http://www.ncbi.nlm.nih.gov/entrez/query.fcgi?cmd=Retrieve&db=pubmed&dopt=Abstract&list_uids=14732345

- **Induction chemotherapy followed by concomitant TFHX chemoradiotherapy with reduced dose radiation in advanced head and neck cancer.**
Author(s): Haraf DJ, Rosen FR, Stenson K, Argiris A, Mittal BB, Witt ME, Brockstein BE, List MA, Portugal L, Pelzer H, Weichselbaum RR, Vokes EE.
Source: Clinical Cancer Research : an Official Journal of the American Association for Cancer Research. 2003 December 1; 9(16 Pt 1): 5936-43.
http://www.ncbi.nlm.nih.gov/entrez/query.fcgi?cmd=Retrieve&db=pubmed&dopt=Abstract&list_uids=14676118

- **Induction chemotherapy followed by radiotherapy in Merkel-cell carcinoma.**
Author(s): Poon D, Yap SP, Mancer K, Quek ST, Soh LT.
Source: The Lancet Oncology. 2004 August; 5(8): 509-10.
http://www.ncbi.nlm.nih.gov/entrez/query.fcgi?cmd=Retrieve&db=pubmed&dopt=Abstract&list_uids=15288240

- **Induction chemotherapy to weekly paclitaxel concurrent with curative radiotherapy in stage IV (M0) unresectable head and neck squamous cell carcinoma: a dose escalation study.**
Author(s): Pergolizzi S, Adamo V, Ferraro G, Sergi C, Santacaterina A, Romeo A, De Renzis C, Zanghi M, Rossello R, Settineri N.
Source: J Chemother. 2004 April; 16(2): 201-5.
http://www.ncbi.nlm.nih.gov/entrez/query.fcgi?cmd=Retrieve&db=pubmed&dopt=Abstract&list_uids=15216957

- **Induction chemotherapy with paclitaxel and cisplatin and CT-based 3D radiotherapy in patients with advanced laryngeal and hypopharyngeal carcinomas--a possibility for organ preservation.**
Author(s): Pfreundner L, Hoppe F, Willner J, Preisler V, Bratengeier K, Hagen R, Helms J, Flentje M.
Source: Radiotherapy and Oncology : Journal of the European Society for Therapeutic Radiology and Oncology. 2003 August; 68(2): 163-70.
http://www.ncbi.nlm.nih.gov/entrez/query.fcgi?cmd=Retrieve&db=pubmed&dopt=Abstract&list_uids=12972311

- **Integrating concurrent navelbine and cisplatin to hyperfractionated radiotherapy in locally advanced non-small cell lung cancer patients treated with induction and consolidation chemotherapy: feasibility and activity results.**
  Author(s): Reguart N, Vinolas N, Casas F, Gimferrer JM, Agusti C, Molina R, Martin-Richard M, Sanchez-Reyes A, Gascon P.
  Source: Lung Cancer (Amsterdam, Netherlands). 2004 July; 45(1): 67-75.
  http://www.ncbi.nlm.nih.gov/entrez/query.fcgi?cmd=Retrieve&db=pubmed&dopt=Abstract&list_uids=15196736

- **Involved-field radiotherapy is equally effective and less toxic compared with extended-field radiotherapy after four cycles of chemotherapy in patients with early-stage unfavorable Hodgkin's lymphoma: results of the HD8 trial of the German Hodgkin's Lymphoma Study Group.**
  Author(s): Engert A, Schiller P, Josting A, Herrmann R, Koch P, Sieber M, Boissevain F, De Wit M, Mezger J, Duhmke E, Willich N, Muller RP, Schmidt BF, Renner H, Muller-Hermelink HK, Pfistner B, Wolf J, Hasenclever D, Loffler M, Diehl V; German Hodgkin's Lymphoma Study Group.
  Source: Journal of Clinical Oncology : Official Journal of the American Society of Clinical Oncology. 2003 October 1; 21(19): 3601-8. Epub 2003 August 11.
  http://www.ncbi.nlm.nih.gov/entrez/query.fcgi?cmd=Retrieve&db=pubmed&dopt=Abstract&list_uids=12913100

- **Irinotecan/cisplatin followed by 5-FU/paclitaxel/radiotherapy and surgery in esophageal cancer.**
  Author(s): Ajani JA, Faust J, Yao J, Komaki R, Stevens C, Swisher S, Putnam JB, Vaporciyan A, Smythe R, Walsh G, Rice D, Roth J.
  Source: Oncology (Huntingt). 2003 September; 17(9 Suppl 8): 20-2.
  http://www.ncbi.nlm.nih.gov/entrez/query.fcgi?cmd=Retrieve&db=pubmed&dopt=Abstract&list_uids=14569843

- **Limited field radiotherapy for early stage, infra-diaphragmatic Hodgkin's lymphoma.**
  Author(s): Harris MA, Radford JA, Deakin DP, James RD, Swindell R, Cowan RA.
  Source: Clin Oncol (R Coll Radiol). 2004 February; 16(1): 53-7.
  http://www.ncbi.nlm.nih.gov/entrez/query.fcgi?cmd=Retrieve&db=pubmed&dopt=Abstract&list_uids=14768756

- **Long-term outcome of phase II trial evaluating chemotherapy, chemoradiotherapy, and surgery for locoregionally advanced esophageal cancer.**
  Author(s): Swisher SG, Ajani JA, Komaki R, Nesbitt JC, Correa AM, Cox JD, Lahoti S, Martin F, Putnam JB, Smythe WR, Vaporciyan AA, Walsh GL, Roth JA.
  Source: International Journal of Radiation Oncology, Biology, Physics. 2003 September 1; 57(1): 120-7.
  http://www.ncbi.nlm.nih.gov/entrez/query.fcgi?cmd=Retrieve&db=pubmed&dopt=Abstract&list_uids=12909224

- **Long-term results of a phase II trial of induction chemotherapy with uracil-ftegafur (UFT), vinorelbine, and cisplatin (UFTVP) followed by radiotherapy concomitant with UFT and carboplatin (RT/UFTJ) in a primary site preservation setting for resectable locally advanced squamous cell carcinoma of larynx and hypopharynx.**
  Author(s): Rivera F, Vega-Villegas ME, Lopez-Brea MF, Garcia-Castano A, de Juan A, Collado A, Galdos P, Rubio A, del Valle A, Rama J, Sanz-Ortiz J.

Source: The Laryngoscope. 2004 July; 114(7): 1163-9.
http://www.ncbi.nlm.nih.gov/entrez/query.fcgi?cmd=Retrieve&db=pubmed&dopt=A
bstract&list_uids=15235341

- **Long-term results of a phase III trial comparing once-daily radiotherapy with twice-daily radiotherapy in limited-stage small-cell lung cancer.**
  Author(s): Schild SE, Bonner JA, Shanahan TG, Brooks BJ, Marks RS, Geyer SM, Hillman SL, Farr GH Jr, Tazelaar HD, Krook JE, Geoffroy FJ, Salim M, Arusell RM, Mailliard JA, Schaefer PL, Jett JR.
  Source: International Journal of Radiation Oncology, Biology, Physics. 2004 July 15; 59(4): 943-51.
  http://www.ncbi.nlm.nih.gov/entrez/query.fcgi?cmd=Retrieve&db=pubmed&dopt=A
  bstract&list_uids=15234027

- **Monitoring individual response to brain-tumour chemotherapy: proton MR spectroscopy in a patient with recurrent glioma after stereotactic radiotherapy.**
  Author(s): Lichy MP, Bachert P, Henze M, Lichy CM, Debus J, Schlemmer HP.
  Source: Neuroradiology. 2004 February; 46(2): 126-9. Epub 2003 December 18.
  http://www.ncbi.nlm.nih.gov/entrez/query.fcgi?cmd=Retrieve&db=pubmed&dopt=A
  bstract&list_uids=14685797

- **Multicenter study differentiated thyroid carcinoma (MSDS). Diminished acceptance of adjuvant external beam radiotherapy.**
  Author(s): Biermann M, Pixberg MK, Schuck A, Heinecke A, Kopcke W, Schmid KW, Dralle H, Willich N, Schober O.
  Source: Nuklearmedizin. 2003 December; 42(6): 244-50.
  http://www.ncbi.nlm.nih.gov/entrez/query.fcgi?cmd=Retrieve&db=pubmed&dopt=A
  bstract&list_uids=14668957

- **Neoadjuvant docetaxel, cisplatin, 5-fluorouracil before concurrent chemoradiotherapy in locally advanced squamous cell carcinoma of the head and neck versus concomitant chemoradiotherapy: a phase II feasibility study.**
  Author(s): Ghi MG, Paccagnella A, D'Amanzo P, Mione CA, Fasan S, Paro S, Mastromauro C, Carnuccio R, Turcato G, Gatti C, Pallini A, Nascimben O, Biason R, Oniga F, Medici M, Rossi F, Fila G.
  Source: International Journal of Radiation Oncology, Biology, Physics. 2004 June 1; 59(2): 481-7.
  http://www.ncbi.nlm.nih.gov/entrez/query.fcgi?cmd=Retrieve&db=pubmed&dopt=A
  bstract&list_uids=15145166

- **Outcome for children with group III rhabdomyosarcoma treated with or without radiotherapy.**
  Author(s): Viswanathan AN, Grier HE, Litman HJ, Perez-Atayde A, Tarbell NJ, Neuberg D, Shamberger RC, Marcus KJ.
  Source: International Journal of Radiation Oncology, Biology, Physics. 2004 March 15; 58(4): 1208-14.
  http://www.ncbi.nlm.nih.gov/entrez/query.fcgi?cmd=Retrieve&db=pubmed&dopt=A
  bstract&list_uids=15001265

- **Outcome of children with centrally reviewed low-grade gliomas treated with chemotherapy with or without radiotherapy on Children's Cancer Group high-grade glioma study CCG-945.**
  Author(s): Fouladi M, Hunt DL, Pollack IF, Dueckers G, Burger PC, Becker LE, Yates AJ, Gilles FH, Davis RL, Boyett JM, Finlay JL.
  Source: Cancer. 2003 September 15; 98(6): 1243-52.
  http://www.ncbi.nlm.nih.gov/entrez/query.fcgi?cmd=Retrieve&db=pubmed&dopt=Abstract&list_uids=12973849

- **Outcome of rectal and sigmoid carcinoma patients receiving adjuvant chemoradiotherapy in Marmara University Hospital.**
  Author(s): Yumuk PF, Abacioglu U, Caglar H, Gumus M, Sengoz M, Turhal NS.
  Source: J Chemother. 2003 December; 15(6): 603-6.
  http://www.ncbi.nlm.nih.gov/entrez/query.fcgi?cmd=Retrieve&db=pubmed&dopt=Abstract&list_uids=14998088

- **Ozone treatment for radiotherapy skin reactions: is there an evidence base for practice?**
  Author(s): Jordan L, Beaver K, Foy S.
  Source: European Journal of Oncology Nursing : the Official Journal of European Oncology Nursing Society. 2002 December; 6(4): 220-7.
  http://www.ncbi.nlm.nih.gov/entrez/query.fcgi?cmd=Retrieve&db=pubmed&dopt=Abstract&list_uids=12849581

- **Paclitaxel and carboplatin concurrent with radiotherapy for primary cervical cancer.**
  Author(s): de Vos FY, Bos AM, Gietema JA, Pras E, Van der Zee AG, de Vries EG, Willemse PH.
  Source: Anticancer Res. 2004 January-February; 24(1): 345-8.
  http://www.ncbi.nlm.nih.gov/entrez/query.fcgi?cmd=Retrieve&db=pubmed&dopt=Abstract&list_uids=15015619

- **Phase I study of 5-fluorouracil and leucovorin by continuous infusion chronotherapy and pelvic radiotherapy in patients with locally advanced or recurrent rectal cancer.**
  Author(s): Parulekar W, de Marsh RW, Wong R, Mendenhall W, Davey P, Zlotecki R, Berry S, Rout WR, Bjarnason GA.
  Source: International Journal of Radiation Oncology, Biology, Physics. 2004 April 1; 58(5): 1487-95.
  http://www.ncbi.nlm.nih.gov/entrez/query.fcgi?cmd=Retrieve&db=pubmed&dopt=Abstract&list_uids=15050328

- **Phase I study of cisplatin, vinorelbine, and concurrent thoracic radiotherapy for unresectable stage III non-small cell lung cancer.**
  Author(s): Sekine I, Noda K, Oshita F, Yamada K, Tanaka M, Yamashita K, Nokihara H, Yamamoto N, Kunitoh H, Ohe Y, Tamura T, Kodama T, Sumi M, Saijo N.
  Source: Cancer Science. 2004 August; 95(8): 691-5.
  http://www.ncbi.nlm.nih.gov/entrez/query.fcgi?cmd=Retrieve&db=pubmed&dopt=Abstract&list_uids=15298734

- **Phase I study of involved-field radiotherapy preceding autologous stem cell transplantation for patients with high-risk lymphoma or Hodgkin's disease.**

Author(s): Dawson LA, Saito NG, Ratanatharathorn V, Uberti JP, Adams PT, Ayash LJ, Reynolds CM, Silver SM, Schipper MJ, Lichter AS, Eisbruch A.
Source: International Journal of Radiation Oncology, Biology, Physics. 2004 May 1; 59(1): 208-18.
http://www.ncbi.nlm.nih.gov/entrez/query.fcgi?cmd=Retrieve&db=pubmed&dopt=Abstract&list_uids=15093918

- **Phase I trial of escalating-dose irinotecan given weekly with cisplatin and concurrent radiotherapy in locally advanced esophageal cancer.**
  Author(s): Ilson DH, Bains M, Kelsen DP, O'Reilly E, Karpeh M, Coit D, Rusch V, Gonen M, Wilson K, Minsky BD.
  Source: Journal of Clinical Oncology : Official Journal of the American Society of Clinical Oncology. 2003 August 1; 21(15): 2926-32.
  http://www.ncbi.nlm.nih.gov/entrez/query.fcgi?cmd=Retrieve&db=pubmed&dopt=Abstract&list_uids=12885811

- **Phase I/II trial of weekly docetaxel and concomitant radiotherapy for squamous cell carcinoma of the head and neck.**
  Author(s): Fujii M, Tsukuda M, Satake B, Kubota A, Kida A, Kohno N, Okami K, Inuyama Y; Japan Cooperative Head and Neck Oncology Group (JCHNOG).
  Source: International Journal of Clinical Oncology / Japan Society of Clinical Oncology. 2004 April; 9(2): 107-12.
  http://www.ncbi.nlm.nih.gov/entrez/query.fcgi?cmd=Retrieve&db=pubmed&dopt=Abstract&list_uids=15108042

- **Phase II study of neoadjuvant carboplatin and paclitaxel followed by radiotherapy and concurrent cisplatin in patients with locoregionally advanced nasopharyngeal carcinoma: therapeutic monitoring with plasma Epstein-Barr virus DNA.**
  Author(s): Chan AT, Ma BB, Lo YM, Leung SF, Kwan WH, Hui EP, Mok TS, Kam M, Chan LS, Chiu SK, Yu KH, Cheung KY, Lai K, Lai M, Mo F, Yeo W, King A, Johnson PJ, Teo PM, Zee B.
  Source: Journal of Clinical Oncology : Official Journal of the American Society of Clinical Oncology. 2004 August 1; 22(15): 3053-60.
  http://www.ncbi.nlm.nih.gov/entrez/query.fcgi?cmd=Retrieve&db=pubmed&dopt=Abstract&list_uids=15284255

- **Phase II study of three-dimensional conformal radiotherapy and concurrent mitomycin-C, vinblastine, and cisplatin chemotherapy for Stage III locally advanced, unresectable, non-small-cell lung cancer.**
  Author(s): Lee SW, Choi EK, Lee JS, Lee SD, Suh C, Kim SW, Kim WS, Ahn SD, Yi BY, Kim JH, Noh YJ, Kim SS, Koh Y, Kim DS, Kim WD.
  Source: International Journal of Radiation Oncology, Biology, Physics. 2003 July 15; 56(4): 996-1004.
  http://www.ncbi.nlm.nih.gov/entrez/query.fcgi?cmd=Retrieve&db=pubmed&dopt=Abstract&list_uids=12829135

- **Phase II trial of cisplatin/etoposide and concurrent radiotherapy followed by paclitaxel/carboplatin consolidation for limited small-cell lung cancer: Southwest Oncology Group 9713.**
  Author(s): Edelman MJ, Chansky K, Gaspar LE, Leigh B, Weiss GR, Taylor SA, Crowley J, Livingston R, Gandara DR.

Source: Journal of Clinical Oncology : Official Journal of the American Society of Clinical Oncology. 2004 January 1; 22(1): 127-32.

http://www.ncbi.nlm.nih.gov/entrez/query.fcgi?cmd=Retrieve&db=pubmed&dopt=Abstract&list_uids=14701775

- **Phase III randomized study of radiotherapy plus procarbazine, lomustine, and vincristine with or without BUdR for treatment of anaplastic astrocytoma: final report of RTOG 9404.**
  Author(s): Prados MD, Seiferheld W, Sandler HM, Buckner JC, Phillips T, Schultz C, Urtasun R, Davis R, Gutin P, Cascino TL, Greenberg HS, Curran WJ Jr.
  Source: International Journal of Radiation Oncology, Biology, Physics. 2004 March 15; 58(4): 1147-52.
  http://www.ncbi.nlm.nih.gov/entrez/query.fcgi?cmd=Retrieve&db=pubmed&dopt=Abstract&list_uids=15001257

- **Preliminary analysis of RTOG 9708: Adjuvant postoperative radiotherapy combined with cisplatin/paclitaxel chemotherapy after surgery for patients with high-risk endometrial cancer.**
  Author(s): Greven K, Winter K, Underhill K, Fontenesci J, Cooper J, Burke T; Radiation Therapy Oncology Group.
  Source: International Journal of Radiation Oncology, Biology, Physics. 2004 May 1; 59(1): 168-73.
  http://www.ncbi.nlm.nih.gov/entrez/query.fcgi?cmd=Retrieve&db=pubmed&dopt=Abstract&list_uids=15093913

- **Preoperative concurrent chemoradiotherapy with cisplatin and docetaxel in patients with locally advanced non-small-cell lung cancer.**
  Author(s): Katayama H, Ueoka H, Kiura K, Tabata M, Kozuki T, Tanimoto M, Fujiwara T, Tanaka N, Date H, Aoe M, Shimizu N, Takemoto M, Hiraki Y.
  Source: British Journal of Cancer. 2004 March 8; 90(5): 979-84.
  http://www.ncbi.nlm.nih.gov/entrez/query.fcgi?cmd=Retrieve&db=pubmed&dopt=Abstract&list_uids=14997193

- **Preoperative hyperfractionated accelerated radiotherapy (HART) and concomitant CPT-11 in locally advanced rectal carcinoma: a phase I study.**
  Author(s): Voelter V, Stupp R, Matter M, Gillet M, Bouzourene H, Leyvraz S, Coucke P.
  Source: International Journal of Radiation Oncology, Biology, Physics. 2003 August 1; 56(5): 1288-94.
  http://www.ncbi.nlm.nih.gov/entrez/query.fcgi?cmd=Retrieve&db=pubmed&dopt=Abstract&list_uids=12873673

- **Preoperative induction of CPT-11 and cisplatin chemotherapy followed by chemoradiotherapy in patients with locoregional carcinoma of the esophagus or gastroesophageal junction.**
  Author(s): Ajani JA, Walsh G, Komaki R, Morris J, Swisher SG, Putnam JB Jr, Lynch PM, Wu TT, Smythe R, Vaporciyan A, Faust J, Cohen DS, Nivers R, Roth JA.
  Source: Cancer. 2004 June 1; 100(11): 2347-54.
  http://www.ncbi.nlm.nih.gov/entrez/query.fcgi?cmd=Retrieve&db=pubmed&dopt=Abstract&list_uids=15160337

- **Primary non-Hodgkin's lymphoma of the CNS treated with CHOD/BVAM or BVAM chemotherapy before radiotherapy: long-term survival and prognostic factors.**
  Author(s): Bessell EM, Graus F, Lopez-Guillermo A, Lewis SA, Villa S, Verger E, Petit J.
  Source: International Journal of Radiation Oncology, Biology, Physics. 2004 June 1; 59(2): 501-8.
  http://www.ncbi.nlm.nih.gov/entrez/query.fcgi?cmd=Retrieve&db=pubmed&dopt=Abstract&list_uids=15145169

- **Radioprotection of normal tissue to improve radiotherapy: the effect of the Bowman Birk protease inhibitor.**
  Author(s): Dittmann KH, Mayer C, Rodemann HP.
  Source: Current Medicinal Chemistry. Anti-Cancer Agents. 2003 September; 3(5): 360-3. Review.
  http://www.ncbi.nlm.nih.gov/entrez/query.fcgi?cmd=Retrieve&db=pubmed&dopt=Abstract&list_uids=12871082

- **Radioprotective effects of vitexina for breast cancer patients undergoing radiotherapy with cobalt-60.**
  Author(s): Hien TV, Huong NB, Hung PM, Duc NB.
  Source: Integrative Cancer Therapies. 2002 March; 1(1): 38-4; Discussion 42-3.
  http://www.ncbi.nlm.nih.gov/entrez/query.fcgi?cmd=Retrieve&db=pubmed&dopt=Abstract&list_uids=14664747

- **Radiotherapy and concurrent low-dose paclitaxel in locally advanced head and neck cancer.**
  Author(s): Lovey J, Koronczay K, Remenar E, Csuka O, Nemeth G.
  Source: Radiotherapy and Oncology : Journal of the European Society for Therapeutic Radiology and Oncology. 2003 August; 68(2): 171-4.
  http://www.ncbi.nlm.nih.gov/entrez/query.fcgi?cmd=Retrieve&db=pubmed&dopt=Abstract&list_uids=12972312

- **Radiotherapy and endothelial cells--(green) tea for two?**
  Author(s): Vuori K.
  Source: Cancer Biology & Therapy. 2003 November-December; 2(6): 650-1.
  http://www.ncbi.nlm.nih.gov/entrez/query.fcgi?cmd=Retrieve&db=pubmed&dopt=Abstract&list_uids=14688469

- **Radiotherapy for advanced Hodgkin's disease.**
  Author(s): Gupta T, Sanghavi V, Laskar S.
  Source: The New England Journal of Medicine. 2003 September 18; 349(12): 1187-8; Author Reply 1187-8.
  http://www.ncbi.nlm.nih.gov/entrez/query.fcgi?cmd=Retrieve&db=pubmed&dopt=Abstract&list_uids=13679537

- **Radiotherapy in the management of giant cell tumor of bone.**
  Author(s): Caudell JJ, Ballo MT, Zagars GK, Lewis VO, Weber KL, Lin PP, Marco RA, El-Naggar AK, Benjamin RS, Yasko AW.

Source: International Journal of Radiation Oncology, Biology, Physics. 2003 September 1; 57(1): 158-65.

http://www.ncbi.nlm.nih.gov/entrez/query.fcgi?cmd=Retrieve&db=pubmed&dopt=Abstract&list_uids=12909228

- **Radiotherapy with concomitant weekly docetaxel for Stages III/IV oropharynx carcinoma. Results of the 98-02 GORTEC Phase II trial.**
  Author(s): Calais G, Bardet E, Sire C, Alfonsi M, Bourhis J, Rhein B, Tortochaux J, Man YT, Auvray H, Garaud P.
  Source: International Journal of Radiation Oncology, Biology, Physics. 2004 January 1; 58(1): 161-6.
  http://www.ncbi.nlm.nih.gov/entrez/query.fcgi?cmd=Retrieve&db=pubmed&dopt=Abstract&list_uids=14697434

- **Radiotherapy with concurrent docetaxel for advanced and recurrent breast cancer.**
  Author(s): Karasawa K, Katsui K, Seki K, Kohno M, Hanyu N, Nasu S, Muramatsu H, Maebayashi K, Mitsuhashi N, Haga S, Kimura T, Takahashi I.
  Source: Breast Cancer. 2003; 10(3): 268-74.
  http://www.ncbi.nlm.nih.gov/entrez/query.fcgi?cmd=Retrieve&db=pubmed&dopt=Abstract&list_uids=12955041

- **Second malignancies after chemotherapy and radiotherapy for Hodgkin disease.**
  Author(s): Chronowski GM, Wilder RB, Levy LB, Atkinson EN, Ha CS, Hagemeister FB, Barista I, Rodriguez MA, Sarris AH, Hess MA, Cabanillas F, Cox JD.
  Source: American Journal of Clinical Oncology : the Official Publication of the American Radium Society. 2004 February; 27(1): 73-80.
  http://www.ncbi.nlm.nih.gov/entrez/query.fcgi?cmd=Retrieve&db=pubmed&dopt=Abstract&list_uids=14758137

- **Shifting from hypofractionated to "conventionally" fractionated thoracic radiotherapy: a single institution's 10-year experience in the management of limited-stage small-cell lung cancer using concurrent chemoradiation.**
  Author(s): Videtic GM, Truong PT, Dar AR, Yu EW, Stitt LW.
  Source: International Journal of Radiation Oncology, Biology, Physics. 2003 November 1; 57(3): 709-16.
  http://www.ncbi.nlm.nih.gov/entrez/query.fcgi?cmd=Retrieve&db=pubmed&dopt=Abstract&list_uids=14529775

- **Stanford V regimen plus consolidative radiotherapy is an effective therapeutic program for bulky or advanced-stage Hodgkin's disease.**
  Author(s): Aversa SM, Salvagno L, Soraru M, Mazzarotto R, Boso C, Gaion F, Chiarion-Sileni V, De Franchis G, Favaretto AG, Crivellari G, Banna GL, Sotti G, Monfardini S.
  Source: Acta Haematologica. 2004; 112(3): 141-7.
  http://www.ncbi.nlm.nih.gov/entrez/query.fcgi?cmd=Retrieve&db=pubmed&dopt=Abstract&list_uids=15345896

- **Ten-year disease-free survival of a small cell lung cancer patient with brain metastasis treated with chemoradiotherapy.**
  Author(s): Niibe Y, Karasawa K, Hayakawa K.

Source: Anticancer Res. 2004 May-June; 24(3B): 2097-100.
http://www.ncbi.nlm.nih.gov/entrez/query.fcgi?cmd=Retrieve&db=pubmed&dopt=A
bstract&list_uids=15274407

- **Tolerance of radiotherapy and chemotherapy in elderly patients with bladder cancer.**
  Author(s): Goffin JR, Rajan R, Souhami L.
  Source: American Journal of Clinical Oncology : the Official Publication of the American
  Radium Society. 2004 April; 27(2): 172-7.
  http://www.ncbi.nlm.nih.gov/entrez/query.fcgi?cmd=Retrieve&db=pubmed&dopt=A
  bstract&list_uids=15057157

- **Treatment of advanced Hodgkin's disease with COPP/ABV/IMEP versus
  COPP/ABVD and consolidating radiotherapy: final results of the German Hodgkin's
  Lymphoma Study Group HD6 trial.**
  Author(s): Sieber M, Tesch H, Pfistner B, Rueffer U, Paulus U, Munker R, Hermann R,
  Doelken G, Koch P, Oertel J, Roller S, Worst P, Bischof H, Glunz A, Greil R, von Kalle K,
  Schalk KP, Hasenclever D, Brosteanu O, Duehmke E, Georgii A, Engert A, Loeffler M,
  Diehl V, Mueller RP, Willich N, Fischer R, Hansmann ML, Stein H, Schober T, Koch B;
  German Hodgkin's Lymphoma Study Group.
  Source: Annals of Oncology : Official Journal of the European Society for Medical
  Oncology / Esmo. 2004 February; 15(2): 276-82.
  http://www.ncbi.nlm.nih.gov/entrez/query.fcgi?cmd=Retrieve&db=pubmed&dopt=A
  bstract&list_uids=14760122

- **Treatment of early clinically staged Hodgkin's disease with a combination of ABVD
  chemotherapy plus limited field radiotherapy.**
  Author(s): Karmiris TD, Grigoriou E, Tsantekidou M, Spanou E, Mihalakeas H,
  Baltadakis J, Apostolidis J, Pagoni M, Karakasis D, Bakiri M, Mitsouli C, Harhalakis N,
  Nikiforakis E.
  Source: Leukemia & Lymphoma. 2003 September; 44(9): 1523-8.
  http://www.ncbi.nlm.nih.gov/entrez/query.fcgi?cmd=Retrieve&db=pubmed&dopt=A
  bstract&list_uids=14565654

- **Treatment of pediatric Hodgkin disease avoiding radiotherapy: excellent outcome
  with the Rotterdam-HD-84-protocol.**
  Author(s): Hakvoort-Cammel FG, Buitendijk S, van den Heuvel-Eibrink M, Hahlen K.
  Source: Pediatric Blood & Cancer. 2004 July; 43(1): 8-16.
  http://www.ncbi.nlm.nih.gov/entrez/query.fcgi?cmd=Retrieve&db=pubmed&dopt=A
  bstract&list_uids=15170884

- **Twice-daily radiotherapy as concurrent boost technique during two chemotherapy
  cycles in neoadjuvant chemoradiotherapy for resectable esophageal carcinoma:
  mature results of phase II study.**
  Author(s): Choi N, Park SD, Lynch T, Wright C, Ancukiewicz M, Wain J, Donahue D,
  Mathisen D.
  Source: International Journal of Radiation Oncology, Biology, Physics. 2004 September 1;
  60(1): 111-22.
  http://www.ncbi.nlm.nih.gov/entrez/query.fcgi?cmd=Retrieve&db=pubmed&dopt=A
  bstract&list_uids=15337546

- **Two-dimensional radiotherapy and docetaxel in treatment of stage III non-small cell lung carcinoma: no good survival due to radiation pneumonitis.**
  Author(s): Dincbas FO, Atalar B, Koca S.
  Source: Lung Cancer (Amsterdam, Netherlands). 2004 February; 43(2): 241-2.
  http://www.ncbi.nlm.nih.gov/entrez/query.fcgi?cmd=Retrieve&db=pubmed&dopt=Abstract&list_uids=14739045

Additional Web Resources

A number of additional Web sites offer encyclopedic information covering CAM and related topics. The following is a representative sample:

- Alternative Medicine Foundation, Inc.: **http://www.herbmed.org/**

- AOL: **http://search.aol.com/cat.adp?id=169&layer=&from=subcats**

- Chinese Medicine: **http://www.newcenturynutrition.com/**

- drkoop.com®: **http://www.drkoop.com/InteractiveMedicine/IndexC.html**

- Family Village: **http://www.familyvillage.wisc.edu/med_altn.htm**

- Google: **http://directory.google.com/Top/Health/Alternative/**

- Healthnotes: **http://www.healthnotes.com/**

- MedWebPlus: **http://medwebplus.com/subject/Alternative_and_Complementary_Medicine**

- Open Directory Project: **http://dmoz.org/Health/Alternative/**

- HealthGate: **http://www.tnp.com/**

- WebMD®Health: **http://my.webmd.com/drugs_and_herbs**

- WholeHealthMD.com: **http://www.wholehealthmd.com/reflib/0,1529,00.html**

- Yahoo.com: **http://dir.yahoo.com/Health/Alternative_Medicine/**

The following is a specific Web list relating to radiotherapy; please note that any particular subject below may indicate either a therapeutic use, or a contraindication (potential danger), and does not reflect an official recommendation:

- **General Overview**

    Breast Cancer
    Source: Healthnotes, Inc.; www.healthnotes.com

    Colorectal Cancer
    Source: Integrative Medicine Communications; www.drkoop.com

    Immune Function
    Source: Healthnotes, Inc.; www.healthnotes.com

Lung Cancer
Source: Healthnotes, Inc.; www.healthnotes.com

Lung Cancer
Source: Integrative Medicine Communications; www.drkoop.com

Proctitis
Source: Integrative Medicine Communications; www.drkoop.com

Rectal Inflammation
Source: Integrative Medicine Communications; www.drkoop.com

- **Chinese Medicine**

  Shengxue Wan
  Alternative names: hengxue Pills; Shengxue Wan (Sheng Xue Wan
  Source: Pharmacopoeia Commission of the Ministry of Health, People's Republic of China

- **Herbs and Supplements**

  Asian Ginseng
  Alternative names: Panax ginseng
  Source: Integrative Medicine Communications; www.drkoop.com

  Chemotherapy
  Source: Healthnotes, Inc.; www.healthnotes.com

  Docetaxel
  Source: Healthnotes, Inc.; www.healthnotes.com

  Fluorouracil
  Source: Healthnotes, Inc.; www.healthnotes.com

  Melatonin
  Source: Prima Communications, Inc.www.personalhealthzone.com

  Methotrexate
  Source: Healthnotes, Inc.; www.healthnotes.com

  Paclitaxel
  Source: Healthnotes, Inc.; www.healthnotes.com

  Panax Ginseng
  Source: Integrative Medicine Communications; www.drkoop.com

  Pentoxifylline
  Source: Healthnotes, Inc.; www.healthnotes.com

General References

A good place to find general background information on CAM is the National Library of Medicine. It has prepared within the MEDLINEplus system an information topic page dedicated to complementary and alternative medicine. To access this page, go to the MEDLINEplus site at **http://www.nlm.nih.gov/medlineplus/alternativemedicine.html**. This Web site provides a general overview of various topics and can lead to a number of general sources.

CHAPTER 4. DISSERTATIONS ON RADIOTHERAPY

Overview

In this chapter, we will give you a bibliography on recent dissertations relating to radiotherapy. We will also provide you with information on how to use the Internet to stay current on dissertations. **IMPORTANT NOTE:** When following the search strategy described below, you may discover <u>non-medical dissertations</u> that use the generic term "radiotherapy" (or a synonym) in their titles. To accurately reflect the results that you might find while conducting research on radiotherapy, <u>we have not necessarily excluded non-medical dissertations</u> in this bibliography.

Dissertations on Radiotherapy

ProQuest Digital Dissertations, the largest archive of academic dissertations available, is located at the following Web address: **http://wwwlib.umi.com/dissertations**. From this archive, we have compiled the following list covering dissertations devoted to radiotherapy. You will see that the information provided includes the dissertation's title, its author, and the institution with which the author is associated. The following covers recent dissertations found when using this search procedure:

- **A system to aid patient positioning during radiotherapy treatment simulation** by Theal, John B., MSc from LAURENTIAN UNIVERSITY OF SUDBURY (CANADA), 2003, 115 pages
  http://wwwlib.umi.com/dissertations/fullcit/MQ85654

- **Ionization chamber response in intensity-modulated radiotherapy beams** by Markovic, Alexander, PhD from THE HERMAN M. FINCH U. OF HEALTH SCIENCES - THE CHICAGO MEDICAL SCH., 2003, 89 pages
  http://wwwlib.umi.com/dissertations/fullcit/3102146

- **Precision radiotherapy in the presence of geometric uncertainties: A Monte Carlo simulation** by Song, William Young-Jae, MSc from UNIVERSITY OF CALGARY (CANADA), 2003, 104 pages
  http://wwwlib.umi.com/dissertations/fullcit/MQ87433

- **The analysis of feasibility and effectiveness of vascular targeting radiotherapy based on a model of tumor growth and angiogenesis** by Ding, Yihong, PhD from UNIVERSITY OF MASSACHUSETTS LOWELL, 2003, 111 pages
  http://wwwlib.umi.com/dissertations/fullcit/3092642

- **Verification of intensity modulated stereotactic radiotherapy using Monte Carlo calculations and EPID dosimetry** by Parker, Brent Christopher, PhD from THE UNIV. OF TEXAS H.S.C. AT HOUSTON GRAD. SCH. OF BIOMED. SCI., 2004, 152 pages
  http://wwwlib.umi.com/dissertations/fullcit/3131487

Keeping Current

Ask the medical librarian at your library if it has full and unlimited access to the *ProQuest Digital Dissertations* database. From the library, you should be able to do more complete searches via **http://wwwlib.umi.com/dissertations**.

CHAPTER 5. PATENTS ON RADIOTHERAPY

Overview

Patents can be physical innovations (e.g. chemicals, pharmaceuticals, medical equipment) or processes (e.g. treatments or diagnostic procedures). The United States Patent and Trademark Office defines a patent as a grant of a property right to the inventor, issued by the Patent and Trademark Office.[8] Patents, therefore, are intellectual property. For the United States, the term of a new patent is 20 years from the date when the patent application was filed. If the inventor wishes to receive economic benefits, it is likely that the invention will become commercially available within 20 years of the initial filing. It is important to understand, therefore, that an inventor's patent does not indicate that a product or service is or will be commercially available. The patent implies only that the inventor has "the right to exclude others from making, using, offering for sale, or selling" the invention in the United States. While this relates to U.S. patents, similar rules govern foreign patents.

In this chapter, we show you how to locate information on patents and their inventors. If you find a patent that is particularly interesting to you, contact the inventor or the assignee for further information. **IMPORTANT NOTE:** When following the search strategy described below, you may discover non-medical patents that use the generic term "radiotherapy" (or a synonym) in their titles. To accurately reflect the results that you might find while conducting research on radiotherapy, we have not necessarily excluded non-medical patents in this bibliography.

Patents on Radiotherapy

By performing a patent search focusing on radiotherapy, you can obtain information such as the title of the invention, the names of the inventor(s), the assignee(s) or the company that owns or controls the patent, a short abstract that summarizes the patent, and a few excerpts from the description of the patent. The abstract of a patent tends to be more technical in nature, while the description is often written for the public. Full patent descriptions contain much more information than is presented here (e.g. claims, references, figures, diagrams, etc.). We will tell you how to obtain this information later in the chapter. The following is an

---

[8]Adapted from the United States Patent and Trademark Office:
http://www.uspto.gov/web/offices/pac/doc/general/whatis.htm.

example of the type of information that you can expect to obtain from a patent search on radiotherapy:

- **Automated calibration for radiation dosimetry using fixed or moving beams and detectors**

  Inventor(s): Ritt; Daniel M. (Colorado Springs, CO)

  Assignee(s): Radiological Imaging Technology, Inc. (Colorado Springs, CO)

  Patent Number: 6,675,116

  Date filed: June 1, 2001

  Abstract: Methods and devices for calibrating a **radiotherapy** system are disclosed. The method includes providing a detection medium that responds to exposure to ionizing radiation, and preparing a calibration dose response pattern by exposing predefined regions of the detection medium to different ionizing radiation dose levels. The method also includes measuring responses of the detection medium in the predefined regions to generate a calibration that relates subsequent responses to ionizing radiation dose. Different dose levels are obtained by differentially shielding portions of the detection medium from the ionizing radiation using, for example, a multi-leaf collimator, a secondary collimator, or an attenuation block. Different dose levels can also be obtained by moving the detection medium between exposures. The disclosed device includes a software routine fixed on a computer-readable medium that is configured to generate a calibration that relates a response of a detection medium to ionizing radiation dose.

  Excerpt(s): The present invention relates to radiation dosimetry, and more particularly to methods and devices for automating radiation dose calibrations associated with **radiotherapy.** An important use of **radiotherapy** is the destruction of tumor cells. In the case of ionizing radiation, tumor destruction depends on the "absorbed dose" or the amount of energy deposited within a tissue mass. Radiation physicists normally express the absorbed dose in cGy units or centigray. One cGy equals 0.01 J/kg. Radiation dosimetry generally describes methods to measure or predict the absorbed dose in various tissues of a patient undergoing **radiotherapy.** Accuracy in predicting and measuring absorbed dose is key to effective treatment and prevention of complications due to over or under exposure to radiation. Many methods exist for measuring and predicting absorbed dose, but most rely on developing a calibration--a curve or a lookup table--that relates the response of a detection medium to absorbed dose. Useful detection media include radiation-sensitive films and three-dimensional gels (e.g., `BANG` and `BANANA` gels) which darken or change color upon exposure to radiation. Other useful detection media include electronic portal-imaging devices and amorphous silicon detector arrays, which generate a signal in response to radiation exposure.

  Web site: http://www.delphion.com/details?pn=US06675116__

- **Collimator for limiting a bundle of high-energy rays**

Inventor(s): Echner; Gernot (Wiesenbach, DE), Ganter; Walter (Walldorf, DE), Pastyr; Otto (Leimen, DE), Schlegel; Wolfgang (Heidelberg, DE)

Assignee(s): Deutsches Krebsforschungszentrum Stiftung Des Oeffentlichen Rechts (Heidelberg, DE)

Patent Number: 6,730,924

Date filed: July 26, 2001

Abstract: The invention relates to a collimator (1) for limiting a bundle of high-energy rays (2), which is emitted by a substantially point-like radiation source (3) and directed towards a treatment object (20) and used in particular for the stereotactic conformation **radiotherapy** of tumors. According to the invention the collimator (1) comprises a plurality of diaphragm leaves (4, 4') which are arranged opposite each other and which are made of a radiation-absorbing material and which, by means of drive mechanisms, can be moved into the optical path in such a way that the contours and/or exposure period of said optical path can be freely defined, the front edges (5, 5') of the diaphragm leaves (4, 4') being parallel to the optical path at all times. Avoiding penumbral shadows with this kind of collimator (1) is made considerably easier if the diaphragm leaves (4, 4') consists of a rear partial element (6, 6') which can be linearly displaced and a front partial element (7, 7') which is hinged to same. Drive means adjust the front partial element (7, 7') in accordance with the prevailing position of the rear partial element (6, 6') in such a way that the front edges (5, 5') are parallel to the optical path at all times.

Excerpt(s): The invention concerns a multiple leaf collimator for limiting a bundle of high-energy rays emitted by a substantially point-like radiation source and directed towards a treatment object and used in particular for the stereotactic conformation **radiotherapy** of tumors, wherein the collimator contains a plurality of opposing collimator leaves made of a radiation-absorbing material which can be moved by drive mechanisms into the optical path such that the contours of said optical path can be freely defined, wherein the front edges of the collimator leaves are always aligned in parallel to the optical path. The treatment devices used today in oncological radiation therapy are provided with collimators which limit high-energy radiation, in most cases high-energy gamma radiation from a linear accelerator, in such a fashion that the rays assume exactly the same shape as the object to be treated. Since irradiation e.g. of a tumor, is implemented from different directions, a high irradiation intensity on the tumor can be effected with only limited exposure to the surrounding tissue. For absorbing high-energy radiation, the collimator must have a thickness of several centimeters, which produces a half shadow when the passage opening has straight walls in the passage direction. Since the rays diverge from the substantially point-like radiation source, the collimator opening is smaller than the actual shape of the tumor so that the collimated rays diverge to have exactly the size of the tumor upon impingement. When the walls of the collimator opening are straight, part of the radiation will not be shielded by the full material thickness due to the inclined path of the radiation. In consequence thereof, either healthy tissue surrounding the tumor is exposed to considerable radiation or the tumor tissue will receive too little dosage. This causes damage which should be prevented. For this reason, one of average skill in the art has tried to develop different collimators which reduce or prevent these half shadows. One suggestion to prevent half shadows which has been described in the literature, consists in providing the collimator leaves (leaves) of a collimator (multi-leaf collimator) with an irregular trapezoidal shape such that their side surfaces and the side surfaces of the outer limits of the collimator opening have the angle of the optical path.

It is, however, more difficult to achieve corresponding alignment of the front edges of the collimator leaves. Many suggestions have been made to solve this problem, none of which is satisfying.

Web site: http://www.delphion.com/details?pn=US06730924__

- **Collimator for radiotherapy apparatus**

  Inventor(s): Brown; Kevin John (Horsham, GB), Williams; Peter (Withington, GB), Wong; John (Royal Oak, MI), Yan; Di (Royal Oak, MI)

  Assignee(s): Elekta AB (Stockholm, SE)

  Patent Number: 6,714,627

  Date filed: May 24, 2001

  Abstract: A **radiotherapy** apparatus comprises a first collimator and a second collimator, the first collimator being a multi-leaf collimator, the second collimator comprising a plurality of slits having a width which is a fraction of the width of the leaves of the first collimator, the first and second collimators being aligned such that each slit of the second collimator is associated with a leaf of the first collimator. A first irradiation is made, during which the first collimator will define the outer edge of the irradiation pattern, and the second collimator will serve to narrow the effective width of each leaf of the first collimator. This narrowing is a simple function of the relative widths of the slits of the second collimator and the leaves of the first. This will leave gaps in between the slits of the second collimator, which can then be filled by moving one or more of the patient, first and second collimators, so as to irradiate an area omitted in the first irradiation. In this second irradiation, the positions of the leaves of the first collimator are adjusted as necessary. This process is then repeated until the entire target area has been irradiated. Suitable values for the fraction are 1/2, 1/3, 1/4, or 1/5.

  Excerpt(s): The present invention relates to a collimator for use in **radiotherapy.** Radiotherapy is routinely employed for the treatment of invasive medical conditions such as cancer. The essential principle of **radiotherapy** is that the applied beam is apt to kill cells in its path. Thus, if the beam is directed at a cancerous or otherwise abnormal area the cells would eventually destroyed. However, it is inevitable that damage will also be caused to surrounding healthy tissue, and if this is not appropriately limited then the side effects for the patient could well be severe. The present invention seeks to provide a collimator in which the irradiation pattern of such a micro multi-leaf collimator can be achieved without the associated engineering difficulties and limited field size.

  Web site: http://www.delphion.com/details?pn=US06714627__

- **Computer assisted radiotherapy dosimeter system and a method therefor**

  Inventor(s): Ding; Wei (Kanata, CA)

  Assignee(s): Thomson & Nielsen Electronics Ltd. (Nepean, CA)

  Patent Number: 6,650,930

  Date filed: October 18, 2001

  Abstract: In order to facilitate the display and evaluation of data acquired while irradiating a body, e.g. a patient undergoing radiation therapy, a dosimetry system has a plurality of sensors for disposition on, in or near the body to be irradiated and connected to a sensor reading instrument which is interfaced with a display system, for example a personal computer, which is arranged to display, in use, one or more representations, for example drawings or photographs, of the body to be irradiated, along with the positions and the dose data for those specific locations where the dosimeter sensors were placed.

Excerpt(s): The invention relates to **radiotherapy** dosimeter systems, especially of the kind which use a plurality of dosimeter sensors distributed in a region to be irradiated and means for monitoring radiation levels detected by the sensors. Radiotherapy treatment of cancer patients involves the use of machines which produce high energy X-rays or high energy electrons. It is common practice to verify the radiation dose delivered to the patient with a dosimetry system such as the Thomson & Nielsen Patient Dose Verification System. There are three different types of dosimetry system used in **radiotherapy.** These are based on (a) film or thermal luminescent dosimeters (TLD), (b) diodes and (c) MOSFETs. Diode and MOSFET systems use electronic dosimeter sensors together with electronic reading systems, whereas film or TLD use chemical or thermal methods of reading the detectors into an electronic reading system.

Web site: http://www.delphion.com/details?pn=US06650930__

- **Delivery system and method for interstitial radiotherapy using hollow seeds**

Inventor(s): Lamoureux; Gary A. (Woodbury, CT), Terwilliger; Richard A. (Southbury, CT)

Assignee(s): IdeaMatrix, Inc. (Estes Park, CO)

Patent Number: 6,786,858

Date filed: April 26, 2002

Abstract: A delivery system and method for interstitial radiation therapy uses a seed strand composed of a plurality of tubular shaped, hollow radioactive seeds with a bore. The seed strand as assembled with a material provided in the bore and between the spaced seeds is axially stiff and radially flexible and is bioabsorbable in living tissue.

Excerpt(s): The present invention relates to systems and methods for delivering a plurality of radioactive sources to a treatment site. In interstitial radiation therapy, one method for treating tumors is to permanently place small, radioactive seeds into the tumor site. This method is currently accomplished by one of the following two procedures: (a) loose seeds are implanted in the target tissue, and/or (b) seeds are contained within a woven or braided absorbable carrier such as braided suture material and implanted in the target tissue. The loose seeds, however, are dependent on the tissue itself to hold each individual seed in place during treatment, and the woven or braided sutures do not assist in the placement of the seeds relative to the target tissue. There have been many developments in brachytherapy (i.e. therapy relating to treating malignant tumors, which use such radioactive seeds). In one technique, hollow metal needles are inserted into the tumor, and the seeds are thereafter inserted into the needles, while the needles are being retracted to deposit the seeds in the tumor. Such devices are shown in U.S. Pat. No. 4,402,308 which is incorporated herein by reference. The most commonly used instruments are the Henschke and Mick devices. The use of such devices has distinct disadvantages. The overall length of such devices is over 20 cm and such devices have significant weight making them difficult to manipulate.

Web site: http://www.delphion.com/details?pn=US06786858__

- **Dynamic respiratory control**

Inventor(s): Kalayjian; Nicholas R. (San Francisco, CA), Robinson; Terry E. (Palo Alto, CA), White; Wallace C. (Menlo Park, CA)

Assignee(s): The Board of Trustees of the Leland Stanford Junior University (Stanford, CA)

Patent Number: 6,631,716

Date filed: July 16, 1999

Abstract: A dynamic respiratory control device includes a fast-response valve capable of dynamically imposing multiple resistive loads on the flow of respiratory gas to and from a patient. The resistive loads are applied in response to measured flow rates, patient lung volumes, and/or mouthpiece pressures. The device can precisely constrain tidal breathing, provide precise volumetric control of the airway, and impose multiple specific inspiratory and/or expiratory loading functions to evaluate respiratory function. The device is useful for pulmonary function testing, CT and MRI imaging of the chest, combined CT imaging/interventional radiology, **radiotherapy** delivery to the thorax/abdomen, and/or as a resistive muscle trainer for weaning patients off ventilators and for respiratory muscle training.

Excerpt(s): This invention relates to systems and methods for respiratory function analysis and control, and in particular to systems and methods for dynamically analyzing and controlling the respiration of a patient. Controlling a patient's respiration is useful for many applications, including pulmonary function testing and evaluation, CT and MRI imaging of the chest, respiratory muscle training, and weaning patients off ventilators. Most currently available systems for controlling and evaluating respiratory function are relatively inflexible, and do not have the capability to precisely and dynamically control respiratory function. Moreover, some available methods of controlling respiratory function can be uncomfortable for the patient, particularly methods requiring the patient to hold his or her breath for extended periods of time. The present invention provides systems and methods for dynamically and accurately controlling a patient's respiratory function. The methods allow substantial flexibility in the evaluation process. The methods further allow limiting patient discomfort during respiratory function control procedures.

Web site: http://www.delphion.com/details?pn=US06631716__

- **Image processing method and apparatus adapted for radiotherapy treatment planning using digitally reconstructed radiograph**

Inventor(s): Kaneki; Kenichi (Nagareyama, JP), Oikawa; Michio (Ebina, JP), Seto; Youichi (Sagamihara, JP), Shimizu; Yusuke (Kashiwa, JP)

Assignee(s): Hitachi Medical Corporation (Tokyo, JP), Hitachi, Ltd. (Tokyo, JP)

Patent Number: 6,549,645

Date filed: June 10, 1998

Abstract: Three-dimensional data is generated by measuring an affected part using a computed tomography unit. Then, color information is allocated so as to correspond to voxel values of the three-dimensional data, and the allocated color information is added up along a ray irradiated from a radiation source. As a result, a digitally reconstructed radiograph (DRR) is generated and displayed.

Excerpt(s): The present invention relates to an image processing method and an apparatus that prepare treatment planning based on three-dimensional data obtained by making measurements on a patient using an X-ray computed tomography (CT) unit in treating diseases such as cancer with radiation. More specifically, the present invention is directed to an image processing method and apparatus adapted for **radiotherapy** treatment planning using digitally reconstructed radiographs (DRRs), which are permeation images generated from three-dimensional data obtained from a tomographic image measurement apparatus. Treatment methods involving injection of beams of radiation such as X-rays and beams of protons onto a focus portion such as cancer are considered effective. To give a patient such a treatment, preliminary treatment planning must be prepared. A **radiotherapy** treatment is generally given under the following procedure. First, part of a patient body including an affected part is measured using an apparatus such as an X-ray CT unit. The affected part is specified from the measured data, and its position and size are grasped. Then, the isocenter is set to the affected part, and conditions such as the direction of irradiation, number of injections and range of irradiation are simulated and adjusted so that radiation can be focused onto the affected part as closely as possible. Then, based on the results of the simulation and adjustment, markings are made on the patient body. Thereafter, the patient is requested to go to the **radiotherapy** treatment unit, positioned on the unit in accordance with the markings, and given the treatment.

Web site: http://www.delphion.com/details?pn=US06549645__

- **Inverse planning for intensity-modulated radiotherapy**

Inventor(s): Johnson; Scott L. (Madison, WI), McNutt; Todd R. (Verona, WI), Tipton; R. Keith (Verona, WI), Ward; R. Terry (Madison, WI)

Assignee(s): Koninklijke Philips Electronics N.V. (Eindhoven, NL)

Patent Number: 6,735,277

Date filed: May 23, 2002

Abstract: A radiation treatment apparatus (10) includes a diagnostic imaging scanner (12) that acquires a diagnostic image of a subject. A contouring processor (54) computes a radiation treatment objective based thereon. A radiation delivery apparatus (60) delivers radiation to the subject. An inverse planning processor (80) computes radiation beamlet parameters conforming with the radiation treatment objective by: grouping the beamlet parameters; assigning a weight to each group (82, 84, 86); optimizing a first group (82) to produce an intermediate dosage objective corresponding to the treatment objective weighted by a weight of the first group (82); and optimizing successive groups (84) to produce with the previously optimized groups (82) an increasing intermediate dosage objective corresponding to the treatment objective weighted by the combined weights of the previous and current groups (82, 84). A conversion processor (90) converts the optimized beamlet parameters into configuration parameters of the radiation delivery apparatus (60).

Excerpt(s): The present invention relates to the irradiating arts. It particularly relates to radiation treatment of a subject using spatially intensity-modulated radiation to deliver targeted and controlled dosage distributions, and will be described with particular reference thereto. However, the invention will also find application in conjunction with controlled delivery of radiation for other applications such as diagnostic imaging as well as in other radiation absorption analyses such as computation of light absorption for optical modeling. Oncological radiation therapy (sometimes called radiotherapy) is used for controlling, reversing, or sometimes even eliminating cancerous growths. Ionizing radiation such as high energy photons (e.g., x-rays or gamma rays), proton or neutron particles, or the like are applied to a cancerous tumor or other cancerous region. The ionizing radiation damages cellular DNA which can kill irradiated cells. Because growing and rapidly multiplying cancer cells are typically more readily damaged by the radiation and less able to repair such damage than are healthy cells, there is usually a beneficially built-in selectivity favoring elimination of cancerous tissue and survival of healthy tissue. However, irradiated healthy tissue is usually also damaged by the **radiotherapy** to at least some extent, and such radiation damage can produce highly detrimental side-effects to the therapy which are preferably minimized or avoided. To reduce damage to healthy tissue, **radiotherapy** typically includes a series of treatments performed over an extended period of time e.g., over several weeks. Serial treatment facilitates beneficial repair of damaged non-cancerous cells between treatments.

Web site: http://www.delphion.com/details?pn=US06735277__

- **Medical preparation for treating arthrosis, arthritis and other rheumatic joint diseases**

Inventor(s): Jordan; Andreas (Berlin, DE)

Assignee(s): MagForce Applications GmbH (DE)

Patent Number: 6,669,623

Date filed: January 23, 2002

Abstract: A medical preparation for treating arthrosis, arthritis and other rheumatic joint diseases comprises a suspension consisting of one-shelled or multi-shelled nanoscalar particles composed of a core containing iron oxide and of an inner shell with groups capable of forming cationic groups or, optionally, of at least one outer shell with neutral and/or anionic groups. Radionuclides and substances, said substances being cytotoxically active when subjected to heat, are bound to the inner shell. The preparation that is injected into the joint cavity and subjected to an alternating electromagnetic field promises an excellent treatment outcome due to the high rate of phagocytosis and the trimodal combinatorial effect of thermotherapy, **radiotherapy** and chemotherapy.

Excerpt(s): Not applicable.

Web site: http://www.delphion.com/details?pn=US06669623__

- **Method and apparatus for calibration of radiation therapy equipment and verification of radiation treatment**

Inventor(s): Mackie; Thomas R. (Madison, WI), McNutt; Todd R. (Madison, WI), Reckwerdt; Paul J. (Madison, WI)

Assignee(s): Wisconsin Alumni Research Foundation (Madison, WI)

Patent Number: 6,636,622

Date filed: January 4, 2002

Abstract: A method of calibration and verification of **radiotherapy** systems deduced radiation beam fluence profiles from the radiation source from a complete model of an extended radiation phantom together with dose information from a portal imaging device. The improved beam fluence profile characterization made with an iterative modeling which includes scatter effects may be used to compute dose profiles in the extended phantom or a patient who has been previously characterized with a CT scan. Deviations from the expected beam fluence profile can be used to detect patient misregistration.

Excerpt(s): This invention relates to radiation therapy equipment for the treatment of tumors or the like and specifically to an improved method of characterizing the radiation beam of such systems and confirming the dose received by the patient using a portal image of radiation exiting the patient. Medical equipment for radiation therapy treats tumorous tissue with high energy radiation. The dose and the placement of the dose must be accurately controlled to insure both that the tumor receives sufficient radiation to be destroyed, and that damage to the surrounding and adjacent non-tumorous tissue is minimized. Internal-source radiation therapy places capsules of radioactive material inside the patient in proximity to the tumorous tissue. Dose and placement are accurately controlled by the physical positioning of the isotope. However, internal-source radiation therapy has the disadvantages of any surgically invasive procedure, including discomfort to the patient and risk of infection.

Web site: http://www.delphion.com/details?pn=US06636622__

- **Method and apparatus for radiotherapy treatment planning**

Inventor(s): Deasy; Joseph O. (St. Louis, MO), Wickerhauser; Mladen Victor (University City, MO)

Assignee(s): Washington University (St. Louis, MO)

Patent Number: 6,792,073

Date filed: May 7, 2001

Abstract: A computationally efficient and accurate procedure for calculating radiation dose distributions within a volume of interest in a patient incorporating variations in patient density and source particle energy, position, direction, and type. The procedure iteratively simulates energy depositions from source particles using the Monte Carlo radiation transport method and then applies methods for reducing noise inherent in Monte Carlo results to obtain an accurate and computationally efficient representation of an actual radiation dose distribution compared to that produced by Monte Carlo methods alone. The invention makes an analogy between real measured data and transformed Monte Carlo generated computer data and then applies data denoising techniques to reduce the noise in the Monte Carlo dose images. Conversely, the present invention can produce a dose distribution having a predetermined noise level in a reduced amount of computation time. Denoising techniques can include digital filtering, wavelet denoising, kernel smoothing and non-parametric regression smoothing.

Excerpt(s): This invention relates generally to accelerating Monte Carlo calculations, and more particularly to determining radiation dose distributions in a patient for **radiotherapy** treatment planning by accelerating Monte Carlo dose distribution calculations through denoising of raw Monte Carlo dose distributions. Medical equipment for radiation therapy treats tumorous (malignant) tissue with high energy radiation. The amount of radiation and its placement must be accurately controlled to ensure that the tumor receives sufficient radiation to be destroyed and that damage to the surrounding and adjacent non-tumorous tissue is minimized. Internal source radiation therapy (referred to as brachytherapy) places capsules of radioactive material inside the patient in proximity to the tumorous tissue. Dose and placement are accurately controlled by the physical positioning of the isotope. However, internal source radiation therapy has disadvantages similar to those present with surgically invasive procedures, which include patient discomfort and risk of infection.

Web site: http://www.delphion.com/details?pn=US06792073__

- **Method and device for delivering radiotherapy**

Inventor(s): Moyers; Michael F. (Colton, CA)

Assignee(s): Loma Linda University Medical Center (Loma Linda, CA)

Patent Number: 6,769,806

Date filed: March 20, 2003

Abstract: A device 10 for aligning a patient for delivering a plurality of radiation beams comprising a patient support surface 12, a coarse alignment subsystem 14 connected to the patient support surface, and a fine alignment subsystem connected to the patient support surface 16. A method of aligning a patient for delivering a plurality of radiation beams from a plurality of device positions comprising compensating for flexion of a radiation beam delivery device within a gantry during movement of the radiation beam delivery device from a first device position to a second device position by using a set of predetermined data describing the flexion behavior of the radiation beam delivery device so that the target tissue within the patient is placed at the beamline center for the radiation beam delivery device at the second device position.

Excerpt(s): The application of radiation is used for a variety of diagnostic and therapeutic purposes. For example, external **radiotherapy** known as "teletherapy" is used to treat approximately half of all patients with cancer in the United States, as well as being used to treat patients with arterio-venous malformations, intraocular subfoveal neovascular membranes and Parkinson's disease, among other diseases and conditions. Generally, teletherapy has been performed using x-ray beams or electron beams. More recently, however, teletherapy has been performed using proton beams due to two characteristics of proton beams. First, proton beams do not scatter as much as either x-ray beams or electron beams. Thus, teletherapy with a proton beam can be applied with a steeper dose gradient near the edge of the proton beam than for an x-ray beam or electron beam. Second, protons lose energy at a more rapid rate as they penetrate tissue, thereby delivering a greater dose at the depth of the target tissue. These two characteristics of proton beams allow the delivery of higher doses to target tissues while minimizing radiation to adjacent normal tissues. The delineation of target tissues from non-target tissues and the selection of beam directions is typically performed using a computerized treatment planning system. The computerized treatment planning system analyzes input information, such as x-ray axial computed tomography and magnetic resonance imaging, and provides output information, such as beam directions, shapes of normal tissue shields for each beam, and patient alignment information for each beam.

Web site: http://www.delphion.com/details?pn=US06769806__

- **Method for breath compensation in radiation therapy**

Inventor(s): Erbel; Stephan (Munchen, DE), Frohlich; Stephan (Aschheim, DE), Schlossbauer; Cornel (Krailling, DE)

Assignee(s): BrainLAB AG (Kirchheim, DE)

Patent Number: 6,731,970

Date filed: July 3, 2001

Abstract: A method for breath compensation in radiation therapy, particularly radiotherapy/radiosurgery, wherein the movement of the target volume inside the patient is detected and tracked in real time during radiation by a movement detector. Adaptation to the movement of the target volume inside the patient is achieved by one or more components of a **radiotherapy** apparatus to compensate for or take into consideration the movement during treatment.

Excerpt(s): The present invention concerns a method for breath compensation in radiation therapy, particularly for breath compensation in **radiotherapy** or radiosurgery. Great improvements have recently been made in the field of **radiotherapy** and radiosurgery, concerning the positioning of patients for the purpose of exposing them to radiation. It is thus possible, by means of prior art navigational and positioning systems comprising markers fixed to the patient which can be detected by a camera system and whose position can be detected with the aid of a computer, to position a patient under an irradiation gantry, e.g. by automatically moving the patient's table such that the volume to be radiated (e.g. a tumour), whose position has been determined in advance by means of a body-section imaging method, can be positioned with utmost accuracy within the path of the radiation. Such exact positioning aims to preserve the patient's healthy tissue surrounding the diseased tissue as much as possible.

Web site: http://www.delphion.com/details?pn=US06731970__

- **Method for preparing a radiation therapy plan**

Inventor(s): Hoban; Peter (Randwick, AU), Mackie; Thomas R. (Madison, WI), Olivera; Gustavo H. (Madison, WI), Reckwerdt; Paul J. (Madison, WI), Shepard; David M. (Madison, WI)

Assignee(s): Wisconsin Alumni Research Foundation (Madison, WI)

Patent Number: 6,560,311

Date filed: March 15, 2001

Abstract: A method for determining a radiation treatment plan for a **radiotherapy** system providing multiple individual rays of intensity modulated radiation iteratively optimized the fluence of an initial set of such rays by a function that requires knowledge of only the prescribed dose and the dose resulting from the particular ray fluences. In this way, the need to store individual dose distributions of each ray are eliminated.

Excerpt(s): The present invention relates generally to radiation therapy planning for the treatment of tumors and suitable for radiation therapy machines providing independent intensity modulated narrow beams of radiation. Radiation therapy involves the treatment of tumorous tissue with high energy radiation according to a treatment plan. The treatment plan controls the radiation's placement and dose level so that the tumorous tissue receives a sufficient dose of radiation while the radiation to surrounding and adjacent non-tumorous tissue is minimal. Intensity modulated radiation therapy (IMRT) treats a patient with multiple rays of radiation each of which may be independently controlled in intensity and/or energy. The rays are directed from different angles about the patient and combine to provide a desired dose pattern. Typically, the radiation source consists of either high-energy X-rays, electrons from certain linear accelerators, or gamma rays from highly focused radioisotopes such as Co.sup.60.

Web site: http://www.delphion.com/details?pn=US06560311__

- **Method for producing or updating radiotherapy plan**

Inventor(s): Erbel; Stephan (Munchen, DE), Frohlich; Stephan (Aschheim, DE)

Assignee(s): BrainLAB AG (Kirchheim/Heimstetten, DE)

Patent Number: 6,792,074

Date filed: July 3, 2001

Abstract: The invention relates to a method for producing or updating a **radiotherapy** plan within the framework of inversely planned **radiotherapy,** wherein an up-to-date **radiotherapy** plan is calculated at least partly on the basis of the results of an already existing, approved, older plan.

Excerpt(s): The present invention relates to the field of **radiotherapy,** in particular radiation therapy or radio-surgery. In particular, it concerns producing or updating **radiotherapy** plans, and here also specifically with **radiotherapy** plans within the framework of inverse **radiotherapy** planning. Work in **radiotherapy** using inverse planning is computer-assisted, pre-set data being entered into a computer system with respect to the desired dosage distribution in the target area and with respect to the organs to be protected. On this basis, the system is supposed to generate a dosage plan which ensures the best possible treatment. Since for medical reasons, the patient's therapy in the extra-cranial area is usually fractionated, i.e. radiation exposure is carried out in a number of sessions spaced out in time, it is not guaranteed that the position of the internal organs and of the target area inside the patient correspond to the positions determined in a previous examination of the patient. For this reason, a dosage distribution found to be correct for an earlier session does not for the most part correspond to a correct dosage distribution for a subsequent session. The correspondence between the positions in the plan and the positions during **radiotherapy,** however, is relatively good if the patient is not relocated between the point in time at which he is subjected to an imaging procedure and the point in time of radiation exposure. If the patient is scanned again before each radiation exposure, however, new positions for the organs and the target volume result, so that an earlier treatment plan cannot in theory be adopted.

Web site: http://www.delphion.com/details?pn=US06792074__

- **Method for protecting cells and tissues from ionizing radiation toxicity with.alpha.,.beta. unsaturated aryl sulfones**

  Inventor(s): Cosenza; Stephen C. (Vorhees, NJ), Helson; Lawrence (Quakertown, PA), Reddy; E. Premkumar (Villanova, PA), Reddy; M. V. Ramana (Upper Darby, PA)

  Assignee(s): Onconova Therapeutics, Inc. (Lawrenceville, NJ), Temple University - Of The Commonwealth System of Higher Education (Philadelphia, PA)

  Patent Number: 6,667,346

  Date filed: February 28, 2002

  Abstract: Pre-treatment with.alpha.,.beta. unsaturated aryl sulfones protects normal cells from the toxic side effects of ionizing radiation. Administration of a radioprotective.alpha.,.beta. unsaturated aryl sulfone compound to a patient prior to anticancer **radiotherapy** reduces the cytotoxic side effects of the radiation on normal cells. The radioprotective effect of the.alpha.,.beta. unsaturated aryl sulfone allows the clinician to safely increase the dosage of anticancer radiation. In some instances, amelioration of toxicity following inadvertent radiation exposure may be mitigated with administration of.alpha.,.beta. unsaturated arylsulfone.

  Excerpt(s): The invention relates to the field of protecting normal cells and tissues from anticipated, planned or inadvertent exposure to ionizing radiation. In particular, the invention relates to radioprotective agents administered to a subject prior to or after exposure to ionizing radiation, such as occurs during anticancer **radiotherapy**. Ionizing radiation has an adverse effect on cells and tissues, primarily through cytotoxic effects. In humans, exposure to ionizing radiation occurs primarily through therapeutic techniques (such as anticancer radiotherapy) or through occupational and environmental exposure. A major source of exposure to ionizing radiation is the administration of therapeutic radiation in the treatment of cancer or other proliferative disorders. Subjects exposed to therapeutic doses of ionizing radiation typically receive between 0.1 and 2 Gy per treatment, and can receive as high as 5 Gy per treatment. Depending on the course of treatment prescribed by the treating physician, multiple doses may be received by a subject over the course of several weeks to several months.

  Web site: http://www.delphion.com/details?pn=US06667346__

- **Radiation recording device**

  Inventor(s): Arndt; Jurgen (Farentuna, SE), Nilsson; Borje (Uppsala, SE)

  Assignee(s): Elekta AB (publ) (Stockholm, SE)

  Patent Number: 6,712,508

  Date filed: June 11, 2002

  Abstract: A device is provided for recording in at least two planes radiation from a **radiotherapy** apparatus. The device comprises a dimensionally stable frame which is adapted to be arranged in a defined position relative to the **radiotherapy** apparatus, an attachment on the frame for a recording means, and a recording means which extends from the attachment at an acute angle to the frame along an axis of rotation and to the center of the frame. The recording means is adapted to assume at least two defined rotational positions on the axis. In addition, the recording means exhibits a surface for supporting a radiation recording unit, which surface is located in a plane that forms an acute angle with the axis of rotation, the plane of the surface when rotating the recording means being adapted to turn on a single pivot point which is fixed relative to the frame.

Excerpt(s): The present invention relates to a device for recording in at least two planes radiation from a **radiotherapy** apparatus in a limited area at which the radiation is directed. In particular, the invention relates to a device for determining the resulting radiation, which from a number of different directions hits a plane or a volume, by recording the radiation on media sensitive to radiation, such as films, semiconductors, ionization chambers, etc., in defined positions and simultaneously or later evaluating recorded radiation data with respect to the distribution of the radiation in time and space by means of a read-out device. The device is especially suited for accurate spatial determination relative to given references of geometrically defined radiation distributions. The device is also suited for quality assurance of a whole precision radiation procedure by allowing target volumes to be simulated, which volumes can be determined as regards shape and position by medical, image-creating equipment, such as magnetic resonance imaging, computer tomography, etc., for planning treatment of precision radiation and for verifying radiation based on planning.

Web site: http://www.delphion.com/details?pn=US06712508__

- **Radiation shield**

Inventor(s): Macklis; Roger M. (Cleveland, OH), Sohn; Jason (Chesterfield, MO), Willoughby; Twyla (Orlando, FL)

Assignee(s): The Cleveland Clinic Foundation (Cleveland, OH)

Patent Number: 6,703,632

Date filed: October 17, 2002

Abstract: A radiation shield is provided for use on patients undergoing **radiotherapy** treatment. The shield is made of a suitable radiation absorbing material for preventing the transmission of high energy radiation to the patient's non-treatment areas. The device may further comprise an exterior surface layer for absorbing low energy photons. The shield is sized and shaped to conform to a patient's anatomy and to provide the necessary amount of absorbing material closest to the beam edge while not interfering with the beam. The shield may further comprise an optional cavity located on the interior surface of the shield which may be lined with a soft compressible material for conforming to a patient's unique anatomy. The shield may be further provided with dosimeters mounted on the exterior surface of the leading edge as well as on the interior surface of the shield. The dosimeters may be connected in a systematic manner with the linear accelerator such that the machine could be automatically switched off or warnings given if the patient is receiving too much radiation scatter dose.

Excerpt(s): The present invention pertains generally to a radiation detecting and shielding device for reducing radiation exposure to healthy tissue of a patient undergoing radiation therapy, as well as detecting the amount of radiation delivered to the patient. More particularly, the invention pertains to protecting the contra-lateral breast or chest wall of a patient undergoing **radiotherapy** as well as sensing the amount of radiation on or near a patient's skin on the non-treated side of the body. Radiation therapy or **radiotherapy** for the chest wall or breast area of a patient has been utilized frequently for the treatment of localized cancer such as breast cancer. A patient typically undergoes a series of radiation treatments in which the treatment area is irradiated with a high energy radiation dose on the order of 25 to 75 Gray (Gy.) units, with a typical treatment dose in the range of 50 to 60 Gy. The most common radiation therapy technique for treating breast cancer utilizes opposing tangential radiation beams. A pair of wedges are often used in conjunction with this technique to obtain a more uniform treatment dose. It is a growing concern among researchers that patients are exposed to scattered radiation in the adjacent region of the radiation field, particularly in the contralateral breast or chest wall in treatment of the breast or chest area. For patients undergoing breast cancer **radiotherapy** treatment, it has been estimated that the contra-lateral breast receives a scattered radiation dose between 5% to 13% of the prescribed treatment dose. Some patients may receive an even higher percentage of the dose depending on the patient's anatomy and the treatment angles utilized. Further, for patients treated with a conventional dose of 50 Gray using traditional tangential fields, the dose to the contra-lateral breast has been estimated to be on the order of 2.5-6.0 Gray at a central axis corresponding to approximately 5 centimeters over the mid-line. Although the effects of this dose of scattered radiation are not yet well understood, one study has suggested that women under 45 years of age who had been treated for breast cancer by radiation therapy had an increased risk by a factor of 1.5 of contralateral breast cancer as compared to controls.

Web site: http://www.delphion.com/details?pn=US06703632__

- **Radiation source wire member for treating cancer and its delivery apparatus**

Inventor(s): Asano; Yuichiro (Tokyo, JP)

Assignee(s): Asano & Associates Corporation (Tokyo, JP), Radiomed Corporation (Tyngsboro, MA)

Patent Number: 6,659,933

Date filed: March 26, 2001

Abstract: A radiation source wire member for **radiotherapy** indwelling in cancer-affected part of the body comprises an indwelling tip end portion having a radiation source of rhodium coil wire partially converted to.sup.103 Pd, and a filament connected to the indwelling portion, the filament having such a length that at least a rear end portion thereof is exposed outside the body after indwelling in the cancer-affected part. An apparatus for delivering the radiation source wire member to the cancer-affected part of the body has a catheter structure comprising (a) an outer tube having an inner diameter permitting the indwelling portion to pass through without resistance, and (b) an inner tube received in the outer tube movably back and forth therein and having an inner diameter not permitting the indwelling portion to pass through but permitting the filament to pass through without resistance.

Excerpt(s): The present invention relates to a radiation source wire member and its delivery apparatus effective in **radiotherapy** of cancers and tumors such as prostate cancer, breast cancer, etc. The number of prostrate cancer patients has been increasing rapidly in Japan because of the recent Westernization of lifestyle and diet. Though the prostrate cancer is likely to provide such symptoms as urination disorder and hematuria, there are so many cases exhibiting no symptoms that it is difficult to find it out at an early stage. The prostate cancer may be cured by the ablation of the affected part and a radiation therapy. However, the former treatment inflicts large pain on the patients, while the latter treatment gives anxiety to them because the other organs are unnecessarily exposed to radiation.

Web site: http://www.delphion.com/details?pn=US06659933__

- **Radiolabeled irreversible inhibitors of epidermal growth factor receptor tyrosine kinase and their use in radioimaging and radiotherapy**

  Inventor(s): Ben-David; Iris (Ashdod, IL), Levitzki; Alexander (Jerusalem, IL), Mishani; Eyal (Mevaseret Zion, IL), Ortu; Gluseppina (Jerusalem, IL), Rozen; Yulia (Jerusalem, IL)

  Assignee(s): Hadasit Medical Research Services and Development Ltd. (Jerusalem, IL), Yissum Research Development Company of the Hebrew University of Jerusalem (Jerusalem, IL)

  Patent Number: 6,562,319

  Date filed: March 12, 2001

  Abstract: Radiolabeled epidermal growth factor receptor tyrosine kinase (EGFR-TK) irreversible inhibitors and their use as biomarkers for medicinal radioimaging such as Positron Emission Tomography (PET) and Single Photon Emission Computed Tomography (SPECT) and as radiopharmaceuticals for **radiotherapy** are disclosed.

  Excerpt(s): The present invention relates to radiolabeled compounds and their use in radioimaging and/or **radiotherapy**. More particularly, the present invention relates to radiolabeled irreversible inhibitors of epidermal growth factor receptor tyrosine kinase (EGFR-TK) and their use as biomarkers for medicinal radioimaging such as Positron Emission Tomography (PET) and Single Photon Emission Computed Tomography (SPECT), and as radiopharmaceuticals for **radiotherapy**. The use of radioactive nuclides for medicinal purposes is well known in the art. Biologically active compounds that bind to specific cell surface receptors or that in other ways modify cellular functions has received some consideration as radiopharmaceuticals, and therefore, when labeled with a radioactive nuclide, such compounds are used as biospecific agents in radioimaging and **radiotherapy**. Positron Emission Tomography (PET), a nuclear medicine imagine technology which allows the three-dimensional, quantitative determination of the distribution of radioactivity within the human body, is becoming an increasingly important tool for the measurement of physiological, biochemical, and pharmacological function at a molecular level, both in healthy and pathological states. PET requires the administration to a subject of a molecule labeled with a positron-emitting nuclide (radiotracer) such as.sup.15 O,.sup.13 N,.sup.11 C and.sup.18 F, which have half-lives of 2, 10, 20, and 110 minutes, respectively.

  Web site: http://www.delphion.com/details?pn=US06562319___

- **Radiotherapy treatment planning with multiple inverse planning results**

  Inventor(s): Frohlich; Stephan (Aschheim, DE)

  Assignee(s): BrainLAB AG (Kirchheim/Heimsteten, DE)

  Patent Number: 6,719,683

  Date filed: October 1, 2001

  Abstract: An inverse planning method and apparatus for **radiotherapy** treatment of a target volume in a body are characterized by using a computer to calculate the results (dose distribution) of multiple treatment solutions (proposed radiation beam arrangements); and simultaneously displaying the calculated results for at least two of the treatment solutions for comparison by a treatment planner to enable the treatment planner to select a desired one of the treatment solutions.

Excerpt(s): The invention herein described relates to **radiotherapy** and more particularly to an apparatus and method for treatment planning for radiotherapeutical procedures. Conformal radiation therapy typically employs a linear accelerator as the source of a radiation beam or beams used to treat a tumor and/or other internal anomaly, herein referred to generally as a target volume. The linear accelerator has a radiation beam source which may be rotated about the patient to direct the radiation beam toward the target volume from different angles. Various means have been employed to control the rotation, intensity, shape and/or direction of the radiation beam in accordance with a predetermined treatment program designed to apply a desired radiation dose to the target area while minimizing the dose of radiation to surrounding healthy tissue and/or adjacent healthy organs, hereinafter referred to generally as a non-target volume. Overall, the goal of conformal radiation therapy is to confine the delivered radiation dose to only the treatment volume while minimizing the dose of radiation to the non-target volume. Accordingly, a treatment plan (also referred to as treatment solution) is desired that optimizes the radiation dose to the target area while minimizing the amount of radiation delivered to the surrounding non-target volume. Existing techniques to optimize treatment planning during radiation oncology include forward treatment planning and the more recent inverse treatment planning. The forward treatment problem is to compute the dose distribution in a tissue given a treatment plan. The inverse treatment problem is to find a treatment plan whose execution will achieve a desired dose distribution.

Web site: http://www.delphion.com/details?pn=US06719683__

- **Seed localization system and method in ultrasound by fluoroscopy and ultrasound fusion**

Inventor(s): Thornton; Kenneth B (Charlottesville, VA)

Assignee(s): Varian Medical Systems, Inc. (Palo Alto, CA)

Patent Number: 6,549,802

Date filed: June 7, 2001

Abstract: A seed localization system and method in which a computer-based system is used to determine the three-dimensional (3D) position of **radiotherapy** seeds with respect to an area of affected tissue, such as the prostate, using ultrasound (US) and fluoroscopy (FL) imaging, so that a **radiotherapy** dose may be calculated. One embodiment the present invention may be used to determine the 3D position of implanted brachytherapy seeds. An alternative embodiment of the invention may be used to determine the 3D position of implanted objects other than brachytherapy seeds. The seed localization system and method includes a graphical user interface useful for assisting a user of the seed localization system in its operation.

Excerpt(s): This invention relates generally to systems and methods for the treatment of cancer using radiation, and, more specifically, to systems and methods for the treatment of cancer using implanted brachytherapy seeds. Brachytherapy, a useful technique for treating cancer, is a radiation treatment using a solid or enclosed radioisotopic source on the surface of the body or a short distance from the area to be treated. With respect to prostate cancer, for example, brachytherapy involves the implantation of **radiotherapy** seeds into the prostate. The effectiveness of the brachytherapy treatment depends, however, on the particularized placement of the implanted brachytherapy seeds to achieve a preferred **radiotherapy** dose. The **radiotherapy** dose administered to the patient may be calculated by observing the three dimensional (3D) positions of the brachytherapy seeds with respect to the affected tissue. Computed tomography (CT) is one technique used to determine the three dimensional locations of the seeds. A common problem with using CT, however, is that many operating rooms do not contain CT equipment. This makes it impossible to evaluate and subsequently adjust the dose of **radiotherapy** while the patient is in the treatment position. For example, if "cold spots" are found after imaging with CT, then the patient must be retreated.

Web site: http://www.delphion.com/details?pn=US06549802__

- **System combining proton beam irradiation and magnetic resonance imaging**

  Inventor(s): Bucholz; Richard D. (St. Louis, MO), Miller; D. Douglas (St. Louis, MO)

  Assignee(s): St. Louis University (St. Louis, MO)

  Patent Number: 6,725,078

  Date filed: January 4, 2001

  Abstract: A system which coordinates proton beam irradiation with an open magnetic resonance imaging (MRI) unit to achieve near-simultaneous, noninvasive localization and **radiotherapy** of various cell lines in various anatomic locations. A reference image of the target aids in determining a treatment plan and repositioning the patient within the MRI unit for later treatments. The patient is located within the MRI unit so that the target and the proton beam are coincident. MRI monitors the location of the target. Target irradiation occurs when the target and the proton beam are coincident as indicated by the MRI monitoring. The patient rotates relative to the radiation source. The target again undergoes monitoring and selective irradiation. The rotation and selective irradiation during MRI monitoring repeats according to the treatment plan.

  Excerpt(s): The present invention relates to systems for localization and **radiotherapy** of various cell lines in various anatomic locations. In particular, this invention relates to a system which coordinates proton beam irradiation with an open magnetic resonance imaging (MRI) unit to achieve near-simultaneous, noninvasive localization and **radiotherapy** of various cell lines in various anatomic locations by maintaining coincidence between the target and the proton beam. Proton beam irradiation therapy treats tumors found in selected locations that are not subject to significant physiologic motion. Examples of such tumors include prostatic cancer, spinal chordomas, and certain retinal or orbital tumors. The proton beam generated by a medical cyclotron has similar biological activity for the destruction of tumors as standard radiation therapy techniques to target a fixed tumor site with minimal radiotoxicity to the surrounding normal tissues. Because protons of a specific energy have a specific penetration depth, adjusting the specific energy of the protons manipulates the distance the proton beam travels into the patient. Because protons deposit most of their energy at the end of the penetration depth, the highest concentration of radiation occurs in the area around the penetration depth. This area is known as the Bragg peak of the proton beam. The focused delivery of protons to a fixed site permits the **radiotherapy** of tumors or the destruction of tissue causing functional problems. However, tumors and tissue located in organs subject to significant physiologic motion cannot be treated without significant collateral radiotoxicity. There is a need for a system which allows proton beam delivery to a target subject to significant physiologic motion that minimizes the collateral damage to the surrounding normal tissues.

  Web site: http://www.delphion.com/details?pn=US06725078__

- **Targeted liposome gene delivery**

Inventor(s): Chang; Esther H. (Chevy Chase, MD), Pirollo; Kathleen (Arlington, VA), Xu; Liang (Arlington, VA)

Assignee(s): Georgetown University (Washington, DC)

Patent Number: 6,749,863

Date filed: January 4, 2001

Abstract: Targeted ligand-liposome-therapeutic molecule complexes (vectors) for the systemic delivery of the therapeutic molecule to various target cell types including cancer cells such as squamous cell carcinoma of the head and neck, breast and prostate tumors. The preferred ligands, folate and transferrin, target the liposome complex and facilitate transient gene transfection. The systemic delivery of complexes containing DNA encoding wild-type p53 to established mouse xenografts markedly sensitized the tumors to **radiotherapy** and chemotherapy. The combination of systemic p53 gene therapy and conventional **radiotherapy** or chemotherapy resulted in total tumor regression and long tern inhibition of recurrence. This cell-specific delivery system was also used in vivo to successfully deliver, via intravenous administration, small DNA molecules (oligonucleotides) resulting in chemosensitivity and xenograft growth inhibition. Other therapeutic molecules, including intact viruses, can be encapsulated in a complex and targeted in accordance with the invention.

Excerpt(s): This invention relates generally to the systemic delivery of a therapeutic molecule via a liposome complex that is targeted to a pre-selected cell type. More specifically, the invention provides compositions and methods for cell-targeted gene transfer and gene therapy for human cancers whereby a therapeutic molecule is delivered to the targeted cancer cell via a ligand/liposome complex. Treatment of cell proliferative disease (e.g. cancer) results in substantial improvement of the efficacy of radiation and chemotherapeutic interventions. The ideal therapeutic for cancer would be one that selectively targets a cellular pathway responsible for the tumor phenotype and would be nontoxic to normal cells. To date, the ideal therapeutic remains just that-- an ideal. While cancer treatments involving gene therapy and anti-sense molecules have substantial promise, there are many issues that need to be addressed before this promise can be realized. Perhaps foremost among the issues associated with macromolecular treatments for cancer and other diseases is the efficient delivery of the therapeutic molecule(s) to the site(s) in the body where they are needed. A variety of nucleic acid delivery systems ("vectors") to treat cancer have been evaluated by others, including viruses and liposomes. The ideal vector for human cancer gene therapy would be one that could be systemically administered and then specifically and efficiently target tumor cells wherever they occur in the body. Viral vector-directed methods show high gene transfer efficiency but are deficient in several areas. The limitations of a viral approach are related to their lack of targeting and to the presence of residual viral elements that can be immunogenic, cytopathic, or recombinogenic.

Web site: http://www.delphion.com/details?pn=US06749863__

- **Tumor radiosensitization using gene therapy**

  Inventor(s): McBride; William H. (Los Angeles, CA)

  Assignee(s): The Regents of the University of California (Oakland, CA)

  Patent Number: 6,551,588

  Date filed: March 24, 2000

Abstract: The invention provides a method of radiosensitizing a tumor in a subject by contacting the tumor with a cytokine or a nucleic acid molecule encoding a cytokine. The invention also provides a method of radiosensitizing a tumor in a subject by administering, at a site other than the tumor, a cell genetically modified to express a cytokine. The invention further provides a method of reducing the severity of a cancer in a subject by administering a cytokine at the site of the tumor or by immunizing the subject at a site other than the tumor with tumor cells genetically modified to express a cytokine, and treating the tumor with **radiotherapy.**

  Excerpt(s): The present invention relates generally to cancer therapy and, more particularly, to compositions and methods for sensitizing a cancer in a subject to radiation therapy. Improved methods and novel agents for treating cancer have resulted in increased survival time and survival rate for patients with various types of cancer. For example, improved surgical and radiotherapeutic procedures result in more effective removal of localized tumors. Surgical methods, however, can be limited due, for example, to the location of a tumor or to dissemination of metastatic tumor cells. **Radiotherapy** also can be limited by these factors, which limits the dose that can be administered. Tumors that are relatively radioresistant will not be cured at such a dose. Immunotherapeutic methods also are being examined as a means to treat a cancer by stimulating the patient's immune response against the cancer. In particular, the role of cytokines, which are cellular factors that can modulate an immune response, is an important factor to consider when planning an immunotherapeutic procedure. For example, expression of a cytokine such as interleukin-2 (IL-2) can increase the proliferation of T cells, which are involved in the cellular immune response against a cancer.

  Web site: http://www.delphion.com/details?pn=US06551588__

- **Use of a Serenoa repens extract for the production of a medicament to treat prostate cancer**

  Inventor(s): Cousse; Henri (Pins Justaret, FR), Fabre; Pierre (Castres, FR), Raynaud; Jean-Pierre (Paris, FR)

  Assignee(s): Pierre Fabre Medicament (Boulogne-Billancourt, FR)

  Patent Number: 6,599,540

  Date filed: September 28, 2001

Abstract: The invention relates to the use of a lipido-sterolic Serenoa repens extract for the production of a medicament which is administered in an isolated manner or in an associated manner, in a simultaneous, separated or staggered manner, with prostatectomy, **radiotherapy** and/or hormonotherapy in order to prevent and/or treat prostate cancer.

  Excerpt(s): The present invention relates to the field of treating prostate cancer which, at the present time, is based on several therapeutic routes dependent on the degree of progress of the disease. The hormonal treatment of metastatic prostate cancer which has crossed the capsule currently relies mainly on several categories of medicinal products which act at different levels on the hypothalamo-gonad axis. The efficacy and limits of hormonal treatments are now more or less defined. These limits are set both by the side effects, in particular vascular effects for estrogens at high doses, and sexual, gastric and pulmonary effects for antiandrogens, and by the emergence of immediate or secondary resistance. The current attitude appears to be focused, at least at the initial phase of the treatment, on total androgenic blockage (inhibition of the testicular secretion of androgens and inhibition of the activity of the residual androgens on the target organ). Specifically, the absence of absolute certainty regarding the advantage of continuing this combination long term occasionally results in a complete androgenic blockage being preferred at the time of starting a treatment with an LHRH agonist, in order to prevent initial flare-ups with subsequent continuation of the agonist alone.

Web site: http://www.delphion.com/details?pn=US06599540__

Patent Applications on Radiotherapy

As of December 2000, U.S. patent applications are open to public viewing.[9] Applications are patent requests which have yet to be granted. (The process to achieve a patent can take several years.) The following patent applications have been filed since December 2000 relating to radiotherapy:

- **Agent for preventing and/or treating cachexia**

  Inventor(s): Iemura, Akihiro; (Fukuoka, JP), Kojiro, Masamichi; (Fukuoka, JP), Yano, Hirohisa; (Fukuoka, JP)

  Correspondence: Testa, Hurwitz & Thibeault, Llp; High Street Tower; 125 High Street; Boston; MA; 02110; US

  Patent Application Number: 20030236191

  Date filed: March 5, 2003

  Abstract: The present invention provides an agent for preventing and/or treating cachesia comprising TCF-II as an effective ingredient. An excellent agent for preventing and treating cachexia caused by cancer, acquired immunodeficient syndrome (AIDS), cardiac diseases, infectious disease, shock, burn, endotoxinemia, organ inflammation, surgery, diabetes, collagen diseases, **radiotherapy,** chemotherapy is provided by the present invention and useful for medicine.

  Excerpt(s): The present invention relates to an agent for preventing and/or treating cachexia comprising Tumor Cytotoxic Factor-II(TCF-II) as an effective ingredient. An excellent agent for preventing and treating cachexia caused by one of the factors selected from the group consisting of cancer, acquired immunodeficient syndrome (AIDS), cardiac diseases, infectious disease, shock, burn, endotoxinemia, organ inflammation, surgery, diabetes, collagen diseases, **radiotherapy,** chemotherapy is provided by the present invention and useful for medicine. Generally, such a disease as cancer, acquired immunodeficiency(AIDS), cardiac disease etc. will accompany with anorexia, weight loss, physical exhaustion, marasmus, dermatrophia, xerosis, anemia, edema, abnormal blood coagulation-fibrinolysis etc. and these pathology is defined as cachexia. After

---

[9] This has been a common practice outside the United States prior to December 2000.

suffering from this systemic marasmus, a patient will eventually die (Tamaguma, M. et.al., Igakuno-ayumi, 149, 371-373(1989)). Further, if **radiotherapy** and/or chemotherapy is carried out for a patient with progressive or terminal cancer for whom curative operation can not be expected, it may lead to extremely lowered biological body defensive function such as immunological function due to specific malnutrition, resulting in shortening life. Therefore, these are serious problems in practical treatment thereof. The cause of cachexia has been so far considered to be triggered by imbalance of nutritional equilibrium between (lowered) nutrition intake and (increased) nutrition consumption and affection of humoric factor mobilized from cancer or lesion on systemic metabolism. From the above situations, positive alimentation is carried out using total parental nutrition in order to supplement extreme nutritional or energetic deficiency and enhance immunological function in the treatment of cachexia. However, in cachexia, intake of energy will be used not for saving patient's life but for proliferation of tumor cell, so that alimentation can not be sufficient treatment. Recently, monokine or cytokine, such as Tumor Necrosis Factor (TNF), mobilized from macrophage is paid attention as cause of cachexia. TNF was found as a factor of affecting tumor cell and elucidated to be secreted by macrophage which is one of immunocytes and has a phagocytic action. Though it was originally expected as anti-cancer drug because of its direct cytotoxic effect and strong anti-tumor activity, recently various kinds of action of TNF have been investigated since it was found that it cause cachexia that is marasmus including weight loss of a patient with cancer or severe infection disease or a ringleader cytokine inducing inflammation. The main actions are (1) osteoclastic action, (2) induction of hyperlipidemia by inhibition of uptake of lipid into cell, (3) induction of production of interleukine 1 and colony stimulation factor, (4) impairment of angioendotherial cell, (5) intervening reaction of exotoxin shock in grave infectious disease. Though an agent for treating cachexia accompanied with cancer, acquired immunodeficient syndrome (AIDS), cardiac diseases, infectious disease, shock, burn, endotoxinemia, organ inflammation, or these diseases themselves or various kinds of inflammatory diseases including chronic rheumatoid arthritis and inflammatory gut disease are expected to be developed, in fact, there is no satisfiable agent at present.

Web site: http://appft1.uspto.gov/netahtml/PTO/search-bool.html

- **Antineoplastic drug**

  Inventor(s): Li, Hongfen; (Beijing, CN)

  Correspondence: Fay, Sharpe, Fagan, Minnich & Mckee, Llp; 1100 Superior Avenue, Seventh Floor; Cleveland; OH; 44114; US

  Patent Application Number: 20040109904

  Date filed: January 29, 2004

  Abstract: A unique class of anti-neoplastic compositions are described. The compositions contain certain Chinese medicinal herbs: Panax ginsing, Poria cocos, Atractylodes macrocephala, Angelic sinensis, Astragalus membranaceus, Curcuma zedoaria, Scutellaria baicalensis, Coptis chinenisis, Glycyrrhiza uralenisis, Crataegus pinatifida, Hordeum vulgare, Schisandra chinensis, Hedyotis diffusa, Ophiophogon japonicus, and Lobelia chinesis lour. Extensive testing indicates an effective treatment rate of 69.7% and 84.3% when used in combination with **radiotherapy** or chemotherapy. The animal trials conducted demonstrate that the anti-neoplastic compositions increase the activity of NK cells, and reduce and prevent metastasis of tumors under stress conditions.

Excerpt(s): The present invention relates to compositions for treatment of cancer and specifically, tumors. More particularly, the present invention is directed to anti-neoplastic compositions comprising a particular combination of herbs. According to the data released by the Ministry of Public Health of China, cancer was ranked as the number one cause of death in urban areas of China in 1990. More than one million patients die from cancer every year in mainland China. In the United States, one person dies from cancer every minute. And in the United States, there are 3 million cancer patients, one-third of which will eventually die from this disease. At present, more than 100 different types of cancer have been identified. Although operation, **radiotherapy** and chemotherapy are used as the main therapeutics, it is well known that the treatment of middle and late stage cancer is very difficult. There are many patients whose cancer has progressed such that they are inoperable. Furthermore, chemotherapy and **radiotherapy** do not always result in the desired effect. Moreover, these treatment strategies have serious side effects, including weakness, anorexia, loss of hair, inhibition of the function of bone marrow hematopoiesis, impairment of liver and kidney and ovary function, etc. After such treatments, patients often relapse because the immune system is extremely suppressed, typically for ten hours after operation. It is therefore pertinent that a new therapeutic strategy is identified to enhance cancer treatment as well as reduce the side effects of operation, chemotherapy and **radiotherapy.**

Web site: http://appft1.uspto.gov/netahtml/PTO/search-bool.html

• **Brachytherapy device and method**

Inventor(s): Apple, Marc G.; (Fort Wayne, IN), Williams, John I.; (Fort Wayne, IN)

Correspondence: Gerald R. Black, ESQ.; Suite 160; 30590 Southfield Road; Southfield; MI; 48076; US

Patent Application Number: 20030233136

Date filed: April 24, 2003

Abstract: The present invention provides a system and method of applying low dose, localized **radiotherapy** which is effective to reduce or eliminate the formation of post-operative scar tissue at surgical sites, such as an epidural site after spinal surgery. In an exemplary embodiment, a device is implantable before closing a surgical site as a barrier, the device being designed to deliver a desired therapeutic amount of energy to particular tissue. The device can be a barrier layer, seed containment unit, radiospike, or catheter. The energy may be provided by the material of the device itself, or may be provided by an external source, such as by circulating radioactive fluid through the device itself. Various embodiments include additional components of the device which deliver drug or chemical agents to targeted tissue and/or shield components to prevent dosage to non-targeted tissue.

Excerpt(s): The present invention generally relates to energy therapy with brachytherapy systems, and the invention more particularly relates to devices and methods for localized treatment to minimize postoperative fibrosis/scarring at a variety of bodily sites, such as an epidural site. It also relates to devices and methods to treat cartilaginous (articular or discal) pathology in order to reduce pain or improve function. Surgical intervention is an established and effective treatment modality to manage acute and chronic spine abnormalities for which direct intervention can mechanically alter and alleviate anatomic dysmorphic elements, secondary injury responses, and functional inhibitions from autoimmune or inflammatory diseases. More specifically, surgical treatment in the form of decompressions (e.g. discectomy, laminotomy, laminectomy) and/or fusion, is often performed on one or more levels of the human spine to ameliorate or alleviate symptoms originating from disc herniation, foraminal and/or central stenosis, instability secondary to post-traumatic, degenerative, congenital, iatrogenic, or idiopathic conditions, epidural fibrosis, adhesive arachnoiditis, and compressive radiculopathy and myelopathy resulting from any form of space occupying lesion. Outcomes may not always be optimal to eliminate pain and/or spinal dysfunction. In fact, delayed recurrent pain and functional decline can often follow initial uncomplicated surgery in an average of 20-25% of patients, and up to as many as 40% of patients in some historical clinical series.

Web site: http://appft1.uspto.gov/netahtml/PTO/search-bool.html

- **CA IX-specific inhibitors**

Inventor(s): Pastorek, Jaromir; (Bratislava, SK), Pastorekova, Silvia; (Bratislava, SK), Scozzafava, Andrea; (Florence, IT), Supuran, Claudiu; (Florence, IT)

Correspondence: Leona L. Lauder; 465 California, Suite 450; San Francisco; CA; 94104-1840; US

Patent Application Number: 20040146955

Date filed: November 26, 2003

Abstract: Therapeutic methods for inhibiting the growth of preneoplastic/neoplastic vertebrate cells that abnormally express MN protein are disclosed. Screening assays are provided for identifying compounds, preferably membrane-impermeant compounds, which inhibit the enzymatic activity of MN protein/polypeptides and that are useful for treating patients with preneoplastic/neoplastic disease. Further methods are disclosed for the preparation of positively-charged, membrane-impermeant heterocyclic sulfonamide CA inhibitors with high affinity for the membrane-bound carbonic anhydrase CA IX. Preferred CA IX-specific inhibitors are aromatic and heterocylic sulfonamides, preferably that are membrane-impermeant. Particularly preferred CA IX-specific inhibitors are pyridinium derivatives of such aromatic and heterocyclic sulfonamides. The CA IX-specific inhibitors of the invention can also be used diagnostically/prognostically for preneoplastic/neoplastic disease, and for imaging use, for example, to detect precancerous cells, tumors and/or metastases. The CA IX-specific inhibitors can be labelled or conjugated to radioisotopes for **radiotherapy.** The CA IX-specific inhibitors may be combined with conventional therapeutic anti-cancer drugs, with other different inhibitors of cancer-related pathways, with bioreductive drugs, or with **radiotherapy** to enhance the efficiency of each treatment. The CA IX-specific inhibitors may also be combined with CA IX-specific antibodies, preferably monoclonal antibodies or biologically active antibody fragments, more preferably humanized or fully human CA IX monoclonal antibodies or biologically active fragments or such monoclonal antibodies. Still further, the CA IX-specific inhibitors can be used for gene therapy coupled to vectors for targeted delivery to preneoplastic/neoplastic cells expressing CA IX on their surfaces.

Excerpt(s): This application claims priority from U.S. Provisional Application Nos. 60/429,089 (filed on Nov. 26, 2002), 60/489,473 (filed on Jul. 22, 2003) and 60/515,140 (filed on Oct. 28, 2003). The present invention is in the general area of medical genetics and in the fields of chemistry, biochemical engineering, and oncology. More specifically, it relates to the use of organic and inorganic compounds, preferably aromatic and heterocyclic sulfonamides, to treat preneoplastic and/or neoplastic diseases by specifically inhibiting the carbonic anhydrase activity of the oncoprotein now known alternatively as the MN protein, the MN/CA IX isoenzyme, the MN/G250 protein or simply MN/CA IX or CA IX or MN. The present invention also relates to methods of treating preneoplastic and/or neoplastic diseases characterized by MN/CA IX overexpression by administering cell membrane-impermeant, inhibitors of MN/CA IX, preferably pyridinium derivatives of aromatic and heterocyclic sulfonamides. The invention further concerns diagnostic/prognostic methods including imaging methods, for preneoplastic/neoplastic diseases, using the disclosed potent CA IX-specific inhibitors, and gene therapy with vectors conjugated to said inhibitors. The instant inventors, Dr. Silvia Pastorekova and Dr. Jaromir Pastorek, with Dr. Jan Zavada ["Zavada et al."], discovered MN/CA IX, a cancer related cell surface protein originally named MN. [73, 123; Zavada et al., U.S. Pat. No. 5,387,676 (Feb. 7, 1995).] Zavada et al., WO 93/18152 (published Sep. 16, 1993) and Zavada et al., WO 95/34650 (published Dec. 21, 1995) disclosed the discovery of the MN gene and protein and the strong association of MN gene expression and tumorigenicity led to the creation of methods that are both diagnostic/prognostic and therapeutic for cancer and precancerous conditions. Zavada et al. disclosed further aspects of the MN/CA IX protein and the MN/CA9 gene in Zavada et al., WO 00/24913 (published May 4, 2000).

Web site: http://appft1.uspto.gov/netahtml/PTO/search-bool.html

- **Cartridge for marker delivery device and marker delivery device**

  Inventor(s): Otsuka, Tetsuya; (Oita, JP)

  Correspondence: Oblon, Spivak, Mcclelland, Maier & Neustadt, P.C.; 1940 Duke Street; Alexandria; VA; 22314; US

  Patent Application Number: 20040097780

  Date filed: November 12, 2003

  Abstract: A new cartridge for a marker delivery device used in **radiotherapy** is provided. The cartridge has a transparent cartridge body that holds the marker inside it and permits external visual observation of the marker, and has an outer tube that is fitted on an outer circumference of the cartridge body, the outer tube is slidable in the longitudinal direction of the cartridge body, with this outer tube's sliding the cartridge body is exposable. The marker delivery device is suitable for implanting the marker in a flexible coil shape, made of X-ray-opaque or ultrasonic-wave opaque metal into the human body. And the cartridge of the device is capable of implanting a coil-shaped marker long enough in size compared with that of tissues, which permits, in marker-assisted ultrasonic imaging, to assess the size of the tissues accurately.

  Excerpt(s): The present invention relates to new and useful improvements in therapeutic material delivery device (vehicle) for delivering (implanting) a therapeutic material such as a coiled or capsulated radioactive source to an organism for **radiotherapy,** for example, of a patient suffering prostate cancer. The present invention also relates to new and useful improvements in marker delivery device for delivering a marker into an objected organ or tissue, prior to implanting a therapeutic material, in order to locate exactly the cancerous part to which **radiotherapy** is to be applied. Radiotherapy (brachytherapy) refers to a treatment made by allowing a radioactive beam to radiate to a morbid tissue suffering a prostate cancer, an esophagus cancer, or the like. **Radiotherapy** includes external beam radiation treatment and close-distance radiation treatment.

  Web site: http://appft1.uspto.gov/netahtml/PTO/search-bool.html

- **Compositions and methods for treating cancer using cytotoxic CD44 antibody immunoconjugates and radiotherapy**

Inventor(s): Adolf, Guenther; (Vienna, AT), Baumann, Michael; (Dresden, DE), Heider, Karl-Heinz; (Stockerau, AT)

Correspondence: Boehringer Ingelheim Corporation; 900 Ridgebury Road; P. O. Box 368; Ridgefield; CT; 06877; US

Patent Application Number: 20040120949

Date filed: November 7, 2003

Abstract: The invention relates to the combined use of antibodies conjugated to cytotoxic compounds and **radiotherapy** in cancer therapy, pharmaceutical compositions comprising such compounds, and methods of cancer treatment. In a preferred embodiment, the antibody is specific for the tumor-associated antigen CD44v6 and is linked to a maytansinoid. The **radiotherapy** may be external beam **radiotherapy** or radioimmunotherapy.

Excerpt(s): The priority benefit of EP 02 024 881.1, filed Nov. 8, 2002 and U.S. Provisional Application No. 60/429,516, filed Nov. 8, 2003 are hereby claimed, both of which are incorporated by reference herein. The invention relates to the combined use of conjugates of antibodies with cytotoxic compounds and **radiotherapy** in cancer therapy, pharmaceutical compositions comprising such compounds, and methods of cancer treatment. There have been numerous attempts to improve the efficacy of anti-neoplastic drugs by conjugating such drugs to antibodies against tumor-associated antigens in order to elevate local concentration of the drug by targeted delivery to the tumor. Many of these approaches have met limited success, and several reasons have been discussed in the literature to explain the failure. For anticancer drugs acting stoichometrically, e.g. doxorubicin or methotrexate, relatively high intracellular concentrations are necessary to exert the required cytotoxicity. These concentrations are thought to be difficult to achieve with many antibody-drug conjugates because of: (a) insufficient potency of many common anticancer drugs, (b) low cell surface concentration of antigen targets, (c) inefficient internalization of antigen-antibody complexes into the target cell, and (d) inefficient release of free drug from the conjugate inside the target cell (Chari, R V J et al., Immunoconjugates containing novel maytansinoids: promising anticancer drugs. Cancer Research 52: 127-31, 1992).

Web site: http://appft1.uspto.gov/netahtml/PTO/search-bool.html

- **Concentrated irradiation type radiotherapy apparatus**

Inventor(s): Ozaki, Masahiro; (Otawara-shi, JP)

Correspondence: Oblon, Spivak, Mcclelland, Maier & Neustadt, P.C.; 1940 Duke Street; Alexandria; VA; 22314; US

Patent Application Number: 20040034269

Date filed: August 14, 2003

Abstract: A concentrated irradiation type **radiotherapy** apparatus comprises a radiation source, a multi-channeled radiation detector, a rotating mechanism, an image reconstruction unit, a multi-leaf collimator disposed between the radiation source and the subject to trim the radioactive rays in arbitrary shapes and including a plurality of first leaves and a plurality of second leaves each disposed to be individually movable forwards/backwards and each having a strip shape and in which types of the first leaves are different from those of the second leaves.

Excerpt(s): This application is based upon and claims the benefit of priority from the prior Japanese Patent Applications No. 2002-236504, filed Aug. 14, 2002; No. 2002-236505, filed Aug. 14, 2002; and No. 2002-236506, filed Aug. 14, 2002, the entire contents of all of which are incorporated herein by reference. The present invention relates to a concentrated irradiation type **radiotherapy** apparatus including an X-ray computer tomography function. An X-ray computer tomography apparatus reconstructs image data based on data transmitted through a subject. Diversion of the X-ray computer tomography apparatus to a concentrated irradiation type **radiotherapy** apparatus has been studied. For this, an X-ray tube is replaced with that having high-dose specifications. A multi-leaf collimator is added before the X-ray tube. The multi-leaf collimator includes a plurality of leaves which can individually move forwards/backwards. By forward/backward control of the leaves, it is possible to trim an X-ray in a shape in accordance with a shape of a treatment object.

Web site: http://appft1.uspto.gov/netahtml/PTO/search-bool.html

- **Delivery for interstitial radiotherapy using hollow seeds**

  Inventor(s): Lamoureux, Gary A.; (Woodbury, CT), Terwilliger, Richard A.; (Southbury, CT)

  Correspondence: Fliesler Meyer, Llp; Four Embarcadero Center; Suite 400; San Francisco; CA; 94111; US

  Patent Application Number: 20040102672

  Date filed: November 18, 2003

  Abstract: A delivery system and method for interstitial radiation therapy uses a seed strand composed of a plurality of tubular shaped, hollow radioactive seeds with a bore. The seed strand as assembled with a material provided in the bore and between the spaced seeds is axially stiff and radially flexible and is bioabsorbable in living tissue.

  Excerpt(s): This application is a divisional application of, and claims priority to U.S. patent application Ser. No. 10/132,930, filed Apr. 26, 2002, which claims priority to U.S. Provisional Patent Application No. 60/336,329, filed Nov. 2, 2001; and U.S. Provisional Patent Application No. 60/360,260 filed Feb. 26, 2002, all of which are incorporated herein by reference. U.S. patent application Ser. No. 10/035,083 entitled "Delivery System and Method for Interstitial Radiation Therapy," by Terwilliger, et al., filed Dec. 28, 2001 (Attorney Docket No. WORLD-01000US1). U.S. Patent Application No. 60/360,241 entitled "Delivery System and Method for Interstitial Radiation Therapy Using Seed Strands Constructed With Preformed Strand Housing," by Terwilliger et al., filed Feb. 26, 2002 (Attorney Docket No. WORLD1000US2).

  Web site: http://appft1.uspto.gov/netahtml/PTO/search-bool.html

- **Device and methods for sequential, regional delivery of multiple cytotoxic agents and directed assembly of wound repair tissues**

Inventor(s): Brekke, John H.; (Duluth, MN), Gubbe, John H.; (Duluth, MN)

Correspondence: Alan D. Kamrath; Rider Bennett, Llp; Suite 2000; 333 South Seventh Street; Minneapolis; MN; 55402; US

Patent Application Number: 20040126426

Date filed: October 21, 2003

Abstract: An implantable delivery system includes a macrostructure formed of bioresorbable material selected from a group of alphahydroxy acids and defined to include an internal architecture of intercommunicating void spaces. A first cytotoxic agent in the preferred form of cisplatin is joined to the macrostructure during formation. A microstructure in the preferred form of a blend of high molecular weight hyaluronic acid conjugated with a second cytotoxic agent in the preferred form of paclitaxel and of pure high molecular weight hyaluronic acid is invested in the void spaces. Thus, when implanted, the paclitaxel and cisplatin are released sequentially, each initially at high level concentrations followed by lower release. **Radiotherapy** can be begun after the release of the paclitaxel has been completed but while the cisplatin is being released.

Excerpt(s): The present invention generally relates to devices and methods for treatment of cancer and particularly breast cancer and specifically to devices and methods for the regional delivery of multiple cytotoxic agents in a programmable, sequential manner and for the directed assembly of wound repair tissues. Every adult is at risk for breast cancer. One in nine women who live to the age of 90 will be treated for breast cancer at some time in her life, and more than 180,000 women in the United States were diagnosed with the disease in 2000. Although breast cancer is rare in men, it does occur: an estimated 1,400 cases will be diagnosed in American men in the year 2002. In 1999, approximately 43,000 women died from the disease according to the American Cancer Society. Breast cancer is the most common form of cancer in women and ranks as the second leading cause of cancer deaths among women of all ages. Breast cancer is the number one cause of cancer death for women aged 29-59. Despite the development of innovative systemic medical therapies for the treatment of breast cancer, local disease control is still a problem. This is also true for other common malignancies such as prostatic carcinoma and colon cancer. Under most current systemic therapy protocols, chemotherapeutic drugs are given to patients systemically as an adjunct to the removal of malignant tumors. Even with preoperative and postoperative radiation therapy, local recurrences often develop. Because of the toxicity of the drugs, the attainable concentration of an active drug in the tumor after systemically-administered chemotherapy is, in part, restricted by the dose-limiting systemic toxicity tolerated by the body. Pre-operative high dose chemotherapy or radiation therapy can adversely affect normal tissue healing, add morbidity and expense and may allow primary tumors that are insensitive to preoperative treatment an opportunity to extend locally, to distant sites, or both.

Web site: http://appft1.uspto.gov/netahtml/PTO/search-bool.html

- **Extract of lentinus lepideus and composition comprising the same having immune enhancing activity**

Inventor(s): Choi, Jeong-June; (Icheon, KR), Jeon, Hyang; (Seoul, KR), Jin, Mirim; (Seoul, KR), Jung, Hyung-Jin; (Seoul, KR), Kim, Sunyoung; (Seoul, KR), Shin, Sung-Seup; (Seoul, KR)

Correspondence: Foley And Lardner; Suite 500; 3000 K Street NW; Washington; DC; 20007; US

Patent Application Number: 20040001856

Date filed: March 10, 2003

Abstract: The present invention is related to pharmaceutical composition comprising an extract of Lentinus lepideus prepared by inventive preparation showing immune enhancing and immune modulating activity.The composition according to the present invention are useful in the prevention or treatment of infectious diseases caused by bacteria or virus and treatment of immune-suppressed patients, suppressed immunity due to anti-cancer therapy such as chemotherapy and **radiotherapy** and the patients suffered from AIDS or cancer and immune enhancing agent. Moreover, present composition can be used in preventing bacterial infection or viral disease such as influenza and also can be used for adjuvants of vaccine.

Excerpt(s): This application is a continuation patent application of U.S. Provisional Application No. 60/362,638 and No. 60/372,056 filed on Mar. 8, 2002 and Apr. 12, 2002, which were now abandoned. The present invention related to an extract of Lentinus lepideus and a composition comprising the same having immune enhancing activity. Mycelia or fruit bodies of various mushrooms have been found to contain biological response modifiers (BRMs). Indeed, various extracts from medicinal mushrooms have been reported to exhibit antiviral, antibiotic, anti-inflammatory, hypoglycemic, and hypotensive activities (Kabir Y et al.; J. Nutr. Sci. Vitaminol. (Tokyo), 33, pp341-346, 1987). The most widely known effects of the compounds isolated from above described fungi are anti-tumor and immune modulating activities of BRMs isolated from Ganoderma lucidum, Lentinus edodes, and Grifola frondosa. For example, oral administration of powdered fruit bodies of Lentinus edodes has been found to be effective in inhibiting carcinoma growth in C3H/He mice (Nanba H and Kuroda H, Chem. Pharm. Bull. (Tokyo), 35, pp2459-2464, 1987). It has been reported that the cytotoxic activity of NK (Natural Killer) and LAK (Lymphokine-Activated Killer) cells was significantly increased by administration of Lentinus edodes (Nanba H and Kuroda H, Chem. Pharm. Bull. (Tokyo), 35, pp2459-2464, 1987; Nanba H et al.; Chem. Pharm. Bull. (Tokyo), 35, pp2453-2458, 1987). In administering mice pretreated with immunosuppressive carcinogen, with mushroom-enriched diet comprising Lentinus edodes, Grifola frondosa, and oyster mushroom, the level of the chemotactic activity of macrophage and the capability of lymphocyte to proliferate in response to mitogen were restored to the normal level (Kurashige S et al.; Immunopharmacol. Immunotoxicol., 19, pp175-183, 1997). A number of such bioactive molecules have been reported in numerous other mushroom species.

Web site: http://appft1.uspto.gov/netahtml/PTO/search-bool.html

- **Gastrin releasing peptide compounds**

Inventor(s): Cappelletti, Enrico; (Sergno, IT), Lattuada, Luciano; (Bussero, IT), Linder, Karen E.; (Kingston, NJ), Marinelli, Ed; (Lawrenceville, NJ), Nanjappan, Palaniappa; (Dayton, NJ), Raju, Natarajan; (Kendall Park, NJ), Swenson, Rolf E.; (Princeton, NJ), Tweedle, Michael; (Princeton, NJ)

Correspondence: Kramer Levin Naftalis & Frankel Llp; Intellectual Property Department; 919 Third Avenue; New York; NY; 10022; US

Patent Application Number: 20040136906

Date filed: January 13, 2003

Abstract: New and improved compounds for use in radiodiagnostic imaging or **radiotherapy** having the formula M-N--O--P-G, wherein M is the metal chelator (in the form complexed with a metal radionuclide or not), N--O--P is the linker, and G is the GRP receptor targeting peptide. Methods for imaging a patient and/or providing **radiotherapy** to a patient using the compounds of the invention are also provided. A method for preparing a diagnostic imaging agent from the compound is further provided. A method for preparing a radiotherapeutic agent is further provided.

Excerpt(s): This invention relates to novel radionuclide-labeled gastrin releasing peptide (GRP) compounds which are useful as diagnostic imaging agents or radiotherapeutic agents. These GRP compounds include the use of novel linkers between a metal chelator and the targeting peptide, which provides for improved pharmacokinetics. The use of radiopharmaceuticals (e.g., diagnostic imaging agents, radiotherapeutic agents) to detect and treat cancer is well known. In more recent years, the discovery of site-directed radiopharmaceuticals for cancer detection and/or treatment has gained popularity and continues to grow as the medical profession better appreciates the specificity, efficacy and utility of such compounds. These newer radiopharmaceutical agents typically consist of a targeting agent connected to a metal chelator, which can be chelated to (e.g., complexed with) a diagnostic metal radionuclide such as, for example, technetium or indium, or a therapeutic metal radionuclide such as, for example, lutetium, yttrium, or rhenium. The role of the metal chelator is to hold (i.e., chelate) the metal radionuclide as the radiopharmaceutical agent is delivered to the desired site. A metal chelator which does not bind strongly to the metal radionuclide would render the radiopharmaceutical agent ineffective for its desired use since the metal radionuclide would therefore not reach its desired site. Thus, further research and development led to the discovery of metal chelators, such as that reported in U.S. Pat. No. 5,662,885 to Pollak et. al., hereby incorporated by reference, which exhibited strong binding affinity for metal radionuclides and the ability to conjugate with the targeting agent. Subsequently, the concept of using a "spacer" to create a physical separation between the metal chelator and the targeting agent was further introduced, for example in U.S. Pat. No. 5,976,495 to Pollak et. al., hereby incorporated by reference.

Web site: http://appft1.uspto.gov/netahtml/PTO/search-bool.html

- **Imaging device for radiation treatment applications**

  Inventor(s): Graf, Ulrich Martin; (Mettmenstetten, CH), Kopels, Robert; (Cupertion, CA), Mansfield, Stan; (Sunnyvale, CA)

  Correspondence: Blakely Sokoloff Taylor & Zafman; 12400 Wilshire Boulevard, Seventh Floor; Los Angeles; CA; 90025; US

  Patent Application Number: 20040068169

  Date filed: October 5, 2002

  Abstract: A **radiotherapy** clinical treatment machine is described having a rotatable gantry and an imaging device with articulating robotic arms to provide variable positioning and clearance for radiation treatment applications. According to one aspect of the invention, a first and a second robotic arms are pivotally coupled to the rotatable gantry, allowing the robotic arms to maneuver independently from the rotatable gantry.

  Excerpt(s): The present invention pertains in general to radiation medicine. In particular, the invention involves imaging devices. A technique to perform radiation therapy uses a **radiotherapy** device to target a radiation treatment beam onto a target volume (e.g., a tumor) of a patient. Such, radiation treatment beams emulate from a treatment radiation source, such as a megavoltage x-ray source. Here, the primary purpose of the x-ray source is to provide a sufficient dose of radiation to treat the target volume. Additionally such a **radiotherapy** device may include a separate imaging device used to image anatomy in the region of the target volume. This imaging device may use an imaging radiation source, such as a kilovoltage x-ray source. A radiation imager or detector is also used to capture the radiation after it passes through the patient. Information obtained from this imager can be used to adjust or verify correct positioning of patient anatomy and particularly of the target volume relative to the treatment beam. The imaging device including an x-ray source and imager may be attached to a gantry that houses the treatment radiation source. One such design is typically embedded in a wall in a treatment area. In another design, the x-ray source and imager are attached inside a large diameter bearing (e.g., a cylinder) that the patient must enter for treatment.

  Web site: http://appft1.uspto.gov/netahtml/PTO/search-bool.html

- **Intensity modulated radiotherapy inverse planning algorithm**

  Inventor(s): Luo, Chunsong; (Miami, FL)

  Correspondence: Venable, Baetjer, Howard And Civiletti, Llp; P.O. Box 34385; Washington; DC; 20043-9998; US

  Patent Application Number: 20040001569

  Date filed: April 29, 2003

  Abstract: A method in a computer for optimizing a dosage of intensity modulated **radiotherapy** (IMRT) comprises the steps of: dividing a three dimensional (3D) volume into a grid of dose voxels, wherein each dose voxel receives a dose of radiation from at least one pencil beam having a pencil beam weight and a gantry angle; selecting a first set of dose voxels from the 3D volume positioned within at least one of a planning target volume (PTV), organs at risk (OAR), and normal tissue in a neighborhood of the PTV; choosing a dose matrix from the first set of dose voxels; constructing a beam weight vector of individual beam weights for each pencil beam at each gantry angle; calculating a transfer matrix representing a dose deposition to the dose voxels from each pencil beam with unit beam weight; inverting the transfer matrix; performing a matrix multiplication of the inverted transfer matrix and the dose matrix and populating the beam weight vector with the results of the matrix multiplication; and iteratively modifying a plurality of doses in the dose matrix within a given range, wherein the range has a specific probability distribution function of acceptable dose values, and repeating the matrix multiplication until the negative weights in the beam weight vector are substantially eliminated, resulting in an optimized set of doses.

Excerpt(s): This application claims the benefit of U.S. Provisional Patent Application No. 60/375,828, Confirmation No. 3165, filed Apr. 29, 2002, of common inventorship and assignee, the contents of which are incorporated by reference in their entirety. The present invention relates generally to optimizing a dosage of intensity modulated **radiotherapy** (IMRT), and more particularly to minimizing the negative beam in IMRT. Intensity modulated **radiotherapy** (IMRT) is a method of treating cancer that is particularly useful when the cancer is entangled with critical organs, such as the spinal cord. IMRT allows for a balanced dose to the target, i.e. the cancerous area, while sparing the surrounding critical organs.

Web site: http://appft1.uspto.gov/netahtml/PTO/search-bool.html

- **Membrane-permeant peptide complexes for medical imaging, diagnostics, and pharmaceutical therapy**

Inventor(s): Piwnica-Worms, David; (Ladue, MO)

Correspondence: Michael T. Marrah; Sonnenschein Nath & Rosenthal; Wacker Drive Station, Sears Tower; P.O. Box #061080; Chicago; IL; 60606-1080; US

Patent Application Number: 20030219375

Date filed: February 18, 2003

Abstract: Methods and compositions for medical imaging, evaluating intracellular processes and components, **radiotherapy** of intracellular targets, and drug delivery by the use of novel cell membrane-permeant peptide conjugate coordination and covalent complexes having target cell specificity are provided. Kits for conjugating radionuclides and other metals to peptide coordination complexes are also provided.

Excerpt(s): This is a divisional and claims the priority of co-pending U.S. application Ser. No. 09/557,465, filed on Apr. 25, 2000, which is incorporated herein by reference as if restated in full. Ser. No. 09/557,465 is a continuance in part of Ser. No. 09/376,093 filed Jun. 18, 1999 and now U.S. Pat. No. 6,348,185 which claims the priority of provisional application Serial No. 60/090,087 filed Jun. 20, 1998. The present invention broadly relates to the field of medicine. More specifically, the present invention relates to the fields of medical imaging, diagnostics, and pharmaceutical therapy. The present invention provides methods and compositions for medical imaging, evaluating intracellular processes, **radiotherapy** of intracellular targets, and drug delivery by the use of novel cell membrane-permeant peptide conjugate coordination and covalent complexes having target cell specificity. The present invention also provides kits for conjugating radionuclides and other metals to the peptide coordination complexes. Radiopharmaceuticals provide vital information that aids in the diagnosis and therapy of a variety of medical diseases (Hom and Katzenellenbogen, Nucl. Med. Biol. 24:485-498, 1997). Data on tissue shape, function, and localization within the body are relayed by use of one of the various radionuclides, which can be either free chemical species, such as the gas.sup.133Xe or the ions.sup.123I.sup.-, and.sup.201Tl.sup.-, covalently or coordinately bound as part of a larger organic or inorganic moiety, the images being generated by the distribution of radioactive decay of the nuclide. Radionuclides that are most useful for medical imaging include.sup.11C (t.sub.1/2 20.3 min),.sup.13N (t.sub.1/2 9.97 min),.sup.15O (t.sub.1/2 2.03 min),.sup.18F (t.sub.1/2 109.7 min),.sup.64Cu (t.sub.1/2 12 h),.sup.68Ga (t.sub.1/2 68 min) for positron emission tomography (PET) and.sup.67Ga (t.sub.1/2 68 min),.sup.99mTc (t.sub.1/2 6 h),.sup.123I (t.sub.1/2 13 h) and.sup.201Tl (t.sub.1/2 73.5 h) for single photon emission computed tomography (SPECT) (Hom and Katzenellenbogen, Nucl. Med. Biol. 24:485-498, 1997).

Web site: http://appft1.uspto.gov/netahtml/PTO/search-bool.html

- **Method and apparatus including use of metalloporphyrins for subsequent optimization of radiosurgery and radiotherapy**

Inventor(s): Adair, Edwin L.; (Castle Pines Village, CO)

Correspondence: Sheridan Ross PC; 1560 Broadway; Suite 1200; Denver; CO; 80202

Patent Application Number: 20040202610

Date filed: April 30, 2004

Abstract: An apparatus and method for subsequent optimization of radiosurgery and **radiotherapy** is provided. The invention includes administering a metalloporphyrin to the patient, and then creating a 3-dimensional mapping of tissue through use of PET or SPECT. Malignant and pre-malignant tissue has an affinity for the metalloporphyrin. During treatment, real-time images are also provided which are compared to the previous 3-dimensional mapping. Creation of the real-time images is also achieved through PET or SPECT wherein a metalloporphyrin is administered to the patient. Total administration of radiation is calculated by summing radiation from the metalloporphyrins and from the radiosurgery/radiotherapy. The amount of radiation delivered by the metalloporphyrins and by the radiosurgery/radiotherapy are adjustable based on a patient's response to the dual delivery.

Excerpt(s): This application is a continuation-in-part of co-pending application Ser. No. 10/176,558, filed on Jun. 21, 2002, entitled "Method of Cancer Screening Primarily Utilizing Non-Invasive Cell Collection, Fluorescence Detection Techniques, and Radio Tracing Detection Techniques", the disclosure of which is hereby incorporated by reference herein. This invention relates to cancer screening and cancer treatment, and more particularly, to the use of metalloporphyrins for subsequent optimization of radiosurgery and/or **radiotherapy.** There are a number of prior art methods and apparatuses which are used in the detection and treatment of cancer. Fluorescent markers have been used to help identify cancerous tissue within a patient. Radio tracers or markers have also been used in the detection and treatment of cancer.

Web site: http://appft1.uspto.gov/netahtml/PTO/search-bool.html

- **METHOD AND ASSEMBLY FOR CONTAINING RADIOACTIVE MATERIALS**

Inventor(s): McDaniel, Benjamin David; (Newport Beach, CA), O'Hara, Michael Dennis; (Stewartsville, NJ)

Correspondence: Audley A. Ciamporcero JR.; Johnson & Johnson; One Johnson & Johnson Plaza; New Brunswick; NJ; 08933-7003; US

Patent Application Number: 20030220534

Date filed: March 14, 2001

Abstract: A radioactive substance absorber is incorporated into an intravascular **radiotherapy** source ribbon assembly to prevent the migration of radioactive matter throughout the assembly container. The radioactive substance absorber comprises carbon in various forms and configurations. The radioactive substance absorber is positioned in proximity to the source core and absorbs radioactive materials which break free from the source core, thereby containing the radioactive material.

Excerpt(s): The present invention relates to brachytherapy devices, and more particularly to a method and assembly for containing the radioisotopes or other radioactive materials utilized in brachytherapy devices. Percutaneous transluminal coronary angioplasty (PTCA) is a therapeutic medical procedure used to increase blood flow through an artery and is the predominant treatment for coronary vessel stenosis. The increasing popularity of the PTCA procedure is attributable to its relatively high success rate and its minimal invasiveness compared with coronary by-pass surgery. Patients treated utilizing PTCA; however, may suffer from restenosis. Restenosis refers to the re-narrowing of an artery after a successful angioplasty procedure. Restenosis usually occurs within the initial six months after an angioplasty. Early attempts to alleviate the effect of restenosis included repeat PTCA procedures or by-pass surgery, with attendant high cost and added patient risk. More recent attempts to prevent restenosis by use of drugs, mechanical devices, and other experimental procedures have limited long term success. Stents, for example, dramatically reduce acute reclosure and slow the effects of smooth muscle cell proliferation by enlarging the maximal luminal diameter, but otherwise do nothing substantial to slow the proliferative response to the angioplasty induced injury.

Web site: http://appft1.uspto.gov/netahtml/PTO/search-bool.html

- **Method for combining proton beam irradiation and magnetic resonance imaging**

Inventor(s): Bucholz, Richard D.; (St. Louis, MO), Miller, D. Douglas; (St. Louis, MO)

Correspondence: Senniger Powers Leavitt And Roedel; One Metropolitan Square; 16th Floor; ST Louis; MO; 63102; US

Patent Application Number: 20040199068

Date filed: April 16, 2004

Abstract: A method which coordinates proton beam irradiation with an open magnetic resonance imaging (MRI) unit to achieve near-simultaneous, noninvasive localization and **radiotherapy** of various cell lines in various anatomic locations. A reference image of the target aids in determining a treatment plan and repositioning the patient within the MRI unit for later treatments. The patient is located within the MRI unit so that the target and the proton beam are coincident. MRI monitors the location of the target. Target irradiation occurs when the target and the proton beam are coincident as indicated by the MRI monitoring. The patient rotates relative to the radiation source. The target again undergoes monitoring and selective irradiation. The rotation and selective irradiation during MRI monitoring repeats according to the treatment plan.

Excerpt(s): This application is a continuation of U.S. application Ser. No. 09/754,852, filed Jan. 4, 2001 which claims benefit of U.S. application serial No. 60/179,271, filed Jan. 31, 2000. The present invention relates to systems for localization and **radiotherapy** of various cell lines in various anatomic locations. In particular, this invention relates to a system which coordinates proton beam irradiation with an open magnetic resonance imaging (MRI) unit to achieve near-simultaneous, noninvasive localization and **radiotherapy** of various cell lines in various anatomic locations by maintaining coincidence between the target and the proton beam. Proton beam irradiation therapy treats tumors found in selected locations that are not subject to significant physiologic motion. Examples of such tumors include prostatic cancer, spinal chordomas, and certain retinal or orbital tumors. The proton beam generated by a medical cyclotron has similar biological activity for the destruction of tumors as standard radiation therapy techniques to target a fixed tumor site with minimal radiotoxicity to the surrounding normal tissues. Because protons of a specific energy have a specific penetration depth, adjusting the specific energy of the protons manipulates the distance the proton beam travels into the patient. Because protons deposit most of their energy at the end of the penetration depth, the highest concentration of radiation occurs in the area around the penetration depth. This area is known as the Bragg peak of the proton beam.

Web site: http://appft1.uspto.gov/netahtml/PTO/search-bool.html

- **Method of imaging cell death in vivo**

  Inventor(s): Blankenberg, Francis G.; (Menlo Park, CA), Green, Allan M.; (Cambridge, MA), Steinmetz, Neil; (Atlantis, FL), Strauss, H. William; (West Harrison, NY)

  Correspondence: Lahive & Cockfield, LLP.; 28 State Street; Boston; MA; 02109; US

  Patent Application Number: 20040170603

  Date filed: March 5, 2004

  Abstract: A method of imaging apoptosis in vivo, using radiolabeled annexin, is described. Methods for tumor **radiotherapy** are also provided.

  Excerpt(s): This application is a divisional application of U.S. patent application Ser. No. 10/114,926 filed Apr. 3, 2002, pending, and claims priority to U.S. Provisional Patent Application Serial No. 60/281,352 filed Apr. 3, 2001. The entire contents of the foregoing applications are incorporated herein by reference. The present invention relates to a method of imaging cell death in vivo. In particular, it relates to the use of radiolabeled annexin to image regions of cell death in a mammal using gamma ray imaging. Amann, E. and Brosius, J., Gene 40:183 (1985).

  Web site: http://appft1.uspto.gov/netahtml/PTO/search-bool.html

- **Monoterpene as a chemopreventive agent for regression of mammalian nervous system cell tumors, use of monoterpene for causing regression and inhibition of nervous system cell tumors, and method for administration of monoterpene perillyl alcohol**

  Inventor(s): Alves Brown, Gilda; (Rio de Janeiro, BR), Da Costa Carvalho, Maria da Gloria; (Rio de Janeiro, BR), Da Fonseca Quirico Dos Santos, Thereza; (Rio de Janeiro, BR), Pereira Da Fonseca, Clovis Orlando; (Rio de Janeiro, BR)

  Correspondence: Jacobson Holman Pllc; 400 Seventh Street N.W.; Suite 600; Washington; DC; 20004; US

  Patent Application Number: 20040087651

  Date filed: December 13, 2002

Abstract: The present invention refers to a composition based on monoterpenes with chemopreventive and chemotherapeutic effects in malignant neoplasias of humans and animals containing from 0,03% to 30% of monoterpenes and 99,97% of solvents. Another objective of the present invention is an application of monoterpenes in inhibition of cell growth and metastasis control of primary tumors being applied in vitro and in vivo gliomas cell lines C6 and U 87 and A172. Further another objective of the present invention refers to a specific methods for applying the composition with chemopreventive and chemotherapeutic effects in humans and animals showing malignant neoplasias by inhalation and nebulization treatment, oral and intratumoral, followed or not by **radiotherapy** with dilutions from 0,03% to 30% of the monoterpene perillyl or its derived metabolites diluted in the solvents specified by the usual techniques.

  Excerpt(s): The present invention relates to treatment for mammalian nervous system cell tumors. In particular, the present invention relates to using of monoterpene perillyl alcohol to inhibit tumor formation and to cause tumor regression. The progress in treating most common solid malignancies has slowed due at least in part to the lack of new effective agents. This has led to a new emphasis on cancer prevention and on developing therapeutic agents with novel mechanisms. Recent data suggest that monoterpenes, a class of non-toxic compounds that act through novel mechanism, may be useful for both chemoprevention and treatment of cancer. These compounds have been shown to exert chemopreventive and chemotherapeutic activities in several tumor models and represent a new class of cancer therapeutic agents.

  Web site: http://appft1.uspto.gov/netahtml/PTO/search-bool.html

- **Multi-mode cone beam CT radiotherapy simulator and treatment machine with a flat panel imager**

  Inventor(s): Colbeth, Richard E.; (Los Altos, CA), Johnsen, Stanley W.; (Palo Alto, CA), Munro, Peter; (Mountain View, CA), Pavkovich, John M.; (Palo Alto, CA), Seppi, Edward J.; (Portola Valley, CA), Shapiro, Edward G.; (Menlo Park, CA)

  Correspondence: Blakely Sokoloff Taylor & Zafman; 12400 Wilshire Boulevard, Seventh Floor; Los Angeles; CA; 90025; US

  Patent Application Number: 20040120452

  Date filed: December 18, 2002

Abstract: A multi-mode cone beam computed tomography **radiotherapy** simulator and treatment machine is disclosed. The **radiotherapy** simulator and treatment machine both include a rotatable gantry on which is positioned a cone-beam radiation source and a flat panel imager. The flat panel imager captures x-ray image data to generate cone-beam CT volumetric images used to generate a therapy patient position setup and a treatment plan.

Excerpt(s): The present invention pertains in general to therapeutic radiology. In particular, the invention involves imaging devices. An objective of radiation therapy is to maximize the amount of radiation to a target volume (e.g., a cancerous tumor) and minimize the amount of radiation to healthy tissues and critical structures. The process of identifying the precise location of the target volume immediately prior to a dose of therapeutic radiation is key to the objective. Since each patient is treated over 30 to 40 fractionated sessions, then the time allowed for each session is relatively short, e.g. 10 to 15 minutes, so the process must be fast as well as accurate. In the case of electronic portal imaging, megavolt therapeutic X-rays emerging from the patient can be used to generate images. However, this method of target location generates images of low contrast and quality, in addition to incidentally damaging healthy tissue. As a result, imaging with megavoltage (MV) radiation is used primarily for portal verification, that is, to confirm that the treatment volume is being radiated.

Web site: http://appft1.uspto.gov/netahtml/PTO/search-bool.html

- **Novel chelating agents and conjugates thereof, their synthesis and use as diagnois and therapeutic agents**

Inventor(s): Hermann, Petr; (Prague, CZ), Lukes, Ivan; (Prague, CZ)

Correspondence: Henry M Feiereisen, Llc; 350 Fifth Avenue; Suite 4714; New York; NY; 10118; US

Patent Application Number: 20040167330

Date filed: January 20, 2004

Abstract: The present invention relates to novel bifunctional chelates that are based on asymmetrical cyclen derivatives. The chelates contain either three acetates and one methylphosphonic arm or three acetates and one methylphosphonic arm enabling to link the chelate through P-alkyl within phosphoric acid derivative or through P--O-alkyl within phosphonic derivative to any organic back-bone suited for targeting. Suitable targeting moieties are monoclonal antibodies, their fragments and recombinant derivatives such as single chain antibodies, diabodies, triabodies, humanized, human or chimeric variants but also peptides, aptamers, spiegelmers, nucleotides, anti sense oligomers and conventional small molecules. These novel bifunctional chelates are suited for the production of kits for the routine labelling of targeting moieties to be used in **radiotherapy** with radiometals such as Yttrium-90, or for Magnetic Resonance Imagining (MRI) using Gadolinium.

Excerpt(s): The present invention relates to novel bifunctional chelates that are based on asymmetrical cyclen derivatives. The chelates contain either three acetates and one methylphosphinic arm or three acetates and one methylphosphonic arm enabling to link the chelate through P-alkyl within phosphinic acid derivative or through P--O-alkyl within phosphonic derivative to any organic backbone suited for targeting. Suitable targeting moieties are monoclonal antibodies, their fragments and recombinant derivatives such as single chain antibodies, diabodies, triabodies, humanized, human or chimeric variants but also peptides, aptamers, spiegelmers, nucleotides, anti sense oligomers and conventional small molecules. These novel bifunctional chelates are suited for the production of kits for the routine labelling of targeting moieties to be used in **radiotherapy** with radiometals such as Yttrium-90, or for Magnetic Resonance Imaging (MRI) using Gadolinium. Polydentate ligands, such as DTPA (diethylenetriaminepentaacetic acid), macrocyclic TETA (1,4,8,11-tetraazacyclotetradecane-1,4,8,11-tetra- acetic acid), and DOTA (1,4,7,10-tetraazacyclododecane-1,4,7,10-tetraaceti- c acid) form thermodynamically and kinetically very stable metal chelate complexes even with labile metal ions as the first-row transition-metal divalent ions or trivalent lanthanides (Lindoy L. F.: Adv. Inorg. Chem. 1998, 45, 75; Wainwright K. P.: Coord. Chem. Rev. 1997, 166, 35; Lincoln S. F.: Coord. Chem. Rev. 1997, 166, 255; Meyer M., Dahaoui-Gindrey V., Lecomte C., Guilard R.: Coord. Chem. Rev. 1998, 178-180, 1313; Hancock R. D., Maumela H., de Sousa A. S.: Coord. Chem. Rev. 1996, 148, 315). The properties of macrocyclic ligands have been elaborated while designing both Gd.sup.3+ based magnetic resonance imaging (MRI) contrast agents (Parker D. in: Comprehensive Supramolecular Chemistry (Lehn J.-M., Ed.), Vol. 10, pp. 487-536. Pergamon Press, Oxford 1996; Aime S., Botta M., Fasano M., Terreno E.: Chem. Soc. Rev. 1998, 27, 19; Caravan P., Ellison J. J., Mc Murry T. J., Laufer R. B.: Chem. Rev. 1999, 99, 2293; Aime S., Botta M., Fasano M., Terreno E.: Acc. Chem. Res. 1999, 32, 941; Botta M.: Eur. J. Inorg. Chem. 2000, 399) as well as diagnostic and/or therapeutic radiopharmaceuticals based on metal radionuclides (Anderson C. J., Welch M. J.: Chem. Rev. 1999, 99, 2219; Volkert W. A., Hoffmann T. J.: Chem. Rev. 1999, 99, 2269; Reichert D. E., Lewis J. S., Anderson C. J.: Coord. Chem. Rev. 1999, 184, 3; Liu S., Edwards D. S.: Biocojugate Chem. 2601, 12, 7). For radiopharmaceutical use, targeting moieties have to be linked to the radio metal chelate complex. The chelate is called bifunctional due to its ability to bind to the targeting moiety on one hand and to complex the radiometal on the other hand. Targeting moieties such as monoclonal antibodies (Mabs) were described by Koehler and Milstein in mid seventies (Koehler G. and Milstein C.: Nature 1975, 256, 495-497). Since then, investigators tried to develop these proteins of unprecedented specificity as diagnostics and therapeutics. Success in the diagnostic area was achieved very fast, but only recently, despite of significant efforts of many research groups, the first therapeutically successful Mabs were approved by FDA and EMEA to treat cancer. So far, the Mabs approved for the therapy of cancer, are recombinantly manipulated chimeric or humanized Mabs inducing their therapeutic effects by interfering with cell surface receptor function (erb B2 receptor: Herceptin) or mediating ADCC and CDC via an appropriate Fc moiety (CD 20: ROCHE-Rituxan).

Web site: http://appft1.uspto.gov/netahtml/PTO/search-bool.html

- **Optimal configuration of photon and electron multileaf collimators in mixed beam radiotherapy**

Inventor(s): Svatos, Michelle Marie; (Oakland, CA)

Correspondence: Siemens Corporation; Attn: Elsa Keller, Legal Administrator; Intellectual Property Department; 170 Wood Avenue South; Iselin; NJ; 08830; US

Patent Application Number: 20040179648

Date filed: March 12, 2003

Abstract: A radiation therapy method that includes directing a beam along a beam path toward a treatment area. Performing a correction process on the beam, the process includes selectively collimating the beam based on a dose that takes into account bremsstrahlung interactions caused by the beam.

Excerpt(s): The present invention relates generally to radiation therapy devices, and more particularly, to a removable electron multileaf collimator for use in a radiation therapy device. Conventional radiation therapy typically involves directing a radiation beam at a tumor in a patient to deliver a predetermined dose of therapeutic radiation to the tumor according to an established treatment plan. This is typically accomplished using a radiation therapy device such as the device described in U.S. Pat. No. 5,668,847 issued Sep. 16, 1997 to Hernandez, the contents of which are incorporated herein for all purposes. The **radiotherapy** treatment of tumors involves three-dimensional treatment volumes which typically include segments of normal, healthy tissue and organs. Healthy tissue and organs are often in the treatment path of the radiation beam. This complicates treatment, because the healthy tissue and organs must be taken into account when delivering a dose of radiation to the tumor. While there is a need to minimize damage to healthy tissue and organs, there is an equally important need to ensure that the tumor receives an adequately high dose of radiation. Cure rates for many tumors are a sensitive function of the dose they receive. Therefore, it is important to closely match the radiation beam's shape and effects with the shape and volume of the tumor being treated.

Web site: http://appft1.uspto.gov/netahtml/PTO/search-bool.html

- **Patient positioning system for radiotherapy/radiosurgery based on magnetically tracking an implant**

Inventor(s): Erbel, Stephan; (Munchen, DE), Frohlich, Stephan; (Aschhem, DE), Vilsmeier, Stefan; (Kufstein, AT)

Correspondence: Renner, Otto, Boisselle & Sklar, Llp; Nineteenth Floor; 1621 Euclid Avenue; Cleveland; OH; 44115-2191; US

Patent Application Number: 20040102698

Date filed: August 4, 2003

Abstract: A method for positioning a patient or detecting a target volume in **radiotherapy** or radiosurgery includes positionally referencing at least one implant in the vicinity of the target volume and inductively stimulating the at least one implant. Emission from the at least one inductively stimulated implant is detected and a position of the at least one implant is determined based on the detected emission. The current position of the target volume is determined based on the determined position of the at least one implant. Further diagnostic, two-dimensional or three-dimensional image data sets can be recorded in accordance with breathing.

Excerpt(s): This application claims priority of U.S. Provisional Application No. 60/464,247, filed on Apr. 21, 2003, which is incorporated herein by reference in its entirety. The present invention relates to a method and a system for exactly positioning a patient in **radiotherapy** and/or radiosurgery and/or for taking into account shifts in internal structures of the patient caused by breathing, both during the actual treatment and while recording the image data necessary for said treatment. In **radiotherapy** and radiosurgery, major progress has been achieved in recent times in dosage planning. The aim is to use higher radiation doses that are applied to a target volume, for example, a tumor, as precisely as possible, without damaging the surrounding regions. Although dosage planning has been shown to be relatively successful, the use of higher doses, which in certain cases are even administered in a single or in a few fractions, is hindered by the fact that the patient or the section of the body to be treated can only be positioned relatively imprecisely. In order to avoid major damage to healthy tissue, exact positioning is essential.

Web site: http://appft1.uspto.gov/netahtml/PTO/search-bool.html

- **Pharmaceutically enhanced low-energy radiosurgery**

  Inventor(s): Morris, Kevin N.; (Denver, CO), Weil, Michael; (Fort Collins, CO)

  Correspondence: Leslie P. Kramer, ESQ.; Dorr, Carson, Sloan & Birney, P.C.; 3010 E. 6th Avenue; Denver; CO; 80206; US

  Patent Application Number: 20040006254

  Date filed: April 1, 2002

  Abstract: Contrast agents developed specifically for x-ray diagnostics provide dose-enhanced **radiotherapy** and radiosurgery. The presence of heavy elements, for example, gold or iron, from these contrast agents, even small quantities, leads to a major dose increase in target tissue when combined with in vivo calibration of the amount of contrast agent. The technique can also be used in combination with other techniques, such as focused x-rays, to achieve further enhancement of therapeutic ratio. The technique is enhanced by employing oil-based contrast agents, which will remain in the target much longer than conventional agents. Through optimization of the equipment it is possible to achieve very large ratios of dose in target to dose in healthy tissue.

  Excerpt(s): This application claims the benefit of U.S. Provisional Application No. 60/057,106, filed Aug. 27, 1997, and further claims the benefit of U.S. patent application Ser. No. 09/140,981, filed Aug. 27, 1998, which is now U.S. Pat. No. 6,125,295, issued Sep. 26, 2000, and further claims the benefit of U.S. patent application Ser. No. 09/550,498, filed Apr. 14, 2000. The present invention relates to the fields of x-ray therapy and x-ray surgery. More specifically, devices and enhanced methods for performing such therapeutic techniques, comprising the use of pharmaceutical contrast agents, are provided. Since early in the twentieth century it has been recognized that the ionizing properties of x-rays allow them to be used for therapeutic and diagnostic purposes. However, treatment of tumors with x-rays is difficult because about the same x-ray dose is required to kill the cancerous cells as kills healthy cells. Therefore, techniques for concentrating the x-ray dose in the target area, with minimum dose to surrounding healthy tissue, are of basic importance in **radiotherapy** and radiosurgery.

  Web site: http://appft1.uspto.gov/netahtml/PTO/search-bool.html

- **Radio-labelled ferrite particles and methods for the manufacture and use thereof**

  Inventor(s): Browitt, Rodney James; (New South Wales, AU), Senden, Timothy John; (New South Wales, AU)

  Correspondence: Birch Stewart Kolasch & Birch; PO Box 747; Falls Church; VA; 22040-0747; US

  Patent Application Number: 20040081617

  Date filed: November 18, 2003

Abstract: A method for the production of radio-labelled ferrite nanoparticles for use in medical imaging and **radiotherapy** comprising the steps of: a) adding an aqueous solution containing Fe.sup.2+ and Fe.sup.3+ ions and at least one radioisotope to an alkaline solution and agitating the mixture to form a precipitate comprising ferrite particles labelled with the at least one radioisotope; and b) isolating and washing the precipitated labelled particles, wherein said radioisotope is a radioisotope which functions as a radiotracer isotope and a **radiotherapy** isotope or said radioisotope includes at least one radiotracer isotope and at least one **radiotherapy** isotope.

Excerpt(s): The present invention relates to radio-labelled ferrite particles and methods of manufacturing same. The invention further relates to uses of such particles for medical imaging and therapy. Ferrimagnetic nanoparticles are known. Such particles have been used previously in hyperthermia therapy for human cancers. The principle used in this case involves the induction of intracellular hyperthermia by external application of an oscillating electromagnetic field after endocytosis of magnetic nanoparticles by tumour cells. This method of treatment has particularly been pursued for treatment of malignant brain tumours and oral cancers. It would be desirable in such applications to quantify localisation of nanoparticles in the target tissues. As such, the inventors have now provided a method of radiolabelling such ferrimagnetic nonoparticles. It has also been found that the labelled nanoparticles may also have a wider usefulness in other applications, thus permitting better imaging of tumours based on the selective rapid uptake of the particles by tumour cells with gamma camera imaging or scintigraphy; localised **radiotherapy** of tumours using high density labelling of the nanoparticles; and radio-guided surgery for more effective resection of poorly defined tumours.

Web site: http://appft1.uspto.gov/netahtml/PTO/search-bool.html

- **Radiosensitivity enhancers in radiotherapy for cancer and nucleic acids and proteins enhancing radiosensitivity**

Inventor(s): Nakagawara, Akira; (Chiba-shi, JP)

Correspondence: Fitch Even Tabin And Flannery; 120 South LA Salle Street; Suite 1600; Chicago; IL; 60603-3406; US

Patent Application Number: 20040115129

Date filed: May 14, 2003

Abstract: A radiosensitivity enhancer comprising as the effective ingredient, a nucleic acid having the base sequence set forth in SEQ ID NO:1 or SEQ ID NO:3, or a protein having the amino acid sequence set forth in SEQ ID NO:2 or SEQ ID NO: 4 is used to enhance the radiosensitivity of a malignant tumor cell with the sensitization effect allowing **radiotherapy** to be effective against a radiation resistant tumor or the malignant tumor of which the radiosensitivity has been lowered.

Excerpt(s): This invention relates to radiosensitivity enhancers, as well as to radiosensitivity-enhancing nucleic acids and proteins in cancer **radiotherapy**. More particularly, it relates to nucleic acid information of genes in the homozygous deletion region that may be commonly present at position 36 on the short arm of chromosome 1 (hereafter referred to as "1p36") of human neuroblastoma, as well as to the therapeutic or diagnostic utility of the nucleic acids and proteins encoded by said nucleic acids (especially, enhancement of the radiosensitivity of cancer cells in the cancer radiotherapy). Conventionally, therapy against cancer (malignant tumor) has been conducted, including surgical treatment, chemotherapy, immunotherapy, hiperthermia treatment, and **radiotherapy.** The **radiotherapy** can be employed alone or in combination with other treatment methods, and the therapy is an effective treatment method since it shows a high local controlling rate in many malignant tumors. The radiosensitivity of tumor cells is known to decrease with lowering oxygen concentration. In order for the **radiotherapy** to be effective, it is assumed that with respect to radiosensitivity, tumor cells are greater than normal cells in the region to be treated. Thus, the development of pharmaceutical agents for enhancing the radiosensitivity of the tumor cells in place of oxygen is progressing. One example of such pharmaceutical agents is referred to as "a hypoxic cell radiation sensitizer"; and it displays no enhancement of the radiosensitivity of peroxic cells (normal cells), but has enhancing effect only on hypoxic cells (tumor cells). Nitroimidazole derivatives are recognized to be the radiation sensitizers, and compounds such as misonidazole and ethanidazole have been developed. However, they have not resulted in the practical use because their nerve toxicity is too strong at the doses providing sensitization activity. Although the combined use of the pharmaceutical agent for enhancing radiosensitivity is desired in the treatment of a radiation resistant tumor, many of the radiosensitivity enhancers (such as radiation sensitizers) experience a problem in their development because of nerve toxicity.

Web site: http://appft1.uspto.gov/netahtml/PTO/search-bool.html

• **Radiotherapy apparatus and collimator set therefor**

Inventor(s): Brown, Kevin John; (West Sussex, GB), Streamer, Ralph Peter; (West Sussex, GB)

Correspondence: Bromberg & Sunstein Llp; 125 Summer Street; Boston; MA; 02110-1618; US

Patent Application Number: 20040013237

Date filed: April 10, 2003

Abstract: A collimator set for a **radiotherapy** apparatus comprises, in sequence, an aperture collimator, a multi-leaf collimator with a pair of opposing arrays of elongate leaves each moveable longitudinally in a Y direction, and a leaf edge collimator, the aperture collimator being adapted to collimate the beam in the X and Y direction to a first extent, and the leaf edge collimator being adapted to further collimate the extent of the beam in the Y direction to a second and therefore lesser extend. This means that to close a pair of opposing leaves, they are moved to their minimum separation, with the gap being convered by the leaf edge collimator. The MLC is after the aperture collimator, so in combination with thin leaves, the MLC leaves will project a much reduced leaf width at the isocentre of the **radiotherapy** apparatus and collimation of the radiation field by fractional leaf widths becomes unnecessary. A **radiotherapy** apparatus comprising a collimator set as defined above is also disclosed.

Excerpt(s): The present invention relates to a **radiotherapy** apparatus, in particular to the arrangement of collimators within the radiation head. In a conventional multi-leaf collimator (MLC), the radiation beam is collimated by an array of thin leaves lying alongside each other which can each be extended longitudinally to define a unique edge. The leaves move in a given direction (Y) and generally there are two sets of additional backup diaphragms orthogonal to this (X). These are solid and move in and out in the X and Y directions. They perform two functions. The X diaphragm allows the field edge to be adjusted in a continuous manner, whereas the leaves alone would only allow discrete adjustments a leaf width at a time. The Y diaphragm reduces the effect of leakage through the leaves. The X diaphragm also shields the gap between leaves that are out of the treatment field and are effectively `closed`. Subsequent to the MLC 22 is a Y collimator. This consists of a pair of jaws 32, 34 which each extend across the width of the multi-leaf array 22 and can be moved in and out in the same Y direction as the leaves 24, 26 of the MLC array 22. These leaves therefore lie behind the leaves of the MLC 22 and limit leakage of radiation between the individual leaves.

Web site: http://appft1.uspto.gov/netahtml/PTO/search-bool.html

- **Radiotherapy apparatus and operating method**

Inventor(s): Brown, Kevin John; (Horsham, GB)

Correspondence: Bromberg & Sunstein Llp; 125 Summer Street; Boston; MA; 02110-1618; US

Patent Application Number: 20040114718

Date filed: November 26, 2003

Abstract: A **radiotherapy** apparatus comprises a source of therapeutic radiation, a source of imaging radiation and a two-dimensional imager for the imaging radiation, a computing means for preparing tomography data from the output of the imager, the therapeutic source being controllable on the basis of feedback from the tomography data, wherein the computing means is arranged to prepare a plurality of intersecting sectional views from the output of the imager, akin to a portal image but with better contrast and the detail of a section rather than that of a projection. This is easier to interpret and visualise a series of sectional than a three dimensional view. Pixels of the images are the result of averaging a plurality of voxels arranged transverse to the section, typically orthogonal and linear. Typically, good results can be achieved using between 5 and 20 voxels. About 10 is suitable, ie between 7 and 15. There is a ideally a display means for showing the sectional views to an operator. The therapeutic source can then be controlled on the basis of instructions from the operator, given via an input means such as a mouse or other pointer, which is preferably correlated to the display. This correlation can be via a superimposed image on the display which is moveable in response to operation of the input means. The superimposed image can derived from one of a previous investigation and a treatment of the patient, so that it corresponds in shape to the area or the image which is being sought. The superimposed image is preferably an outline so that the underlying image is clear.

Excerpt(s): The present invention relates to a **radiotherapy** apparatus and a method by which it can be operated and controlled. Existing **radiotherapy** apparatus seeks to direct a beam of radiation to a tumour within a patient in order to cause the death of cancerous cells. By its nature, the radiation is harmful and efforts are therefore made to limit the application of the radiation to healthy areas of the patient. Typically, these involve the use of collimators for the beam, and directional techniques in which the beam is directed toward the tumour from a variety of directions, thereby maximising the dose at the tumour site and minimising it in adjacent areas. Such techniques depend on the operator being aware of the position of the tumour. This knowledge will usually be gained from previous investigations and from off-line analysis carried out after the treatment for use in refining subsequent treatments. However, soft tissue is apt to move randomly even over short periods of time, and this places a limitation on the use of historic information.

Web site: http://appft1.uspto.gov/netahtml/PTO/search-bool.html

- **Radiotherapy apparatus equipped with an articulable gantry for positioning an imaging unit**

Inventor(s): Graf, Ulrich Martin; (Mettmenstetten, CH)

Correspondence: Blakely Sokoloff Taylor & Zafman; 12400 Wilshire Boulevard, Seventh Floor; Los Angeles; CA; 90025; US

Patent Application Number: 20040024300

Date filed: November 2, 2001

Abstract: An apparatus including a first radiation source attached to a first gantry, at least one second radiation source, a second gantry that is rotatable; and an imager attached to an articulable end of the second gantry.

Excerpt(s): The present invention pertains in general to oncology radiation therapy. In particular, the invention involves an X-ray and electron **radiotherapy** machine used in radiation treatment applications. The use of linear accelerators for the generation of either electron radiation or X-ray radiation is well known. After generating a stream of electrons, components in the **radiotherapy** machine can convert the electrons to X-rays, a flattening filter can broaden the X-ray beam, the beam can be shaped with a multileaf collimator, and a dose chamber can be arranged at the exit of an accelerator. A detector is mounted and is mechanically or electronically scanned synchronously with the mechanically or electronically scanned paraxial X-ray beam, providing continuous monitoring of alignment of the patient's anatomy. These systems typically provide either static fixed field radiation therapy or fully dynamic intensity modulated radiation therapy (IMRT) used by the medical community in the treatment of cancer. One of the challenges inherent in **radiotherapy** treatment is the accurate positioning of the tumor in the radiation field. The main sources of the problem result from the fact that there is a natural motion of organs inside the body, which can range, for example, from approximately a millimeter in the case of the brain inside the skull, to several centimeters for the organs in the trunk above the diaphragm. Another factor relates to changes which occur in the tumor over time because of successful treatment. Over the course of treatment and as the tumor shrinks in volume, normal tissue which had been displaced returns to its original position within the treatment volume.

Web site: http://appft1.uspto.gov/netahtml/PTO/search-bool.html

- **Radiotherapy device**

Inventor(s): Hara, Kenji; (Hiroshima, JP), **Kamino**, Yuichiro; (Aichi, JP), Mihara, Kazumasa; (Hiroshima, JP), Wakamoto, Ikuo; (Hiroshima, JP), Yamashita, Ichiro; (Hiroshima, JP)

Correspondence: Armstrong, Kratz, Quintos, Hanson & Brooks, Llp; 1725 K Street, NW; Suite 1000; Washington; DC; 20006; US

Patent Application Number: 20040037390

Date filed: May 9, 2003

Abstract: The **radiotherapy** apparatus in the present invention includes a bed, a radiation irradiating head, head swing mechanisms, a precise inspection unit and a control unit. The bed carries a subject. The radiation irradiating head irradiates a treatment radiation to a treatment field of the subject. The head swing mechanisms, which are coupled to the radiation irradiating head, swings the head of the radiation irradiating head so that the treatment radiation emitted from the radiation irradiating head pursues the motion of the treatment field. The precise inspection unit obtains a diagnosis image containing the treatment field. The control unit controls the positions of the head swing mechanisms so that an irradiation field of the radiation irradiating head pursues the treatment field, based on the diagnosis image, the position of the radiation irradiating head and the state of the swung head. Then, the control unit controls the radiation irradiating head so that the treatment radiation is irradiated from the radiation irradiating head, after the positional control of the head swing mechanisms.

Excerpt(s): The present invention relates to a **radiotherapy** apparatus, and more particularly to a **radiotherapy** apparatus used for a stereotactic **radiotherapy.** A **radiotherapy** apparatus for treating a cancer and a tumor by using radiation has been well known. As a three-dimensional irradiation **radiotherapy** apparatus for carrying out an irradiation at a stereotactic multiple arc, there are a radiosurgery treating apparatus, a linac (medical linear accelerator) treating apparatus and the like. Here, the stereotactic multiple arc irradiation designates the **radiotherapy** method that intensively irradiates the radiation to a small focus from many directions and thereby improves the treatment effect, and further minimizes the exposure amount of ambient tissues. Its power is exerted on the treatment for a primary benign brain tumor, a single metastatic brain tumor whose size is 3 cm or less, a small lesion inside a brain such as a cranial base metastasis whose operation is difficult, an artery malformation, a vein malformation or the like.

Web site: http://appft1.uspto.gov/netahtml/PTO/search-bool.html

- **Residual map segmentation method for multi-leaf collimator-intensity modulated radiotherapy**

Inventor(s): Chang, Sha; (Chapel Hill, NC)

Correspondence: Jenkins & Wilson, PA; 3100 Tower Blvd; Suite 1400; Durham; NC; 27707; US

Patent Application Number: 20040190680

Date filed: March 28, 2003

Abstract: In a method for sequentially generating segment fields for use in delivering intensity modulated **radiotherapy** an input continuous intensity map is generated. A segment field is generated directly from the input intensity map. A residual continuous intensity map is generated that is based on the respective photon fluence contributions from the input intensity map and a fractionally intensity map corresponding to the segment field. These steps are repeated for a number of iterations to generate a like number of additional segment fields and residual maps derived therefrom. In each iteration, the residual map generated in the previous iteration is used as the input intensity map.

Excerpt(s): The present invention generally relates to intensity-modulated **radiotherapy** (IMRT). More particularly, the invention relates to the optimized configuration of multi-leaf collimator leaves for delivery of IMRT. For any given radiation treatment procedure, a common goal is to deliver an adequate, therapeutically effective dosage of radiation to the tumor while minimizing potentially damaging dosage exposure to nearby critical organs and other tissues (termed organs at risk or OAR). Intensity-modulated **radiotherapy** (IMRT) is a popular new technology to customize radiation treatment in accordance with this goal for each patient. The most widely available apparatus for delivering IMRT procedures for cancer patients is a medical linear accelerator (LINAC). LINAC-based IMRT treatment apparatuses are described in, for example, U.S. Pat. Nos. 5,663,999; 6,134,296; 6,240,161; 6,240,162; 6,330,300; 6,335,961; 6,349,129; 6,353,655; 6,449,335; 6,473,490; and 6,477,229, the respective contents of which are incorporated herein in their entireties. Compared to conventional LINAC-based **radiotherapy** treatments, an IMRT treatment delivers a variable intensity distribution, or intensity map, within a treatment portal. The intensity maps are normally designed by a dose optimization algorithm, whose objective is defined by the radiation oncologist for the patient to meet a set of dose distribution criteria. The criteria often involve the tumor volume and structures of nearby organs at risk (OAR). The intensity maps, sometimes along with other treatment parameters, are used as variables by the dose optimization algorithm to design the optimal treatment. The dose optimization algorithms generally are an integral part of treatment planning systems, and can be implemented in treatment planning software (TPS).

Web site: http://appft1.uspto.gov/netahtml/PTO/search-bool.html

- **Retrievable, shielded radiotherapy implant**

  Inventor(s): Mawad, Michel E.; (Houston, TX)

  Correspondence: Conley Rose, P.C.; P. O. Box 3267; Houston; TX; 77253-3267; US

  Patent Application Number: 20040158116

  Date filed: February 10, 2004

Abstract: A **radiotherapy** device comprises a radioactive wire adapted to deliver an intended dosage of radiation to a lesion or other selected body tissues. The radioactive wire comprises an inner core about which is disposed an outer buffer layer of platinum or other suitable metal of high atomic number. The buffer layer preferably comprises a thin, continuous wire wrapped about the inner core. The **radiotherapy** device may be made into a variety of shapes, such as a straight wire, a helical coil, or other more complex shape, and it may be provided with an elastic memory. The device may be adapted for attachment to a delivery wire for controlled placement, as through a delivery catheter or microcatheter, at the treatment site. When accurate positioning of the device is not necessary, it can simply be injected through the delivery catheter or microcatheter, and in that event a delivery wire is not needed. The device may be provided with mechanically or electrically releasable means for attachment to the delivery wire during delivery, and for releasing the device at the treatment site. The device may be provided with a shoulder, hook, or other suitable gripping means on its distal end, which can be lassoed by a microsnare device for retrieving the device from the body.

Excerpt(s): The present invention relates to the field of **radiotherapy** devices, and more particularly to the field of implantable, permanent or retrievable **radiotherapy** devices. More particularly still, the present invention relates to the field of shielded radioactive wires adapted for implantation at the site of a lesion or other selected body tissue for treatment of cancer or other pathological condition. At present, external beam **radiotherapy** is widely utilized in the treatment of cancer and more recently, in the treatment of vascular malformations particularly those affecting the Central Nervous System. **Radiotherapy** is used as an adjunct to surgical excision and chemotherapy, or as the sole form of treatment. External beam **radiotherapy** can be either nonfocused or stereotactic using a gamma knife apparatus or a linear accelerator. Both of these radiotherapy modalities are limited by the undesirable side effect of radiation necrosis they produce in the normal tissue surrounding the lesion to be irradiated.

Web site: http://appft1.uspto.gov/netahtml/PTO/search-bool.html

- **System for predicting susceptibility of human oropharyngeal squamous cell carcinoma to radiotherapy**

  Inventor(s): Allal, Abdelkarim S.; (Carouge, CH), Boehringer-Wyss, Nicole; (Geneva, CH), Clarkson, Stuart G.; (Geneva, CH)

  Correspondence: John Moetteli, ESQ.; Moetteli & Associe, Sarl; Case Postale 486; Geneva 12; Ch-1211; CH

  Patent Application Number: 20040185444

  Date filed: March 18, 2003

  Abstract: The present invention is a gene expression system for prognosticating susceptibility of a human oropharyngeal squamous cell carcinoma (SCC) to radiotherapy. A selection of human gene fragments is disclosed which are useful, when utilized in a gene expression procedure, for detecting nucleotide sequences in a human SCC sample the over/under expression of which is predictive of the SCC's susceptibility to radiotherapy. Further, a sub-selection of five genes (FLJ11342, H08808, TOP1, DLD and EIF4A2) is identified, which showed a particularly distinct pattern wherein all susceptible (controlled) tumor biopsies were under-expressed and all unsusceptible (not-controlled) tumor samples were over-expressed.

  Excerpt(s): The present invention is in the field of organic compounds useful for testing susceptibility of cancer cells to radiotherapy. More specifically, the present invention relates to an array of human gene fragments useful in detecting nucleotide sequences in a human tumor biopsy sample, which nucleotide sequences are predictive of the tumor's susceptibility or response to radiotherapy. TGF-.beta.: transforming growth factor.beta. In patients with head and neck carcinomas, as in the majority of cancer patients, indicators of oncological outcome are based traditionally on clinical and pathological features such as tumor size/stage, extent of lymph node involvement, and anatomical subsite. However, even after careful evaluation of these factors, predicting the clinical outcome remains hazardous, particularly for tumors of the same stage and sublocation. Moreover, patients with advanced disease are often treated with a combination of radiotherapy (RT) and chemotherapy and many of them suffer from the acute toxicity without commensurate benefit from such combination regimens. Thus, there is a clear need to identify additional prognostic factors, which can differentiate between those patients that potentially can benefit from combining RT with chemotherapy, and those for whom the invasiveness an RT regimen portends little benefit. Such prognostic factors, particularly those related to biological parameters, would permit development of individualized strategies that lead to improved results by a shift away from radiation-based therapy and toward surgery and/or new target-specific biological agents as more appropriate.

  Web site: http://appft1.uspto.gov/netahtml/PTO/search-bool.html

- **Treatment of spinal metastases**

Inventor(s): Patrick, Timothy J.; (Alpharetta, GA), Ramey, Carribeth B.; (Suwanee, GA), Winkler, Rance A.; (Atlanta, GA)

Correspondence: Nutter Mcclennen & Fish Llp; World Trade Center West; 155 Seaport Boulevard; Boston; MA; 02210-2604; US

Patent Application Number: 20040167372

Date filed: February 20, 2004

Abstract: A **radiotherapy** system, and preferably a brachytherapy system, for delivering radiation to tissue surrounding an interstitial space is provided. While the system can be used for a variety of purposes, the system is preferably used to treat spinal metastases. In general, the system includes a catheter member having a proximal end, a distal end, and an inner lumen extending therethrough, and a structural support adapted to fit within an interstitial space in load bearing portion of a patient's body and having an internal space for removably receiving the distal end of the catheter member. At least one anchoring element can be disposed proximate to the distal end of the catheter. The anchoring element is preferably adapted to fit within the internal space in the structural support so as to anchor the distal end of the catheter therein. The system further includes a radiation source disposable within the internal space of the structural support through the lumen in the catheter for delivering radiation to tissue surrounding the interstitial space.

Excerpt(s): The invention relates generally to apparatus for use in treating proliferative tissue disorders, and more particularly to an apparatus for the treatment of such disorders in the body by the application of radiation. Malignant tumors are often treated by surgical resection of the tumor to remove as much of the tumor as possible. Infiltration of the tumor cells into normal tissue surrounding the tumor, however, can limit the therapeutic value of surgical resection because the infiltration can be difficult or impossible to treat surgically. Radiation therapy can be used to supplement surgical resection by targeting the residual tumor margin after resection, with the goal of reducing its size or stabilizing it. Radiation therapy, or surgical excision followed by radiation therapy, is commonly used to treat spinal metastases. Metastases are tumors that have grown in a location that is remote from the site that the tumor started, and spinal metastases result from the spread of cancer cells into a patient's vertebral column. Radiation therapy can be administered through one of several methods, or a combination of methods, including external-beam radiation, stereotactic radiosurgery, and permanent or temporary interstitial brachytherapy. The term "brachytherapy," as used herein, refers to radiation therapy delivered by a spatially confined radioactive material inserted into the body at or near a tumor or other proliferative tissue disease site. Owing to the proximity of the radiation source, brachytherapy offers the advantage of delivering a more localized dose to the target tissue region.

Web site: http://appft1.uspto.gov/netahtml/PTO/search-bool.html

- **Tumor dose enhancement using modified photon beams and contrast media**

Inventor(s): Martin, Monty A.; (Vancouver, CA), Riccio, Silvia A.; (North Vancouver, CA), Robar, James; (Halifax, CA)

Correspondence: Oyen, Wiggs, Green & Mutala; 480 - The Station; 601 West Cordova Street; Vancouver; BC; V6b 1g1; CA

Patent Application Number: 20040082855

Date filed: July 18, 2003

Abstract: A method of **radiotherapy** includes irradiating a treatment volume containing a high atomic number contrast medium with a photon beam characterized by a peak energy of at least 1 MeV and a mean energy in excess of 250 keV. The irradiation may be provided by a beam from a linear accelerator operating without a flattening filter. The linear accelerator may have multiple modes including one or more modes for operating with a flattening filter and one or modes for operating without a flattening filter.

Excerpt(s): This application claims the benefit of the filing date of application Ser. No. 60/396,714 filed on 19 Jul. 2002, which is hereby incorporated herein by reference in its entirety. The invention relates to **radiotherapy**. A principle goal of **radiotherapy** (which includes radiosurgery) is to deliver a desired well-defined dose of radiation to a treatment volume within a subject. The volume may, for example, be the volume of a malignant or benign tumor. At the same time it is desirable to minimize the dose delivered to surrounding tissues so as to spare the surrounding tissues from radiation-induced damage. This is especially important in cases where the treatment volume is closely adjacent to structures which are susceptible to radiation-induced damage such as the brainstem.

Web site: http://appft1.uspto.gov/netahtml/PTO/search-bool.html

- **Use of n-acetyl-d-glucosamine in the manufacture of pharmaceutical useful for suppressing side-effect of radiotherapy and chemotherapy**

Inventor(s): Liu, Junkang; (Chongqing, CN), Xu, Qiwang; (Chongqing, CN), Yuan, Zetao; (Chongqing, CN)

Correspondence: Ladas & Parry; 26 West 61st Street; New York; NY; 10023; US

Patent Application Number: 20040077596

Date filed: December 17, 2003

Abstract: The present invention has disclosed a use of N-acetyl-D-glucosamine in the manufacture of a medicament for inhibiting the side effect of radio-chemical therapy, the medicament with N-acetyl-D-glucosamine as main active component can be used to inhibit the side effect of radio-chemical therapy of cancer patients, with an effective rate up to 85%.

Excerpt(s): The present invention relates to the use of N-acetyl-D-glucosamine and pharmaceutical acceptable salts thereof in the manufacture of a medicament for inhibiting the side effect of radio-chemical therapy. After accepting radio-chemical treatment, patients with neoplasm often have marrow inhibition, hemogram variation, anemia, leucocyte reduction, protein synthesis inhibition and other reflections in dysfunction of metabolism, and they will be quickly accompanied with systematical side effects of radio-chemical therapy: nausea, vomiting, lack energy, appetite decreasing, loss of the hair and so on, the severer may have acute exhaustion or respiratory distress;

as leucocytes decreasing may lead to immune dysfunction, systematical infection is likely to happen; furthermore, with the disturbance of the production of immune cells, most of the patients with neoplasm are finally dead from the whole body exhaustion, cachexia, infection and so on, these are almost resulted from the side effect of radio-chemical therapy. Therefore the control of side effect of radio-chemical therapy is contributed to the long period therapy of neoplasm and to strengthen the support ability of neoplasm patient to the therapy; at the same time, lighten the patient's pain in the course of treatment, and avoid a serious of complication caused by neoplasm. At present, supporting therapies commonly used clinically are mainly symptomatic treatments: for instance, when the patient lacks energy.quadrature. administration of energy mixture is adopted; when water electrolyte is disordered, supplying water electrolyte is adopted; when vomiting is serious, anti-vomiting medicine is administrated; when the patient is infected, anti-inflammation therapy is used, and so on. The effects of these symptomatic treatments do not have good effect. The side effect after radio-chemical therapy almost happens to the each patient with neoplasm who has been treated, making them suffered from pain, and this is a big problem in the neoplasm treatment. Therefore, a medicament capable of inhibiting the side effect caused by radio-chemical therapy is quite needed in the field of neoplasm treatment. In the research of "bio-waves" theory, the present inventor has set up a bacterial wave growth model. Through researching, it is known that this wave is of its intrinsic regulation mechanism: some chemical substances are able to participate the regulation in the bio-wave process, so as to transform an abnormal periodic slow wave into a normal physiological chaotic quick wave, and this kind of substances are known as promoting wave factors. Through separating, purifying and identifying, it is determined that one of the factors is N-acetyl-D-glucosamine, the promoting wave function of which is shown in lubricating and protecting the cell. Many biochemical and physiological process of human body need the participation of the promoting wave factors, and it would lead to an abnormal state, if this kind of promoting wave factors is lacked in the living body.

Web site: http://appft1.uspto.gov/netahtml/PTO/search-bool.html

Keeping Current

In order to stay informed about patents and patent applications dealing with radiotherapy, you can access the U.S. Patent Office archive via the Internet at the following Web address: **http://www.uspto.gov/patft/index.html**. You will see two broad options: (1) Issued Patent, and (2) Published Applications. To see a list of issued patents, perform the following steps: Under "Issued Patents," click "Quick Search." Then, type "radiotherapy" (or synonyms) into the "Term 1" box. After clicking on the search button, scroll down to see the various patents which have been granted to date on radiotherapy.

You can also use this procedure to view pending patent applications concerning radiotherapy. Simply go back to **http://www.uspto.gov/patft/index.html**. Select "Quick Search" under "Published Applications." Then proceed with the steps listed above.

CHAPTER 6. BOOKS ON RADIOTHERAPY

Overview

This chapter provides bibliographic book references relating to radiotherapy. In addition to online booksellers such as **www.amazon.com** and **www.bn.com**, excellent sources for book titles on radiotherapy include the Combined Health Information Database and the National Library of Medicine. Your local medical library also may have these titles available for loan.

Book Summaries: Federal Agencies

The Combined Health Information Database collects various book abstracts from a variety of healthcare institutions and federal agencies. To access these summaries, go directly to the following hyperlink: **http://chid.nih.gov/detail/detail.html**. You will need to use the "Detailed Search" option. To find book summaries, use the drop boxes at the bottom of the search page where "You may refine your search by." Select the dates and language you prefer. For the format option, select "Monograph/Book." Now type "radiotherapy" (or synonyms) into the "For these words:" box. You should check back periodically with this database which is updated every three months. The following is a typical result when searching for books on radiotherapy:

- **Communication Disorders in Childhood Cancer**

  Source: London, United Kingdom: Whurr Publishers Ltd. 1999. 219 p.

  Contact: Available from Taylor and Francis, Inc. 7625 Empire Drive, Florence, KY 41042. (800) 634-7064. Fax (800) 248-4724. PRICE: $47.95 plus shipping and handling. ISBN: 1861561156.

  Summary: As the treatments become more effective, an increasing number of children displaying communication deficits as a consequence of treatment for childhood cancer have begun to appear in the caseloads of speech pathologists and other health professionals. This book offers an overview of the communication impairments that occur in association with the two most common forms of childhood cancer, namely leukemia and brain tumor. The treatments offered for these conditions, such as **radiotherapy** and chemotherapy, may have some long term adverse effects on brain structure and function leading to the development of a number of complications, including cognitive deficits as well as speech and language disorders. The book includes nine chapters, that cover the cancers themselves (leukemia and brain tumors), the effects of treatment for pediatric cancer on brain structure and function, language disorders in children treated for brain tumors, language recovery following treatment for pediatric brain tumors, variability in patterns of language impairment in children following treatment for posterior fossa tumor, language disorders in children treated for acute lymphoblastic leukemia, discourse abilities of children treated for neoplastic conditions, motor speech disorders in children treated for brain tumors, and the assessment and treatment of speech and language disorders occurring subsequent to cancer therapy in children. Each chapter includes extensive references and the textbook concludes with a subject index.

- **Understanding Your Prostate Problems**

Source: Woollahra, New South Wales, Australia: Health Books, Gore and Osment Publications. 1993. 64 p.

Contact: Available from Health Books, Gore and Osment Publications, Private Box 427, 150 Queen Street, Woollahra, NSW 2025, Australia. (02) 361-5244. Fax (02) 360-7558. PRICE: $9.95 (as of 1995). ISBN: 1875531459.

Summary: This health education book is designed to help readers understand the function of the prostate, prostatic diseases, and treatment options for prostate problems. Eleven chapters cover topics including the anatomy and physiology of the prostate; prostatic enlargement; prostate cancer; other prostate problems, including prostatitis, urethral stricture, and urinary stones; diagnostic tests used to confirm or screen for prostate problems; prostate surgery; other types of treatment, include drug therapy, laser treatments, transurethral resection, stents, catheters, hyperthermia, and balloon dilatation; **radiotherapy** for prostate cancer; hormone therapy for prostate cancer; chemotherapy for prostate cancer; and suggestions for patient self-care. The book is written in easy-to-read language, with simple illustrations; a brief glossary concludes the volume.

- **Medical Problems in Dentistry. 4th ed**

Source: Woburn, MA: Butterworth-Heinemann. 1998. 570 p.

Contact: Available from Butterworth-Heinemann. 225 Wildwood Avenue, Woburn, MA 01801-2041. (800) 366-2665 or (781) 904-2500. Fax (800) 446-6520 or (781) 933-6333. E-mail: orders@bhusa.com. Website: www.bh.com. PRICE: $110.00. ISBN: 0723610568.

Summary: This text covers the general medical and surgical conditions relevant to the oral health care sciences. In providing a basis for the understanding of how these disorders influence oral health and oral health care, the text helps dental staff become aware of a variety of medical problems. Twenty-seven chapters cover medical history and assessment, perioperative care, cardiovascular disease, disorders of hemostasis, anemia, malignant disease, cytotoxic chemotherapy and **radiotherapy,** respiratory disorders, gastrointestinal disorders, liver disease, infections and infection control, skin diseases, genitourinary and renal disease, endocrine conditions, metabolic conditions and nutrition, musculoskeletal disorders, neurologic disorders, psychiatric disorders, headache and orofacial pain, immunodeficiencies, immunologically mediated disease, maxillofacial trauma and head injury, patients with disabilities, children and the elderly, chemical dependence, reactions to drugs and materials, drug interactions, emergencies, and socioeconomic, ethnic and geographic health issues. One appendix addresses miscellaneous uncommon or rare disorders of possible relevance to dentistry, not included elsewhere in the text. Each chapter includes references and a subject index concludes the volume.

- **Smith's General Urology. Fifteenth Edition**

Source: Columbus, OH: McGraw-Hill, Inc. 2000. 868 p.

Contact: Available from McGraw-Hill. Medical Publishing. 1221 P.O. Box 182615, Columbus, OH 43272-5046. (800) 262-4729. PRICE: $54.95;plus shipping and handling. ISBN: 0838586074.

Summary: This textbook offers a practical and concise guide to the understanding, diagnosis, and treatment of urologic diseases. The text includes 47 chapters covering the anatomy of the genitourinary tract, embryology of the genitourinary system, symptoms of disorders of the genitourinary tract, physical examination of the genitourinary tract, urologic laboratory examination, radiology of the urinary tract, vascular interventional radiology, percutaneous endourology and ureterorenoscopy, laparoscopic surgery, radionuclide imaging, retrograde instrumentation of the urinary tract, urinary obstruction and stasis, vesicoureteral reflux (return of urine through the ureters to the kidney), bacterial infections, specific infections, sexually transmitted diseases, urinary stone (urolithiasis) disease, extracorporeal shock wave lithotripsy (ESWL, used to break up stones), injuries to the genitourinary tract, immunology and immunotherapy of urologic cancers, urothelial carcinoma (cancers of the bladder, ureter, and renal pelvis), renal parenchymal neoplasms (growths in the body of the kidney), neoplasms of the prostate gland, genital tumors, urinary diversion and bladder substitution, urologic laser surgery, chemotherapy of urologic tumors, **radiotherapy** of urologic tumors, neuropathic (arising from the nervous system) bladder disorders, urodynamic studies, urinary incontinence (involuntary loss of urine), disorders of the adrenal glands, disorders of the kidneys, diagnosis of medical renal diseases, oliguria (acute renal failure, lack of urination), chronic renal failure (CRF) and dialysis, renal transplantation, disorders of the ureter and ureteropelvic junction, disorders of the bladder and prostate (and seminal vesicles), disorders of the penis and male urethra, disorders of the female urethra, disorders of the testis and scrotum (and spermatic cord), skin diseases of the external genitalia, abnormalities of sexual determination and differentiation, renovascular hypertension, male infertility, and male sexual dysfunction. Each chapter concludes with references categorized by subject; the text concludes with an appendix of normal laboratory values and a subject index. The text features over 400 illustrations, including CT scans, radionuclide imaging scans, and x rays.

- **Clinical Maxillofacial Prosthetics**

Source: Chicago, IL: Quintessence Publishing Co, Inc. 2000. 316 p.

Contact: Available from Quintessence Publishing Co, Inc. 551 Kimberly Drive, Carol Stream, IL 60188-9981. (800) 621-0387 or (630) 682-3223. Fax (630) 682-3288. E-mail: quintpub@aol.com. Website: www.quintpub.com. PRICE: $138.00 plus shipping and handling. ISBN: 0867153911.

Summary: This textbook offers an indepth review of prosthodontic (the construction of artificial appliances that replace missing teeth or restore parts of the face) procedures as they are applied in the maxillofacial (jaw) situation. The subspecialty of maxillofacial prosthetics is frequently practiced by prosthodontists and occasionally by general dentists in a hospital environment; the text offers a user's guide to commonly occurring maxillofacial prosthetic challenges. The 19 chapters in the text cover the psychological management of the maxillofacial prosthetic patient, reimbursement considerations, the radiation therapy patient, resin bonding for maxillofacial prostheses, early management of cleft lip and palate, the edentulous (without teeth) maxillectomy (removal of the upper jaw) patient, the dentate (with teeth) maxillectomy patient, the soft palate defect, the use of the palatal lift, the impact of endoosseous (using the patient's own bone) implants, diagnostic considerations, prosthodontic rehabilitation of the mandibulectomy (removal of the lower jaw) patient, implant rehabilitation of the mandible compromised by **radiotherapy,** prosthodontic rehabilitation following total and partial glossectomy, treatment of upper airway sleep disorder patients with dental devices, facial prosthesis fabrication, fabrication of custom ocular (eye) prostheses, and craniofacial osseointegration. Each chapter offers full color photographs and references; a subject index concludes the text.

Book Summaries: Online Booksellers

Commercial Internet-based booksellers, such as Amazon.com and Barnes&Noble.com, offer summaries which have been supplied by each title's publisher. Some summaries also include customer reviews. Your local bookseller may have access to in-house and commercial databases that index all published books (e.g. Books in Print®). **IMPORTANT NOTE:** Online booksellers typically produce search results for medical and non-medical books. When searching for "radiotherapy" at online booksellers' Web sites, you may discover non-medical books that use the generic term "radiotherapy" (or a synonym) in their titles. The following is indicative of the results you might find when searching for "radiotherapy" (sorted alphabetically by title; follow the hyperlink to view more details at Amazon.com):

- **A Guide to radiotherapy nursing (Livingstone nursing texts);** ISBN: 0443006830; http://www.amazon.com/exec/obidos/ASIN/0443006830/icongroupinterna

- **A Guide to the Radiotherapy and Oncology Department** by Thomas J. Deeley; ISBN: 0723605068; http://www.amazon.com/exec/obidos/ASIN/0723605068/icongroupinterna

- **Accidental Overexposure of Radiotherapy Patients in San Jose, Costa Rica;** ISBN: 9203027998; http://www.amazon.com/exec/obidos/ASIN/9203027998/icongroupinterna

- **Advanced Techniques for Radiotherapy (Euro Courses : Advanced Scientific Techniques, Vol 2)** by Marco Castiglioni, Argeo A. Benco; ISBN: 079231588X; http://www.amazon.com/exec/obidos/ASIN/079231588X/icongroupinterna

- **Californium-252: Isotope for 21st Century Radiotherapy : Proceedings of the NATO Advanced Research Workshop On: Californium-252, Isotope for 21st Cent. nership Sub-Series 3, High Technology, V. 29)** by Jcek G. Wierzbicki, et al; ISBN: 0792345436; http://www.amazon.com/exec/obidos/ASIN/0792345436/icongroupinterna

- **Central Axis Depth Dose Data for Use in Radiotherapy (British Journal of Radiology Supplement, No 17);** ISBN: 0905749111; http://www.amazon.com/exec/obidos/ASIN/0905749111/icongroupinterna

- **Chemotherapy and Radiotherapy of Gastrointestinal Tumors (Crystals)** by Klein; ISBN: 0387109382; http://www.amazon.com/exec/obidos/ASIN/0387109382/icongroupinterna

- **Clinical Radiotherapy Physics** by Subramania Jayaraman, Lawrence H. Lanzl; ISBN: 3540402845;
  http://www.amazon.com/exec/obidos/ASIN/3540402845/icongroupinterna

- **Clinical Radiotherapy Physics: Treatment Planning and Radiation Safety** by Subramania Jayaraman, et al; ISBN: 0849340179;
  http://www.amazon.com/exec/obidos/ASIN/0849340179/icongroupinterna

- **Combined effects of chemotherapy and radiotherapy on normal tissue tolerance (Frontiers of radiation therapy and oncology)**; ISBN: 3805529325;
  http://www.amazon.com/exec/obidos/ASIN/3805529325/icongroupinterna

- **Combined Radiotherapy and Chemotherapy in Clinical Oncology** by Horwich; ISBN: 0340551593;
  http://www.amazon.com/exec/obidos/ASIN/0340551593/icongroupinterna

- **Computers in Radiotherapy and Oncology** by R.F. Mould; ISBN: 0852747802;
  http://www.amazon.com/exec/obidos/ASIN/0852747802/icongroupinterna

- **Computers in Radiotherapy Planning (Medical Computing Series)** by Raymond G. Wood; ISBN: 0471099945;
  http://www.amazon.com/exec/obidos/ASIN/0471099945/icongroupinterna

- **Concepts in cancer care: A practical explanation of radiotherapy and chemotherapy for primary care physicians** by Jay Scott Cooper; ISBN: B0006D5DEY;
  http://www.amazon.com/exec/obidos/ASIN/B0006D5DEY/icongroupinterna

- **Determination of Absorbed Dose in a Patient Irradiated by Beams of X or Gamma Rays in Radiotherapy Procedures (ICRU report)** by Not Applicable; ISBN: 0913394432;
  http://www.amazon.com/exec/obidos/ASIN/0913394432/icongroupinterna

- **Diagnostic roentgenology of radiotherapy change**; ISBN: 0683049798;
  http://www.amazon.com/exec/obidos/ASIN/0683049798/icongroupinterna

- **Directory of high-energy radiotherapy centres** by International Atomic Energy Agency; ISBN: 9201120761;
  http://www.amazon.com/exec/obidos/ASIN/9201120761/icongroupinterna

- **Dosimetry in Radiotherapy/Isp760 2: Proceedings of an International Symposium on Dosimetry in Radiotherapy (Proceedings Series (International Atomic Energy Agency).)** by International Symposium on Dosimetry in Radiotherapy; ISBN: 9200101887;
  http://www.amazon.com/exec/obidos/ASIN/9200101887/icongroupinterna

- **Equipment, Workload, and Staffing for Radiotherapy in the UK 1992-1997** by Royal College Of Radiologists; ISBN: 1872599354;
  http://www.amazon.com/exec/obidos/ASIN/1872599354/icongroupinterna

- **Handbook of Radiotherapy Physics: Theory and Practice** by P. Mayles, et al; ISBN: 0750308605;
  http://www.amazon.com/exec/obidos/ASIN/0750308605/icongroupinterna

- **High dose rate intracavitary radiotherapy using the RALSTRON (Hokkaido University Medical Library series)** by Masaru Wakabayashi; ISBN: B0006CIL08;
  http://www.amazon.com/exec/obidos/ASIN/B0006CIL08/icongroupinterna

- **Intercomparison of radiotherapy treatment planning systems using calculated and measured dose distributions for external photon and electron beams (STUK-A)**; ISBN: 9514743326;
  http://www.amazon.com/exec/obidos/ASIN/9514743326/icongroupinterna

- **Intraoperative radiotherapy (SuDoc HE 20.3173/3:In 8)** by Tyvin A. Rich; ISBN: B000103HO0;
http://www.amazon.com/exec/obidos/ASIN/B000103HO0/icongroupinterna

- **Investigation of an Accidental Exposure of Radiotherapy Patients in Panama: Report of a Team of Experts, 26 May-1 June 2001**; ISBN: 9201017014;
http://www.amazon.com/exec/obidos/ASIN/9201017014/icongroupinterna

- **Joint U.S.-Scandinavian Symposium on Future Directions of Computer-Aided Radiotherapy : proceedings (SuDoc HE 20.3152:C 73/3)** by U.S. Dept of Health and Human Services; ISBN: B00010IQXM;
http://www.amazon.com/exec/obidos/ASIN/B00010IQXM/icongroupinterna

- **Kilovoltage X-Ray Beam Dosimetry for Radiotherapy and Radiobiology (Symposium Proceedings / American Association of Physicists i)** by Chang-Ming Charlie Ma (Other Contributor); ISBN: 1888340169;
http://www.amazon.com/exec/obidos/ASIN/1888340169/icongroupinterna

- **Lessons Learned from Accidental Exposures in Radiotherapy (Safety Report Ser. Series, 17)** by Not Applicable; ISBN: 9201002009;
http://www.amazon.com/exec/obidos/ASIN/9201002009/icongroupinterna

- **Lung Cancer: Diagnostic Procedures and Therapeutic Management With Special Reference to Radiotherapy (Medical Radiology)** by C.W. Scarantino; ISBN: 0387131760;
http://www.amazon.com/exec/obidos/ASIN/0387131760/icongroupinterna

- **Making Your Radiotherapy Service More Patient Friendly**; ISBN: 1872599508;
http://www.amazon.com/exec/obidos/ASIN/1872599508/icongroupinterna

- **Malignant diseases in children (Modern radiotherapy & oncology)** by Thomas J Deeley; ISBN: 0407278702;
http://www.amazon.com/exec/obidos/ASIN/0407278702/icongroupinterna

- **Normal Tissue Reactions in Radiotherapy and Oncology: International Symposium, Marburg, Germany, April 14-16, 2000 (Frontiers of Radiation Therapy and Oncology, Vol 37)** by Wolfgang Dorr, et al; ISBN: 3805572840;
http://www.amazon.com/exec/obidos/ASIN/3805572840/icongroupinterna

- **Nuclear and Atomic Data for Radiotherapy and Related Radiobiology (Panel Proceedings Series)**; ISBN: 9201310870;
http://www.amazon.com/exec/obidos/ASIN/9201310870/icongroupinterna

- **Nutrition and Radiotherapy (NT Clinical Monographs)** by Sue Holmes; ISBN: 190249931X;
http://www.amazon.com/exec/obidos/ASIN/190249931X/icongroupinterna

- **Physics Aspects of Quality Control in Radiotherapy (IPEM Report)** by W.P.M. Mayles; ISBN: 090418191X;
http://www.amazon.com/exec/obidos/ASIN/090418191X/icongroupinterna

- **Poly-radiomodification in the Radiotherapy of Tumors/Thermoradio-therapy in the USSR/Oxybaro- and Hypoxyradiotherapy (Soviet Medical Reviews Series, Section F)** by S. P. Yarmonenko, et al; ISBN: 3718652285;
http://www.amazon.com/exec/obidos/ASIN/3718652285/icongroupinterna

- **Practical Radiotherapy Planning** by Jane Dobbs, et al; ISBN: 0340706317;
http://www.amazon.com/exec/obidos/ASIN/0340706317/icongroupinterna

- **Practical Radiotherapy Planning**; ISBN: 0713146265;
http://www.amazon.com/exec/obidos/ASIN/0713146265/icongroupinterna

- **Precision Radiotherapy Planning (Oncologic: Multidisciplinary Decisions in Oncology,)** by James M. Slater; ISBN: 0080274706;
  http://www.amazon.com/exec/obidos/ASIN/0080274706/icongroupinterna

- **Proton Radiotherapy Accelerators** by Wioletta Wieszczycka, Waldemar Henryk Schaf; ISBN: 9810245289;
  http://www.amazon.com/exec/obidos/ASIN/9810245289/icongroupinterna

- **Quality Assurance in Radiotherapy Physics: Proceedings of an American College of Medical Physics Symposium, May 1991** by George Starkschall; ISBN: 0944838219;
  http://www.amazon.com/exec/obidos/ASIN/0944838219/icongroupinterna

- **Radiotherapy and TNM classification of cancer of the larynx: A study based on 1447 cases seen at the Radiotherapy clinic of Helsinki during 1936-1961, (Acta radiologica. Supplementum)** by Pentti J Taskinen; ISBN: B0006D1WT4;
  http://www.amazon.com/exec/obidos/ASIN/B0006D1WT4/icongroupinterna

- **Scientific Basis of Modern Radiotherapy (British Institute Radiology Report Ser. : No. 19)** by N.J. McNally; ISBN: 0905749200;
  http://www.amazon.com/exec/obidos/ASIN/0905749200/icongroupinterna

- **Secondary Neoplasias Following Chemotherapy, Radiotherapy and Immunosuppression: Secondary Neoplasias After Organ Transplants and Radiotherapy** by W. Queisser, et al; ISBN: 380557116X;
  http://www.amazon.com/exec/obidos/ASIN/380557116X/icongroupinterna

- **Seeing through you: Radiography and radiotherapy (My life and my work series)** by Elizabeth Lawson; ISBN: 0852257597;
  http://www.amazon.com/exec/obidos/ASIN/0852257597/icongroupinterna

- **Selected topics in physics of radiotherapy and imaging: Invited talks presented at the Asian Regional Conference on Medical Physics, 8-12 December 1986, at Bhabha Atomic Research Centre, Bombay;** ISBN: 0074518836;
  http://www.amazon.com/exec/obidos/ASIN/0074518836/icongroupinterna

- **Simplified Radiotherapy for Technicians** by Barbara Howl; ISBN: 0398023182;
  http://www.amazon.com/exec/obidos/ASIN/0398023182/icongroupinterna

- **Surgery, radiotherapy and chemotherapy of cancer (Proceedings, XI International Cancer Congress; v. 5);** ISBN: 0444151710;
  http://www.amazon.com/exec/obidos/ASIN/0444151710/icongroupinterna

- **Systemic Radiotherapy With Monoclonal Antibodies: Options and Problems (Recent Results in Cancer Research, Vol 141)** by M.-L Sautter-Bihl, et al; ISBN: 3540602097;
  http://www.amazon.com/exec/obidos/ASIN/3540602097/icongroupinterna

- **Targeted Radiotherapy (IPEM Report)** by John S. Fleming, A. C. Perkins; ISBN: 0904181979;
  http://www.amazon.com/exec/obidos/ASIN/0904181979/icongroupinterna

- **Testing of radiotherapy dosimeters in accordance with IEC specification (STUK)** by Hannu Järvinen; ISBN: 9514698703;
  http://www.amazon.com/exec/obidos/ASIN/9514698703/icongroupinterna

- **The Design of Radiotherapy Treatment Room Facilities (Report)** by B. Stedeford, et al; ISBN: 0904181855;
  http://www.amazon.com/exec/obidos/ASIN/0904181855/icongroupinterna

- **The Physics of Radiotherapy X-Rays from Linear Accelerators** by Peter Metcalfe, et al;
  ISBN: 0944838766;
  http://www.amazon.com/exec/obidos/ASIN/0944838766/icongroupinterna

- **The Q Book: The Physics of Radiotherapy X-Rays Problems & Solutions** by Peter
  Metcalfe, et al; ISBN: 0944838863;
  http://www.amazon.com/exec/obidos/ASIN/0944838863/icongroupinterna

- **The Radiotherapy of Malignant Disease** by Eric C. Easson (Other Contributor); ISBN:
  0387131043;
  http://www.amazon.com/exec/obidos/ASIN/0387131043/icongroupinterna

- **The Radiotherapy of Malignant Disease** by R. C. S. Pointon (Other Contributor); ISBN:
  3540196226;
  http://www.amazon.com/exec/obidos/ASIN/3540196226/icongroupinterna

- **The Radiotherapy of Malignant Disease**; ISBN: 3540131043;
  http://www.amazon.com/exec/obidos/ASIN/3540131043/icongroupinterna

- **The World Market for X-Ray, Radiography, or Radiotherapy Apparatus: A 2004
  Global Trade Perspective [DOWNLOAD: PDF]**; ISBN: B0001342XM;
  http://www.amazon.com/exec/obidos/ASIN/B0001342XM/icongroupinterna

- **Topical Reviews in Radiotherapy and Oncology (Topical Reviews)** by Thomas J.
  Deeley (Editor); ISBN: 0723605386;
  http://www.amazon.com/exec/obidos/ASIN/0723605386/icongroupinterna

- **Tumors of the central nervous system: Modern radiotherapy in multi-disciplinary
  management**; ISBN: 089352137X;
  http://www.amazon.com/exec/obidos/ASIN/089352137X/icongroupinterna

- **Urological Complications of Pelvic Surgery and Radiotherapy (Societe Internationale
  D'Urologie Reports)** by Michael A. S. Jewett; ISBN: 1899066144;
  http://www.amazon.com/exec/obidos/ASIN/1899066144/icongroupinterna

- **Use of Computers in External Beam Radiotherapy Procedures With High-Energy
  Photons and Electrons (Icru Report No. 42)** by Icru Staff; ISBN: 091339436X;
  http://www.amazon.com/exec/obidos/ASIN/091339436X/icongroupinterna

Chapters on Radiotherapy

In order to find chapters that specifically relate to radiotherapy, an excellent source of abstracts is the Combined Health Information Database. You will need to limit your search to book chapters and radiotherapy using the "Detailed Search" option. Go to the following hyperlink: **http://chid.nih.gov/detail/detail.html**. To find book chapters, use the drop boxes at the bottom of the search page where "You may refine your search by." Select the dates and language you prefer, and the format option "Book Chapter." Type "radiotherapy" (or synonyms) into the "For these words:" box. The following is a typical result when searching for book chapters on radiotherapy:

- **Implant Rehabilitation of the Mandible Compromised by Radiotherapy**

  Source: in Taylor, T.D., ed. Clinical Maxillofacial Prosthetics. Chicago, IL: Quintessence Publishing Co, Inc. 2000. p. 189-203.

Contact: Available from Quintessence Publishing Co, Inc. 551 Kimberly Drive, Carol Stream, IL 60188-9981. (800) 621-0387 or (630) 682-3223. Fax (630) 682-3288. E-mail: quintpub@aol.com. Website: www.quintpub.com. PRICE: $138.00 plus shipping and handling. ISBN: 0867153911.

Summary: This chapter is from a textbook that offers an indepth review of prosthodontic (the construction of artificial appliances that replace missing teeth or restore parts of the face) procedures as they are applied in the maxillofacial (jaw) situation. This chapter covers implant rehabilitation of the mandible (lower jaw) compromised by radiation therapy (**radiotherapy**). The author discusses treatment sequence, post tumor treatment considerations, preimplant treatment prostheses, preimplant and postimplant hyperbaric oxygen treatment, surgical stents, placement and modification of treatment prostheses, abutment connection surgery, prosthesis modification, preliminary impression, the final impression, maxillomandibular relationship records, tooth arrangement, framework fabrication and fitting, tooth arrangement and process, prosthesis placement, and follow up and maintenance. The author discusses some of the philosophical controversies regarding treatment protocols, then covers one protocol in detail. The chapter is illustrated with full color and black and white photographs and radiographs. 16 figures. 3 references.

- **Cytotoxic Chemotherapy and Radiotherapy**

  Source: in Scully, C. and Cawson, R.A. Medical Problems in Dentistry. 4th ed. Woburn, MA: Butterworth-Heinemann. 1998. p. 145-153.

  Contact: Available from Butterworth-Heinemann. 225 Wildwood Avenue, Woburn, MA 01801-2041. (800) 366-2665 or (781) 904-2500. Fax (800) 446-6520 or (781) 933-6333. E-mail: orders@bhusa.com. Website: www.bh.com. PRICE: $110.00. ISBN: 0723610568.

  Summary: This chapter on cytotoxic chemotherapy and **radiotherapy** (radiation therapy) is from a text that covers the general medical and surgical conditions relevant to the oral health care sciences. Topics include the complications of cytotoxic chemotherapy, including infections, ulcers and mucositis, lip cracking, bleeding, xerostomia (dry mouth), and delayed and abnormal development of the teeth and jaws; the dental management of patients on cytotoxic chemotherapy; the complications of radiation therapy involving the oral cavity or salivary glands, including mucositis, xerostomia and infections, radiation caries and dental hypersensitivity, loss of taste, trismus (reduction of mouth opening), osteoradionecrosis (bone death) and osteomyelitis (bone marrow infection), and craniofacial defects; and the dental management of patients receiving **radiotherapy** to the head and neck. Extensive tables summarize the various chemotherapeutic agents and their main uses. The chapter includes a lengthy summary of the points covered. 1 figure. 4 tables. 37 references.

- **Management of the Patient Undergoing Radiotherapy or Chemotherapy**

  Source: in Peterson, L.J., et al., eds. Contemporary Oral and Maxillofacial Surgery. 3rd ed. St. Louis, MO: Mosby-Year Book, Inc. 1998. p. 456-468.

  Contact: Available from Mosby-Year Book, Inc. 11830 Westline Industrial Drive, St. Louis, MO 63146. PRICE: $69.00. ISBN: 0815166990.

  Summary: This chapter on management of the patient undergoing **radiotherapy** (radiation therapy) or chemotherapy is from a textbook that provides a comprehensive description of the basic oral surgery procedures that the general practitioner performs in his or her office. The basic techniques of evaluation, diagnosis, and medical management are described in sufficient detail to allow immediate clinical application. The first section covers radiation effects on oral mucosa, radiation effects on salivary glands, the treatment of xerostomia (dry mouth), radiation effects on bone, other effects of radiation, evaluation of the dentition before radiation therapy, preparation of the dentition for radiation therapy, maintenance after irradiation, a method of performing preirradiation extractions, the interval between preirradiation extractions and the beginning of **radiotherapy,** impacted third molar removal before **radiotherapy,** a method of dealing with carious teeth (those with cavities) after radiation therapy, tooth extraction after radiation therapy, denture considerations, the use of dental implants in patients who have been irradiated, and the management of patients who develop osteoradionecrosis. The second section focuses on the dental management of patients on systemic chemotherapy for malignant disease (cancer). Topics include the effects on the oral mucosa, on the hematopoietic system, on the oral microbiology, general dental management, and the treatment of oral candidiasis. The chapter is illustrated with black and white photographs and radiographs. 14 figures. 32 references.

CHAPTER 7. PERIODICALS AND NEWS ON RADIOTHERAPY

Overview

In this chapter, we suggest a number of news sources and present various periodicals that cover radiotherapy.

News Services and Press Releases

One of the simplest ways of tracking press releases on radiotherapy is to search the news wires. In the following sample of sources, we will briefly describe how to access each service. These services only post recent news intended for public viewing.

PR Newswire

To access the PR Newswire archive, simply go to **http://www.prnewswire.com/**. Select your country. Type "radiotherapy" (or synonyms) into the search box. You will automatically receive information on relevant news releases posted within the last 30 days. The search results are shown by order of relevance.

Reuters Health

The Reuters' Medical News and Health eLine databases can be very useful in exploring news archives relating to radiotherapy. While some of the listed articles are free to view, others are available for purchase for a nominal fee. To access this archive, go to **http://www.reutershealth.com/en/index.html** and search by "radiotherapy" (or synonyms). The following was recently listed in this archive for radiotherapy:

- **Cisplatin with radiotherapy helps preserve bladder**
  Source: Reuters Industry Breifing
  Date: October 14, 2004

- **Hodgkin's disease radiotherapy tied to later heart problems**
  Source: Reuters Medical News
  Date: August 11, 2004

- **Focused radiotherapy safely controls pediatric ependymoma**
Source: Reuters Medical News
Date: August 10, 2004

- **Internet information on intensity-modulated radiotherapy deemed poor**
Source: Reuters Industry Breifing
Date: August 06, 2004

- **Adjuvant, salvage radiotherapy comparable after prostate cancer surgery**
Source: Reuters Industry Breifing
Date: June 10, 2004

- **Adjuvant single-shot carboplatin equal to radiotherapy in early seminoma**
Source: Reuters Industry Breifing
Date: June 08, 2004

- **Temozolomide plus radiotherapy ups survival in glioblastoma multiforme**
Source: Reuters Medical News
Date: June 07, 2004

- **Gene therapy potentiates radiotherapy in tumors**
Source: Reuters Medical News
Date: May 24, 2004

- **Breast radiotherapy linked to heart disease deaths**
Source: Reuters Health eLine
Date: March 18, 2004

- **Early salvage radiotherapy treats "incurable" recurrent prostate cancer**
Source: Reuters Industry Breifing
Date: March 16, 2004

- **Childhood radiotherapy rarely tied to subsequent melanoma**
Source: Reuters Medical News
Date: November 28, 2003

- **Utilization of radiotherapy for breast cancer suboptimal**
Source: Reuters Medical News
Date: November 12, 2003

- **Targeted high-dose radiotherapy benefits inoperable lung cancer patients**
Source: Reuters Medical News
Date: November 12, 2003

- **Stereotactic radiotherapy effective for pediatric brain tumors**
Source: Reuters Medical News
Date: October 22, 2003

- **Single-fraction radiotherapy effectively treats painful bone metastases**
Source: Reuters Medical News
Date: October 20, 2003

- **New test for reaction to radiotherapy treatment**
Source: Reuters Industry Breifing
Date: September 22, 2003

- **Lymphocyte apoptosis assay predicts late radiotherapy toxicity**
Source: Reuters Medical News
Date: September 22, 2003

- **Accelerated radiotherapy may benefit cancer patients**
  Source: Reuters Health eLine
  Date: September 19, 2003

- **Accelerated radiotherapy improves head and neck cancer outcomes**
  Source: Reuters Medical News
  Date: September 18, 2003

- **Adding 5-FU to preoperative radiotherapy improves rectal cancer outcomes**
  Source: Reuters Medical News
  Date: September 17, 2003

- **Limited-field radiotherapy provides adequate local control for early breast cancer**
  Source: Reuters Medical News
  Date: August 19, 2003

- **TSH use before radiotherapy for thyroid cancer reduces iodine isotope half-life**
  Source: Reuters Medical News
  Date: July 18, 2003

- **Molecular markers point to radiotherapy outcome in prostate cancer**
  Source: Reuters Medical News
  Date: May 02, 2003

- **Low-iodide diet enhances efficacy of radiotherapy for thyroid cancer**
  Source: Reuters Medical News
  Date: April 30, 2003

The NIH

Within MEDLINEplus, the NIH has made an agreement with the New York Times Syndicate, the AP News Service, and Reuters to deliver news that can be browsed by the public. Search news releases at **http://www.nlm.nih.gov/medlineplus/alphanews_a.html**. MEDLINEplus allows you to browse across an alphabetical index. Or you can search by date at the following Web page: **http://www.nlm.nih.gov/medlineplus/newsbydate.html**. Often, news items are indexed by MEDLINEplus within its search engine.

Business Wire

Business Wire is similar to PR Newswire. To access this archive, simply go to **http://www.businesswire.com/**. You can scan the news by industry category or company name.

Market Wire

Market Wire is more focused on technology than the other wires. To browse the latest press releases by topic, such as alternative medicine, biotechnology, fitness, healthcare, legal, nutrition, and pharmaceuticals, access Market Wire's Medical/Health channel at **http://www.marketwire.com/mw/release_index?channel=MedicalHealth**. Or simply go to Market Wire's home page at **http://www.marketwire.com/mw/home**, type "radiotherapy" (or synonyms) into the search box, and click on "Search News." As this service is technology oriented, you may wish to use it when searching for press releases covering diagnostic procedures or tests.

Search Engines

Medical news is also available in the news sections of commercial Internet search engines. See the health news page at Yahoo (**http://dir.yahoo.com/Health/News_and_Media/**), or you can use this Web site's general news search page at **http://news.yahoo.com/**. Type in "radiotherapy" (or synonyms). If you know the name of a company that is relevant to radiotherapy, you can go to any stock trading Web site (such as **http://www.etrade.com/**) and search for the company name there. News items across various news sources are reported on indicated hyperlinks. Google offers a similar service at **http://news.google.com/**.

BBC

Covering news from a more European perspective, the British Broadcasting Corporation (BBC) allows the public free access to their news archive located at **http://www.bbc.co.uk/**. Search by "radiotherapy" (or synonyms).

Newsletter Articles

Use the Combined Health Information Database, and limit your search criteria to "newsletter articles." Again, you will need to use the "Detailed Search" option. Go directly to the following hyperlink: **http://chid.nih.gov/detail/detail.html**. Go to the bottom of the search page where "You may refine your search by." Select the dates and language that you prefer. For the format option, select "Newsletter Article." Type "radiotherapy" (or synonyms) into the "For these words:" box. You should check back periodically with this database as it is updated every three months. The following is a typical result when searching for newsletter articles on radiotherapy:

- **Stereotactic Radiation and Head and Neck Cancer**

    Source: News from SPOHNC. News from Support for People with Oral and Head and Neck Cancer, Inc. 10(7): 1-3, 7. April 2001.

    Contact: Available from Support for People with Oral and Head and Neck Cancer, Inc. (SPOHNC). P.O. Box 53, Locust Valley, NY 11560-0053. (516) 759-5333. E-mail: info@spohnc.org. Website: www.spohnc.org.

    Summary: The goal of the oncologist (cancer doctor) is to cure the patient with head and neck cancer with minimal cosmetic alteration while preserving the ability to swallow, speak, and articulate normally. This article explains the technique of stereotactic radiation and its use in treating patients with head and neck cancer. The authors stress that the primary advantage of stereotactic radiation is that it allows delivery of tightly shaped (conformal) radiation around the tumor, thereby sparing surrounding organs. The authors explain the differences between stereotactic radiosurgery (SRS) in which one large dose of radiation is delivered, from stereotactic **radiotherapy** (SRT) during which multiple smaller doses are given over a prolonged period. Other topics include the importance of treatment setup, gamma knife versus linear accelerator based treatment, the indications for stereotactic radiation, the treatment planning process, the side effects of treatment, expected results, and the limitations of stereotactic radiation (including small margin for error, tumor size limits, increased daily setup time, and increased labor sensitivity).

- **Nasopharyngeal Carcinoma**

  Source: News from SPOHNC. News from Support for People with Oral and Head and Neck Cancer, Inc. 11(2): 1-3. October 2001.

  Contact: Available from Support for People with Oral and Head and Neck Cancer, Inc. (SPOHNC). P.O. Box 53, Locust Valley, NY 11560-0053. (516) 759-5333. E-mail: info@spohnc.org. Website: www.spohnc.org.

  Summary: This article, from a newsletter for people with oral and head and neck cancer, reviews nasopharyngeal cancer. The nasopharynx is an open chamber located behind the nasal cavity and below the base of the skull. The authors discuss the etiology (cause) and risk factors, clinical presentation (symptoms), routes of spread, physical and diagnostic evaluation, staging, complications, and treatment recommendations. The most common side effects occurring during and shortly after treatment are breakdown of the mucosa of the pharynx, dry mouth (xerostomia), and reddening (erythema) of the skin. The most common long term side effect is xerostomia, although its incidence decreases tremendously with IMRT (intensity modulated radiation therapy). Trismus (difficulty opening the mouth) may occur. The authors note that patients who present with early T1-2 N0-1 staged disease are good candidates for external beam **radiotherapy** alone. Combined modality treatment is recommended for all other lesions. 20 references.

Academic Periodicals covering Radiotherapy

Numerous periodicals are currently indexed within the National Library of Medicine's PubMed database that are known to publish articles relating to radiotherapy. In addition to these sources, you can search for articles covering radiotherapy that have been published by any of the periodicals listed in previous chapters. To find the latest studies published, go to **http://www.ncbi.nlm.nih.gov/pubmed**, type the name of the periodical into the search box, and click "Go."

If you want complete details about the historical contents of a journal, you can also visit the following Web site: **http://www.ncbi.nlm.nih.gov/entrez/jrbrowser.cgi**. Here, type in the name of the journal or its abbreviation, and you will receive an index of published articles. At **http://locatorplus.gov/**, you can retrieve more indexing information on medical periodicals (e.g. the name of the publisher). Select the button "Search LOCATORplus." Then type in the name of the journal and select the advanced search option "Journal Title Search."

CHAPTER 8. RESEARCHING MEDICATIONS

Overview

While a number of hard copy or CD-ROM resources are available for researching medications, a more flexible method is to use Internet-based databases. Broadly speaking, there are two sources of information on approved medications: public sources and private sources. We will emphasize free-to-use public sources.

U.S. Pharmacopeia

Because of historical investments by various organizations and the emergence of the Internet, it has become rather simple to learn about the medications recommended for radiotherapy. One such source is the United States Pharmacopeia. In 1820, eleven physicians met in Washington, D.C. to establish the first compendium of standard drugs for the United States. They called this compendium the U.S. Pharmacopeia (USP). Today, the USP is a non-profit organization consisting of 800 volunteer scientists, eleven elected officials, and 400 representatives of state associations and colleges of medicine and pharmacy. The USP is located in Rockville, Maryland, and its home page is located at **http://www.usp.org/**. The USP currently provides standards for over 3,700 medications. The resulting USP DI® Advice for the Patient® can be accessed through the National Library of Medicine of the National Institutes of Health. The database is partially derived from lists of federally approved medications in the Food and Drug Administration's (FDA) Drug Approvals database, located at **http://www.fda.gov/cder/da/da.htm**.

While the FDA database is rather large and difficult to navigate, the Phamacopeia is both user-friendly and free to use. It covers more than 9,000 prescription and over-the-counter medications. To access this database, simply type the following hyperlink into your Web browser: **http://www.nlm.nih.gov/medlineplus/druginformation.html**. To view examples of a given medication (brand names, category, description, preparation, proper use, precautions, side effects, etc.), simply follow the hyperlinks indicated within the United States Pharmacopeia (USP).

Commercial Databases

In addition to the medications listed in the USP above, a number of commercial sites are available by subscription to physicians and their institutions. Or, you may be able to access these sources from your local medical library.

Mosby's Drug Consult™

Mosby's Drug Consult™ database (also available on CD-ROM and book format) covers 45,000 drug products including generics and international brands. It provides prescribing information, drug interactions, and patient information. Subscription information is available at the following hyperlink: **http://www.mosbysdrugconsult.com/**.

PDR*health*

The PDR*health* database is a free-to-use, drug information search engine that has been written for the public in layman's terms. It contains FDA-approved drug information adapted from the Physicians' Desk Reference (PDR) database. PDR*health* can be searched by brand name, generic name, or indication. It features multiple drug interactions reports. Search PDR*health* at **http://www.pdrhealth.com/drug_info/index.html**.

Other Web Sites

Drugs.com (**www.drugs.com**) reproduces the information in the Pharmacopeia as well as commercial information. You may also want to consider the Web site of the Medical Letter, Inc. (**http://www.medletter.com/**) which allows users to download articles on various drugs and therapeutics for a nominal fee.

Researching Orphan Drugs

Although the list of orphan drugs is revised on a daily basis, you can quickly research orphan drugs that might be applicable to radiotherapy by using the database managed by the National Organization for Rare Disorders, Inc. (NORD), at **http://www.rarediseases.org/**. Scroll down the page, and on the left toolbar, click on "Orphan Drug Designation Database." On this page (**http://www.rarediseases.org/search/noddsearch.html**), type "radiotherapy" (or synonyms) into the search box, and click "Submit Query." When you receive your results, note that not all of the drugs may be relevant, as some may have been withdrawn from orphan status. Write down or print out the name of each drug and the relevant contact information. From there, visit the Pharmacopeia Web site and type the name of each orphan drug into the search box at **http://www.nlm.nih.gov/medlineplus/druginformation.html**. You may need to contact the sponsor or NORD for further information.

NORD conducts "early access programs for investigational new drugs (IND) under the Food and Drug Administration's (FDA's) approval 'Treatment INDs' programs which allow for a limited number of individuals to receive investigational drugs before FDA marketing approval." If the orphan product about which you are seeking information is approved for marketing, information on side effects can be found on the product's label. If the product is not approved, you may need to contact the sponsor.

The following is a list of orphan drugs currently listed in the NORD Orphan Drug Designation Database for radiotherapy:

- **Temoporfin (trade name: Foscan)**
  http://www.rarediseases.org/nord/search/nodd_full?code=1000

If you have any questions about a medical treatment, the FDA may have an office near you. Look for their number in the blue pages of the phone book. You can also contact the FDA through its toll-free number, 1-888-INFO-FDA (1-888-463-6332), or on the World Wide Web at **www.fda.gov**.

APPENDICES

APPENDIX A. PHYSICIAN RESOURCES

Overview

In this chapter, we focus on databases and Internet-based guidelines and information resources created or written for a professional audience.

NIH Guidelines

Commonly referred to as "clinical" or "professional" guidelines, the National Institutes of Health publish physician guidelines for the most common diseases. Publications are available at the following by relevant Institute[10]:

- Office of the Director (OD); guidelines consolidated across agencies available at **http://www.nih.gov/health/consumer/conkey.htm**

- National Institute of General Medical Sciences (NIGMS); fact sheets available at **http://www.nigms.nih.gov/news/facts/**

- National Library of Medicine (NLM); extensive encyclopedia (A.D.A.M., Inc.) with guidelines: **http://www.nlm.nih.gov/medlineplus/healthtopics.html**

- National Cancer Institute (NCI); guidelines available at **http://www.cancer.gov/cancerinfo/list.aspx?viewid=5f35036e-5497-4d86-8c2c-714a9f7c8d25**

- National Eye Institute (NEI); guidelines available at **http://www.nei.nih.gov/order/index.htm**

- National Heart, Lung, and Blood Institute (NHLBI); guidelines available at **http://www.nhlbi.nih.gov/guidelines/index.htm**

- National Human Genome Research Institute (NHGRI); research available at **http://www.genome.gov/page.cfm?pageID=10000375**

- National Institute on Aging (NIA); guidelines available at **http://www.nia.nih.gov/health/**

---

[10] These publications are typically written by one or more of the various NIH Institutes.

- National Institute on Alcohol Abuse and Alcoholism (NIAAA); guidelines available at http://www.niaaa.nih.gov/publications/publications.htm

- National Institute of Allergy and Infectious Diseases (NIAID); guidelines available at http://www.niaid.nih.gov/publications/

- National Institute of Arthritis and Musculoskeletal and Skin Diseases (NIAMS); fact sheets and guidelines available at http://www.niams.nih.gov/hi/index.htm

- National Institute of Child Health and Human Development (NICHD); guidelines available at http://www.nichd.nih.gov/publications/pubskey.cfm

- National Institute on Deafness and Other Communication Disorders (NIDCD); fact sheets and guidelines at http://www.nidcd.nih.gov/health/

- National Institute of Dental and Craniofacial Research (NIDCR); guidelines available at http://www.nidr.nih.gov/health/

- National Institute of Diabetes and Digestive and Kidney Diseases (NIDDK); guidelines available at http://www.niddk.nih.gov/health/health.htm

- National Institute on Drug Abuse (NIDA); guidelines available at http://www.nida.nih.gov/DrugAbuse.html

- National Institute of Environmental Health Sciences (NIEHS); environmental health information available at http://www.niehs.nih.gov/external/facts.htm

- National Institute of Mental Health (NIMH); guidelines available at http://www.nimh.nih.gov/practitioners/index.cfm

- National Institute of Neurological Disorders and Stroke (NINDS); neurological disorder information pages available at http://www.ninds.nih.gov/health_and_medical/disorder_index.htm

- National Institute of Nursing Research (NINR); publications on selected illnesses at http://www.nih.gov/ninr/news-info/publications.html

- National Institute of Biomedical Imaging and Bioengineering; general information at http://grants.nih.gov/grants/becon/becon_info.htm

- Center for Information Technology (CIT); referrals to other agencies based on keyword searches available at http://kb.nih.gov/www_query_main.asp

- National Center for Complementary and Alternative Medicine (NCCAM); health information available at http://nccam.nih.gov/health/

- National Center for Research Resources (NCRR); various information directories available at http://www.ncrr.nih.gov/publications.asp

- Office of Rare Diseases; various fact sheets available at http://rarediseases.info.nih.gov/html/resources/rep_pubs.html

- Centers for Disease Control and Prevention; various fact sheets on infectious diseases available at http://www.cdc.gov/publications.htm

NIH Databases

In addition to the various Institutes of Health that publish professional guidelines, the NIH has designed a number of databases for professionals.[11] Physician-oriented resources provide a wide variety of information related to the biomedical and health sciences, both past and present. The format of these resources varies. Searchable databases, bibliographic citations, full-text articles (when available), archival collections, and images are all available. The following are referenced by the National Library of Medicine:[12]

- **Bioethics:** Access to published literature on the ethical, legal, and public policy issues surrounding healthcare and biomedical research. This information is provided in conjunction with the Kennedy Institute of Ethics located at Georgetown University, Washington, D.C.: **http://www.nlm.nih.gov/databases/databases_bioethics.html**

- **HIV/AIDS Resources:** Describes various links and databases dedicated to HIV/AIDS research: **http://www.nlm.nih.gov/pubs/factsheets/aidsinfs.html**

- **NLM Online Exhibitions:** Describes "Exhibitions in the History of Medicine": **http://www.nlm.nih.gov/exhibition/exhibition.html**. Additional resources for historical scholarship in medicine: **http://www.nlm.nih.gov/hmd/hmd.html**

- **Biotechnology Information:** Access to public databases. The National Center for Biotechnology Information conducts research in computational biology, develops software tools for analyzing genome data, and disseminates biomedical information for the better understanding of molecular processes affecting human health and disease: **http://www.ncbi.nlm.nih.gov/**

- **Population Information:** The National Library of Medicine provides access to worldwide coverage of population, family planning, and related health issues, including family planning technology and programs, fertility, and population law and policy: **http://www.nlm.nih.gov/databases/databases_population.html**

- **Cancer Information:** Access to cancer-oriented databases: **http://www.nlm.nih.gov/databases/databases_cancer.html**

- **Profiles in Science:** Offering the archival collections of prominent twentieth-century biomedical scientists to the public through modern digital technology: **http://www.profiles.nlm.nih.gov/**

- **Chemical Information:** Provides links to various chemical databases and references: **http://sis.nlm.nih.gov/Chem/ChemMain.html**

- **Clinical Alerts:** Reports the release of findings from the NIH-funded clinical trials where such release could significantly affect morbidity and mortality: **http://www.nlm.nih.gov/databases/alerts/clinical_alerts.html**

- **Space Life Sciences:** Provides links and information to space-based research (including NASA): **http://www.nlm.nih.gov/databases/databases_space.html**

- **MEDLINE:** Bibliographic database covering the fields of medicine, nursing, dentistry, veterinary medicine, the healthcare system, and the pre-clinical sciences: **http://www.nlm.nih.gov/databases/databases_medline.html**

---

[11] Remember, for the general public, the National Library of Medicine recommends the databases referenced in MEDLINE*plus* (**http://medlineplus.gov/** or **http://www.nlm.nih.gov/medlineplus/databases.html**).

[12] See **http://www.nlm.nih.gov/databases/databases.html**.

- **Toxicology and Environmental Health Information (TOXNET):** Databases covering toxicology and environmental health: **http://sis.nlm.nih.gov/Tox/ToxMain.html**

- **Visible Human Interface:** Anatomically detailed, three-dimensional representations of normal male and female human bodies: **http://www.nlm.nih.gov/research/visible/visible_human.html**

The NLM Gateway[13]

The NLM (National Library of Medicine) Gateway is a Web-based system that lets users search simultaneously in multiple retrieval systems at the U.S. National Library of Medicine (NLM). It allows users of NLM services to initiate searches from one Web interface, providing one-stop searching for many of NLM's information resources or databases.[14] To use the NLM Gateway, simply go to the search site at **http://gateway.nlm.nih.gov/gw/Cmd**. Type "radiotherapy" (or synonyms) into the search box and click "Search." The results will be presented in a tabular form, indicating the number of references in each database category.

Results Summary

Category	Items Found
Journal Articles	166650
Books / Periodicals / Audio Visual	2361
Consumer Health	1413
Meeting Abstracts	185
Other Collections	82
Total	170691

HSTAT[15]

HSTAT is a free, Web-based resource that provides access to full-text documents used in healthcare decision-making.[16] These documents include clinical practice guidelines, quick-reference guides for clinicians, consumer health brochures, evidence reports and technology assessments from the Agency for Healthcare Research and Quality (AHRQ), as well as AHRQ's Put Prevention Into Practice.[17] Simply search by "radiotherapy" (or synonyms) at the following Web site: **http://text.nlm.nih.gov**.

---

[13] Adapted from NLM: **http://gateway.nlm.nih.gov/gw/Cmd?Overview.x**.

[14] The NLM Gateway is currently being developed by the Lister Hill National Center for Biomedical Communications (LHNCBC) at the National Library of Medicine (NLM) of the National Institutes of Health (NIH).

[15] Adapted from HSTAT: **http://www.nlm.nih.gov/pubs/factsheets/hstat.html**.

[16] The HSTAT URL is **http://hstat.nlm.nih.gov/**.

[17] Other important documents in HSTAT include: the National Institutes of Health (NIH) Consensus Conference Reports and Technology Assessment Reports; the HIV/AIDS Treatment Information Service (ATIS) resource documents; the Substance Abuse and Mental Health Services Administration's Center for Substance Abuse Treatment (SAMHSA/CSAT) Treatment Improvement Protocols (TIP) and Center for Substance Abuse Prevention (SAMHSA/CSAP) Prevention Enhancement Protocols System (PEPS); the Public Health Service (PHS) Preventive Services Task Force's *Guide to Clinical Preventive Services*; the independent, nonfederal Task Force on Community Services' *Guide to Community Preventive Services*; and the Health Technology Advisory Committee (HTAC) of the Minnesota Health Care Commission (MHCC) health technology evaluations.

Coffee Break: Tutorials for Biologists[18]

Coffee Break is a general healthcare site that takes a scientific view of the news and covers recent breakthroughs in biology that may one day assist physicians in developing treatments. Here you will find a collection of short reports on recent biological discoveries. Each report incorporates interactive tutorials that demonstrate how bioinformatics tools are used as a part of the research process. Currently, all Coffee Breaks are written by NCBI staff.[19] Each report is about 400 words and is usually based on a discovery reported in one or more articles from recently published, peer-reviewed literature.[20] This site has new articles every few weeks, so it can be considered an online magazine of sorts. It is intended for general background information. You can access the Coffee Break Web site at the following hyperlink: **http://www.ncbi.nlm.nih.gov/Coffeebreak/**.

Other Commercial Databases

In addition to resources maintained by official agencies, other databases exist that are commercial ventures addressing medical professionals. Here are some examples that may interest you:

- **CliniWeb International:** Index and table of contents to selected clinical information on the Internet; see **http://www.ohsu.edu/cliniweb/**.

- **Medical World Search:** Searches full text from thousands of selected medical sites on the Internet; see **http://www.mwsearch.com/**.

---

[18] Adapted from **http://www.ncbi.nlm.nih.gov/Coffeebreak/Archive/FAQ.html**.

[19] The figure that accompanies each article is frequently supplied by an expert external to NCBI, in which case the source of the figure is cited. The result is an interactive tutorial that tells a biological story.

[20] After a brief introduction that sets the work described into a broader context, the report focuses on how a molecular understanding can provide explanations of observed biology and lead to therapies for diseases. Each vignette is accompanied by a figure and hypertext links that lead to a series of pages that interactively show how NCBI tools and resources are used in the research process.

APPENDIX B. PATIENT RESOURCES

Overview

Official agencies, as well as federally funded institutions supported by national grants, frequently publish a variety of guidelines written with the patient in mind. These are typically called "Fact Sheets" or "Guidelines." They can take the form of a brochure, information kit, pamphlet, or flyer. Often they are only a few pages in length. Since new guidelines on radiotherapy can appear at any moment and be published by a number of sources, the best approach to finding guidelines is to systematically scan the Internet-based services that post them.

Patient Guideline Sources

The remainder of this chapter directs you to sources which either publish or can help you find additional guidelines on topics related to radiotherapy. Due to space limitations, these sources are listed in a concise manner. Do not hesitate to consult the following sources by either using the Internet hyperlink provided, or, in cases where the contact information is provided, contacting the publisher or author directly.

The National Institutes of Health

The NIH gateway to patients is located at **http://health.nih.gov/**. From this site, you can search across various sources and institutes, a number of which are summarized below.

Topic Pages: MEDLINEplus

The National Library of Medicine has created a vast and patient-oriented healthcare information portal called MEDLINEplus. Within this Internet-based system are "health topic pages" which list links to available materials relevant to radiotherapy. To access this system, log on to **http://www.nlm.nih.gov/medlineplus/healthtopics.html**. From there you can either search using the alphabetical index or browse by broad topic areas. Recently, MEDLINEplus listed the following when searched for "radiotherapy":

Brain Cancer
http://www.nlm.nih.gov/medlineplus/braincancer.html

Cancer
http://www.nlm.nih.gov/medlineplus/cancer.html

Prostate Cancer
http://www.nlm.nih.gov/medlineplus/prostatecancer.html

Radiation Exposure
http://www.nlm.nih.gov/medlineplus/radiationexposure.html

Within the health topic page dedicated to radiotherapy, the following was listed:

- Treatment

    Epoetin Treatment
    Source: American Society of Clinical Oncology
    http://www.asco.org/ac/1%2C1003%2C_12-002214-00_18-0024517-00_19-0024518-00_20-001%2C00.asp

- Coping

    Radiation Therapy Effects
    Source: American Cancer Society
    http://www.cancer.org/docroot/MBC/MBC_2x_RadiationEffects.asp?sitearea=MBC

- Children

    Interventional Radiology for Children
    Source: Society of Interventional Radiology
    http://www.sirweb.org/patPub/forChildren.shtml

    Radiation Therapy
    Source: Nemours Foundation
    http://kidshealth.org/parent/system/doctor/radiation.html

- From the National Institutes of Health

    Radiation Therapy and You: A Guide to Self-Help during Cancer Treatment
    Source: National Cancer Institute
    http://www.cancer.gov/cancerinfo/radiation-therapy-and-you/

- Latest News

    New Method May Improve Therapy Prostate Cancer
    Source: 10/22/2004, Reuters Health
    http://www.nlm.nih.gov//www.nlm.nih.gov/medlineplus/news/fullstory_20821.html

    Radiation Not Needed After Chemo Cures Hodgkin's
    Source: 10/05/2004, Reuters Health
    http://www.nlm.nih.gov//www.nlm.nih.gov/medlineplus/news/fullstory_20506

.html

Rectal Cancer Chemo, Radiation Best Before Surgery
Source: 10/20/2004, Reuters Health
http://www.nlm.nih.gov//www.nlm.nih.gov/medlineplus/news/fullstory_20757
.html

- Organizations

    International Radiosurgery Support Association
    http://www.irsa.org/

    National Cancer Institute
    http://www.cancer.gov/

    Radiation Therapy Oncology Group
    http://www.rtog.org/index.html

    Radiology Info
    Source: American College of Radiology, Radiological Society of North America
    http://www.radiologyinfo.org/

    Society of Interventional Radiology
    http://www.sirweb.org/

- Research

    Radiation for Childhood Cancer May Affect Future Pregnancies
    Source: American Cancer Society
    http://www.cancer.org/docroot/NWS/content/NWS_2_1x_Radiation_For_Childh
    ood_Cancer_May_Affect_Future_Pregnancies.asp

    Single-Dose Radiation Cost Effective for Cancer Bone Pain
    Source: American Cancer Society
    http://www.cancer.org/docroot/NWS/content/NWS_2_1x_Single-
    Dose_Radiation_Cost_Effective_For_Cancer_Bone_Pain.asp

You may also choose to use the search utility provided by MEDLINEplus at the following Web address: **http://www.nlm.nih.gov/medlineplus/**. Simply type a keyword into the search box and click "Search." This utility is similar to the NIH search utility, with the exception that it only includes materials that are linked within the MEDLINEplus system (mostly patient-oriented information). It also has the disadvantage of generating unstructured results. We recommend, therefore, that you use this method only if you have a very targeted search.

The Combined Health Information Database (CHID)

CHID Online is a reference tool that maintains a database directory of thousands of journal articles and patient education guidelines on radiotherapy. CHID offers summaries that describe the guidelines available, including contact information and pricing. CHID's general Web site is **http://chid.nih.gov/**. To search this database, go to **http://chid.nih.gov/detail/detail.html**. In particular, you can use the advanced search options to look up pamphlets, reports, brochures, and information kits. The following was recently posted in this archive:

- **We Have Walked in Your Shoes: Radiation Therapy and Chemotherapy for the Oral and Head and Neck Cancer Patient: Part II**

  Source: Locust Valley, New York: SPOHNC (Support for People with Oral and Head and Neck Cancer, Inc.). 2002. 20 p.

  Contact: Available from SPOHNC (Support for People with Oral and Head and Neck Cancer, Inc.). P. O. Box 53, Locust Valley, New York, 11560-0053. (800) 377-0928. Fax: (516) 671-8794. Website: www.spohnc.org. Email: info@spohnc.org. PRICE: Full-text available online at no charge; Single copy free; $5.00 for shipping and handling.

  Summary: Cancer patients and their families face many challenges in learning to live with their disease. Having access to helpful information and support services may help people to cope with their individual circumstances. This booklet is the second component of the SPOHNC (Support for People with Oral and Head and Neck Cancer) Patient Information Folder. The booklet contains basic information about two treatments for oral and head and neck cancer: radiation therapy and chemotherapy. Written in a question and answer format, the booklet covers standard radiation therapy, hyperfractionated radiation therapy, brachytherapy (radiation implant therapy), three dimensional conformal radiation therapy, intensity modulated radiation therapy (IMRT), 3D stereotactic radiation therapy, chemotherapy, the use of radiation therapy and chemotherapy at the same time, fast neutron **radiotherapy,** proton therapy, how to maintain a healthy mouth, pretreatment considerations, and the oral complications of radiation therapy and chemotherapy, including dry mouth (xerostomia), loss or change of taste, mucositis, bleeding in the mouth, trismus (loss of elasticity in the muscles that open and close the mouth), infections of the tongue, osteoradionecrosis (bone death, usually in the jaw bones), difficulties in swallowing and eating, difficulties in maintaining proper nutrition, and fatigue. The booklet also includes a list of oral and head and neck cancer resources and web site addresses, as well as related publications. A glossary of acronyms and medical terms concludes the booklet. Readers are encouraged to contact the organization (www.spohnc.org or 800-377-0928) for more information.

The National Guideline Clearinghouse™

The National Guideline Clearinghouse™ offers hundreds of evidence-based clinical practice guidelines published in the United States and other countries. You can search this site located at **http://www.guideline.gov/** by using the keyword "radiotherapy" (or synonyms). The following was recently posted:

- **2002 update of recommendations for the use of chemotherapy and radiotherapy protectants: clinical practice guidelines of the American Society of Clinical Oncology**

  Source: American Society of Clinical Oncology - Medical Specialty Society; 1999 October (revised 2002 Jun); 9 pages

  http://www.guideline.gov/summary/summary.aspx?doc_id=3348&nbr=2574&string=radiotherapy

- **Accelerated radiotherapy for locally advanced squamous cell carcinoma of the head and neck**

  Source: Practice Guidelines Initiative - State/Local Government Agency [Non-U.S.]; 2000 November 27 (updated online 2002 Oct); 19 pages

  http://www.guideline.gov/summary/summary.aspx?doc_id=3764&nbr=2990&string=radiotherapy

- **Combined modality radiotherapy and chemotherapy in the non-surgical management of localized carcinoma of the esophagus**

  Source: Practice Guidelines Initiative - State/Local Government Agency [Non-U.S.]; 2003 August 18; 22 pages

  http://www.guideline.gov/summary/summary.aspx?doc_id=4264&nbr=3264&string=radiotherapy

- **Hyperfractionated radiotherapy for locally advanced squamous cell carcinoma of the head and neck**

  Source: Practice Guidelines Initiative - State/Local Government Agency [Non-U.S.]; 2000 November 27 (revised online 2003 Jan); 13 pages

  http://www.guideline.gov/summary/summary.aspx?doc_id=3601&nbr=2827&string=radiotherapy

- **Management of brain metastases: role of radiotherapy alone or in combination with other treatment modalities**

  Source: Practice Guidelines Initiative - State/Local Government Agency [Non-U.S.]; 2004 March 30; 35 pages

  http://www.guideline.gov/summary/summary.aspx?doc_id=4983&nbr=3529&string=radiotherapy

- **Postoperative adjuvant radiotherapy and/or chemotherapy for resected stage II or III rectal cancer**

  Source: Practice Guidelines Initiative - State/Local Government Agency [Non-U.S.]; 1998 September 5 (updated online 2001 Dec); Various pagings

  http://www.guideline.gov/summary/summary.aspx?doc_id=3282&nbr=2508&string=radiotherapy

- **The role of chemotherapy with radiotherapy in the management of patients with newly diagnosed locally advanced squamous cell or undifferentiated nasopharyngeal cancer**

  Source: Practice Guidelines Initiative - State/Local Government Agency [Non-U.S.]; 2003 July 22 (revised 2004 Mar); 20 pages

  http://www.guideline.gov/summary/summary.aspx?doc_id=4981&nbr=3527&string=radiotherapy

- **The role of thoracic radiotherapy as an adjunct to standard chemotherapy in limited-stage small cell lung cancer**

  Source: Practice Guidelines Initiative - State/Local Government Agency [Non-U.S.]; 1999 October 8 (updated online 2003 Jan); 20 pages

  http://www.guideline.gov/summary/summary.aspx?doc_id=3765&nbr=2991&string=radiotherapy

- **The use of conformal radiotherapy and the selection of radiation dose in T1 or T2 prostate cancer**

  Source: Practice Guidelines Initiative - State/Local Government Agency [Non-U.S.]; 2002 October; 23 pages

  http://www.guideline.gov/summary/summary.aspx?doc_id=3461&nbr=2687&string=radiotherapy

- **The use of preoperative radiotherapy in the management of patients with clinically resectable rectal cancer**

  Source: Practice Guidelines Initiative - State/Local Government Agency [Non-U.S.]; 2002 December (revised 2004 Jan); 23 pages

  http://www.guideline.gov/summary/summary.aspx?doc_id=4783&nbr=3461&string=radiotherapy

- **Use of preoperative chemotherapy with or without postoperative radiotherapy in technically resectable stage IIIA non-small cell lung cancer**

  Source: Practice Guidelines Initiative - State/Local Government Agency [Non-U.S.]; 1997 September 15 (updated online 2002 Apr); 14 pages

  http://www.guideline.gov/summary/summary.aspx?doc_id=3281&nbr=2507&string=radiotherapy

The NIH Search Utility

The NIH search utility allows you to search for documents on over 100 selected Web sites that comprise the NIH-WEB-SPACE. Each of these servers is "crawled" and indexed on an ongoing basis. Your search will produce a list of various documents, all of which will relate in some way to radiotherapy. The drawbacks of this approach are that the information is not organized by theme and that the references are often a mix of information for professionals and patients. Nevertheless, a large number of the listed Web sites provide useful background information. We can only recommend this route, therefore, for relatively rare or specific disorders, or when using highly targeted searches. To use the NIH search utility, visit the following Web page: **http://search.nih.gov/index.html**.

Additional Web Sources

A number of Web sites are available to the public that often link to government sites. These can also point you in the direction of essential information. The following is a representative sample:

- AOL: http://search.aol.com/cat.adp?id=168&layer=&from=subcats

- Family Village: http://www.familyvillage.wisc.edu/specific.htm

- Google: http://directory.google.com/Top/Health/Conditions_and_Diseases/

- Med Help International: http://www.medhelp.org/HealthTopics/A.html

- Open Directory Project: http://dmoz.org/Health/Conditions_and_Diseases/

- Yahoo.com: http://dir.yahoo.com/Health/Diseases_and_Conditions/

- WebMD®Health: http://my.webmd.com/health_topics

Finding Associations

There are several Internet directories that provide lists of medical associations with information on or resources relating to radiotherapy. By consulting all of associations listed in this chapter, you will have nearly exhausted all sources for patient associations concerned with radiotherapy.

The National Health Information Center (NHIC)

The National Health Information Center (NHIC) offers a free referral service to help people find organizations that provide information about radiotherapy. For more information, see the NHIC's Web site at http://www.health.gov/NHIC/ or contact an information specialist by calling 1-800-336-4797.

Directory of Health Organizations

The Directory of Health Organizations, provided by the National Library of Medicine Specialized Information Services, is a comprehensive source of information on associations. The Directory of Health Organizations database can be accessed via the Internet at http://www.sis.nlm.nih.gov/Dir/DirMain.html. It is composed of two parts: DIRLINE and Health Hotlines.

The DIRLINE database comprises some 10,000 records of organizations, research centers, and government institutes and associations that primarily focus on health and biomedicine. To access DIRLINE directly, go to the following Web site: http://dirline.nlm.nih.gov/. Simply type in "radiotherapy" (or a synonym), and you will receive information on all relevant organizations listed in the database.

Health Hotlines directs you to toll-free numbers to over 300 organizations. You can access this database directly at http://www.sis.nlm.nih.gov/hotlines/. On this page, you are given the option to search by keyword or by browsing the subject list. When you have received your search results, click on the name of the organization for its description and contact information.

The Combined Health Information Database

Another comprehensive source of information on healthcare associations is the Combined Health Information Database. Using the "Detailed Search" option, you will need to limit your search to "Organizations" and "radiotherapy". Type the following hyperlink into your Web browser: **http://chid.nih.gov/detail/detail.html**. To find associations, use the drop boxes at the bottom of the search page where "You may refine your search by." For publication date, select "All Years." Then, select your preferred language and the format option "Organization Resource Sheet." Type "radiotherapy" (or synonyms) into the "For these words:" box. You should check back periodically with this database since it is updated every three months.

The National Organization for Rare Disorders, Inc.

The National Organization for Rare Disorders, Inc. has prepared a Web site that provides, at no charge, lists of associations organized by health topic. You can access this database at the following Web site: **http://www.rarediseases.org/search/orgsearch.html**. Type "radiotherapy" (or a synonym) into the search box, and click "Submit Query."

APPENDIX C. FINDING MEDICAL LIBRARIES

Overview

In this Appendix, we show you how to quickly find a medical library in your area.

Preparation

Your local public library and medical libraries have interlibrary loan programs with the National Library of Medicine (NLM), one of the largest medical collections in the world. According to the NLM, most of the literature in the general and historical collections of the National Library of Medicine is available on interlibrary loan to any library. If you would like to access NLM medical literature, then visit a library in your area that can request the publications for you.[21]

Finding a Local Medical Library

The quickest method to locate medical libraries is to use the Internet-based directory published by the National Network of Libraries of Medicine (NN/LM). This network includes 4626 members and affiliates that provide many services to librarians, health professionals, and the public. To find a library in your area, simply visit **http://nnlm.gov/members/adv.html** or call 1-800-338-7657.

Medical Libraries in the U.S. and Canada

In addition to the NN/LM, the National Library of Medicine (NLM) lists a number of libraries with reference facilities that are open to the public. The following is the NLM's list and includes hyperlinks to each library's Web site. These Web pages can provide information on hours of operation and other restrictions. The list below is a small sample of

---

[21] Adapted from the NLM: **http://www.nlm.nih.gov/psd/cas/interlibrary.html**.

libraries recommended by the National Library of Medicine (sorted alphabetically by name of the U.S. state or Canadian province where the library is located)[22]:

- **Alabama:** Health InfoNet of Jefferson County (Jefferson County Library Cooperative, Lister Hill Library of the Health Sciences), **http://www.uab.edu/infonet/**

- **Alabama:** Richard M. Scrushy Library (American Sports Medicine Institute)

- **Arizona:** Samaritan Regional Medical Center: The Learning Center (Samaritan Health System, Phoenix, Arizona), **http://www.samaritan.edu/library/bannerlibs.htm**

- **California:** Kris Kelly Health Information Center (St. Joseph Health System, Humboldt), **http://www.humboldt1.com/~kkhic/index.html**

- **California:** Community Health Library of Los Gatos, **http://www.healthlib.org/orgresources.html**

- **California:** Consumer Health Program and Services (CHIPS) (County of Los Angeles Public Library, Los Angeles County Harbor-UCLA Medical Center Library) - Carson, CA, **http://www.colapublib.org/services/chips.html**

- **California:** Gateway Health Library (Sutter Gould Medical Foundation)

- **California:** Health Library (Stanford University Medical Center), **http://www-med.stanford.edu/healthlibrary/**

- **California:** Patient Education Resource Center - Health Information and Resources (University of California, San Francisco), **http://sfghdean.ucsf.edu/barnett/PERC/default.asp**

- **California:** Redwood Health Library (Petaluma Health Care District), **http://www.phcd.org/rdwdlib.html**

- **California:** Los Gatos PlaneTree Health Library, **http://planetreesanjose.org/**

- **California:** Sutter Resource Library (Sutter Hospitals Foundation, Sacramento), **http://suttermedicalcenter.org/library/**

- **California:** Health Sciences Libraries (University of California, Davis), **http://www.lib.ucdavis.edu/healthsci/**

- **California:** ValleyCare Health Library & Ryan Comer Cancer Resource Center (ValleyCare Health System, Pleasanton), **http://gaelnet.stmarys-ca.edu/other.libs/gbal/east/vchl.html**

- **California:** Washington Community Health Resource Library (Fremont), **http://www.healthlibrary.org/**

- **Colorado:** William V. Gervasini Memorial Library (Exempla Healthcare), **http://www.saintjosephdenver.org/yourhealth/libraries/**

- **Connecticut:** Hartford Hospital Health Science Libraries (Hartford Hospital), **http://www.harthosp.org/library/**

- **Connecticut:** Healthnet: Connecticut Consumer Health Information Center (University of Connecticut Health Center, Lyman Maynard Stowe Library), **http://library.uchc.edu/departm/hnet/**

---

[22] Abstracted from **http://www.nlm.nih.gov/medlineplus/libraries.html**.

- **Connecticut:** Waterbury Hospital Health Center Library (Waterbury Hospital, Waterbury), **http://www.waterburyhospital.com/library/consumer.shtml**

- **Delaware:** Consumer Health Library (Christiana Care Health System, Eugene du Pont Preventive Medicine & Rehabilitation Institute, Wilmington), **http://www.christianacare.org/health_guide/health_guide_pmri_health_info.cfm**

- **Delaware:** Lewis B. Flinn Library (Delaware Academy of Medicine, Wilmington), **http://www.delamed.org/chls.html**

- **Georgia:** Family Resource Library (Medical College of Georgia, Augusta), **http://cmc.mcg.edu/kids_families/fam_resources/fam_res_lib/frl.htm**

- **Georgia:** Health Resource Center (Medical Center of Central Georgia, Macon), **http://www.mccg.org/hrc/hrchome.asp**

- **Hawaii:** Hawaii Medical Library: Consumer Health Information Service (Hawaii Medical Library, Honolulu), **http://hml.org/CHIS/**

- **Idaho:** DeArmond Consumer Health Library (Kootenai Medical Center, Coeur d'Alene), **http://www.nicon.org/DeArmond/index.htm**

- **Illinois:** Health Learning Center of Northwestern Memorial Hospital (Chicago), **http://www.nmh.org/health_info/hlc.html**

- **Illinois:** Medical Library (OSF Saint Francis Medical Center, Peoria), **http://www.osfsaintfrancis.org/general/library/**

- **Kentucky:** Medical Library - Services for Patients, Families, Students & the Public (Central Baptist Hospital, Lexington), **http://www.centralbap.com/education/community/library.cfm**

- **Kentucky:** University of Kentucky - Health Information Library (Chandler Medical Center, Lexington), **http://www.mc.uky.edu/PatientEd/**

- **Louisiana:** Alton Ochsner Medical Foundation Library (Alton Ochsner Medical Foundation, New Orleans), **http://www.ochsner.org/library/**

- **Louisiana:** Louisiana State University Health Sciences Center Medical Library-Shreveport, **http://lib-sh.lsuhsc.edu/**

- **Maine:** Franklin Memorial Hospital Medical Library (Franklin Memorial Hospital, Farmington), **http://www.fchn.org/fmh/lib.htm**

- **Maine:** Gerrish-True Health Sciences Library (Central Maine Medical Center, Lewiston), **http://www.cmmc.org/library/library.html**

- **Maine:** Hadley Parrot Health Science Library (Eastern Maine Healthcare, Bangor), **http://www.emh.org/hll/hpl/guide.htm**

- **Maine:** Maine Medical Center Library (Maine Medical Center, Portland), **http://www.mmc.org/library/**

- **Maine:** Parkview Hospital (Brunswick), **http://www.parkviewhospital.org/**

- **Maine:** Southern Maine Medical Center Health Sciences Library (Southern Maine Medical Center, Biddeford), **http://www.smmc.org/services/service.php3?choice=10**

- **Maine:** Stephens Memorial Hospital's Health Information Library (Western Maine Health, Norway), **http://www.wmhcc.org/Library/**

- **Manitoba, Canada:** Consumer & Patient Health Information Service (University of Manitoba Libraries), http://www.umanitoba.ca/libraries/units/health/reference/chis.html

- **Manitoba, Canada:** J.W. Crane Memorial Library (Deer Lodge Centre, Winnipeg), http://www.deerlodge.mb.ca/crane_library/about.asp

- **Maryland:** Health Information Center at the Wheaton Regional Library (Montgomery County, Dept. of Public Libraries, Wheaton Regional Library), http://www.mont.lib.md.us/healthinfo/hic.asp

- **Massachusetts:** Baystate Medical Center Library (Baystate Health System), http://www.baystatehealth.com/1024/

- **Massachusetts:** Boston University Medical Center Alumni Medical Library (Boston University Medical Center), http://med-libwww.bu.edu/library/lib.html

- **Massachusetts:** Lowell General Hospital Health Sciences Library (Lowell General Hospital, Lowell), http://www.lowellgeneral.org/library/HomePageLinks/WWW.htm

- **Massachusetts:** Paul E. Woodard Health Sciences Library (New England Baptist Hospital, Boston), http://www.nebh.org/health_lib.asp

- **Massachusetts:** St. Luke's Hospital Health Sciences Library (St. Luke's Hospital, Southcoast Health System, New Bedford), http://www.southcoast.org/library/

- **Massachusetts:** Treadwell Library Consumer Health Reference Center (Massachusetts General Hospital), http://www.mgh.harvard.edu/library/chrcindex.html

- **Massachusetts:** UMass HealthNet (University of Massachusetts Medical School, Worchester), http://healthnet.umassmed.edu/

- **Michigan:** Botsford General Hospital Library - Consumer Health (Botsford General Hospital, Library & Internet Services), http://www.botsfordlibrary.org/consumer.htm

- **Michigan:** Helen DeRoy Medical Library (Providence Hospital and Medical Centers), http://www.providence-hospital.org/library/

- **Michigan:** Marquette General Hospital - Consumer Health Library (Marquette General Hospital, Health Information Center), http://www.mgh.org/center.html

- **Michigan:** Patient Education Resouce Center - University of Michigan Cancer Center (University of Michigan Comprehensive Cancer Center, Ann Arbor), http://www.cancer.med.umich.edu/learn/leares.htm

- **Michigan:** Sladen Library & Center for Health Information Resources - Consumer Health Information (Detroit), http://www.henryford.com/body.cfm?id=39330

- **Montana:** Center for Health Information (St. Patrick Hospital and Health Sciences Center, Missoula)

- **National:** Consumer Health Library Directory (Medical Library Association, Consumer and Patient Health Information Section), http://caphis.mlanet.org/directory/index.html

- **National:** National Network of Libraries of Medicine (National Library of Medicine) - provides library services for health professionals in the United States who do not have access to a medical library, http://nnlm.gov/

- **National:** NN/LM List of Libraries Serving the Public (National Network of Libraries of Medicine), http://nnlm.gov/members/

- **Nevada:** Health Science Library, West Charleston Library (Las Vegas-Clark County Library District, Las Vegas), http://www.lvccld.org/special_collections/medical/index.htm

- **New Hampshire:** Dartmouth Biomedical Libraries (Dartmouth College Library, Hanover), http://www.dartmouth.edu/~biomed/resources.htmld/conshealth.htmld/

- **New Jersey:** Consumer Health Library (Rahway Hospital, Rahway), http://www.rahwayhospital.com/library.htm

- **New Jersey:** Dr. Walter Phillips Health Sciences Library (Englewood Hospital and Medical Center, Englewood), http://www.englewoodhospital.com/links/index.htm

- **New Jersey:** Meland Foundation (Englewood Hospital and Medical Center, Englewood), http://www.geocities.com/ResearchTriangle/9360/

- **New York:** Choices in Health Information (New York Public Library) - NLM Consumer Pilot Project participant, http://www.nypl.org/branch/health/links.html

- **New York:** Health Information Center (Upstate Medical University, State University of New York, Syracuse), http://www.upstate.edu/library/hic/

- **New York:** Health Sciences Library (Long Island Jewish Medical Center, New Hyde Park), http://www.lij.edu/library/library.html

- **New York:** ViaHealth Medical Library (Rochester General Hospital), http://www.nyam.org/library/

- **Ohio:** Consumer Health Library (Akron General Medical Center, Medical & Consumer Health Library), http://www.akrongeneral.org/hwlibrary.htm

- **Oklahoma:** The Health Information Center at Saint Francis Hospital (Saint Francis Health System, Tulsa), http://www.sfh-tulsa.com/services/healthinfo.asp

- **Oregon:** Planetree Health Resource Center (Mid-Columbia Medical Center, The Dalles), http://www.mcmc.net/phrc/

- **Pennsylvania:** Community Health Information Library (Milton S. Hershey Medical Center, Hershey), http://www.hmc.psu.edu/commhealth/

- **Pennsylvania:** Community Health Resource Library (Geisinger Medical Center, Danville), http://www.geisinger.edu/education/commlib.shtml

- **Pennsylvania:** HealthInfo Library (Moses Taylor Hospital, Scranton), http://www.mth.org/healthwellness.html

- **Pennsylvania:** Hopwood Library (University of Pittsburgh, Health Sciences Library System, Pittsburgh), http://www.hsls.pitt.edu/guides/chi/hopwood/index_html

- **Pennsylvania:** Koop Community Health Information Center (College of Physicians of Philadelphia), http://www.collphyphil.org/kooppg1.shtml

- **Pennsylvania:** Learning Resources Center - Medical Library (Susquehanna Health System, Williamsport), http://www.shscares.org/services/lrc/index.asp

- **Pennsylvania:** Medical Library (UPMC Health System, Pittsburgh), http://www.upmc.edu/passavant/library.htm

- **Quebec, Canada:** Medical Library (Montreal General Hospital), http://www.mghlib.mcgill.ca/

- **South Dakota:** Rapid City Regional Hospital Medical Library (Rapid City Regional Hospital), **http://www.rcrh.org/Services/Library/Default.asp**

- **Texas:** Houston HealthWays (Houston Academy of Medicine-Texas Medical Center Library), **http://hhw.library.tmc.edu/**

- **Washington:** Community Health Library (Kittitas Valley Community Hospital), **http://www.kvch.com/**

- **Washington:** Southwest Washington Medical Center Library (Southwest Washington Medical Center, Vancouver), **http://www.swmedicalcenter.com/body.cfm?id=72**

ONLINE GLOSSARIES

The Internet provides access to a number of free-to-use medical dictionaries. The National Library of Medicine has compiled the following list of online dictionaries:

- ADAM Medical Encyclopedia (A.D.A.M., Inc.), comprehensive medical reference: **http://www.nlm.nih.gov/medlineplus/encyclopedia.html**

- MedicineNet.com Medical Dictionary (MedicineNet, Inc.): **http://www.medterms.com/Script/Main/hp.asp**

- Merriam-Webster Medical Dictionary (Inteli-Health, Inc.): **http://www.intelihealth.com/IH/**

- Multilingual Glossary of Technical and Popular Medical Terms in Eight European Languages (European Commission) - Danish, Dutch, English, French, German, Italian, Portuguese, and Spanish: **http://allserv.rug.ac.be/~rvdstich/eugloss/welcome.html**

- On-line Medical Dictionary (CancerWEB): **http://cancerweb.ncl.ac.uk/omd/**

- Rare Diseases Terms (Office of Rare Diseases): **http://ord.aspensys.com/asp/diseases/diseases.asp**

- Technology Glossary (National Library of Medicine) - Health Care Technology: **http://www.nlm.nih.gov/nichsr/ta101/ta10108.htm**

Beyond these, MEDLINEplus contains a very patient-friendly encyclopedia covering every aspect of medicine (licensed from A.D.A.M., Inc.). The ADAM Medical Encyclopedia can be accessed at **http://www.nlm.nih.gov/medlineplus/encyclopedia.html**. ADAM is also available on commercial Web sites such as drkoop.com (**http://www.drkoop.com/**) and Web MD (**http://my.webmd.com/adam/asset/adam_disease_articles/a_to_z/a**).

Online Dictionary Directories

The following are additional online directories compiled by the National Library of Medicine, including a number of specialized medical dictionaries:

- Medical Dictionaries: Medical & Biological (World Health Organization): **http://www.who.int/hlt/virtuallibrary/English/diction.htm#Medical**

- MEL-Michigan Electronic Library List of Online Health and Medical Dictionaries (Michigan Electronic Library): **http://mel.lib.mi.us/health/health-dictionaries.html**

- Patient Education: Glossaries (DMOZ Open Directory Project): **http://dmoz.org/Health/Education/Patient_Education/Glossaries/**

- Web of Online Dictionaries (Bucknell University): **http://www.yourdictionary.com/diction5.html#medicine**

RADIOTHERAPY DICTIONARY

The definitions below are derived from official public sources, including the National Institutes of Health [NIH] and the European Union [EU].

3-dimensional: 3-D. A graphic display of depth, width, and height. Three-dimensional radiation therapy uses computers to create a 3-dimensional picture of the tumor. This allows doctors to give the highest possible dose of radiation to the tumor, while sparing the normal tissue as much as possible. [NIH]

Abdomen: That portion of the body that lies between the thorax and the pelvis. [NIH]

Abdominal: Having to do with the abdomen, which is the part of the body between the chest and the hips that contains the pancreas, stomach, intestines, liver, gallbladder, and other organs. [NIH]

Aberrant: Wandering or deviating from the usual or normal course. [EU]

Ablation: The removal of an organ by surgery. [NIH]

Acceptor: A substance which, while normally not oxidized by oxygen or reduced by hydrogen, can be oxidized or reduced in presence of a substance which is itself undergoing oxidation or reduction. [NIH]

Acetylcholine: A neurotransmitter. Acetylcholine in vertebrates is the major transmitter at neuromuscular junctions, autonomic ganglia, parasympathetic effector junctions, a subset of sympathetic effector junctions, and at many sites in the central nervous system. It is generally not used as an administered drug because it is broken down very rapidly by cholinesterases, but it is useful in some ophthalmological applications. [NIH]

Acetylcysteine: The N-acetyl derivative of cysteine. It is used as a mucolytic agent to reduce the viscosity of mucous secretions. It has also been shown to have antiviral effects in patients with HIV due to inhibition of viral stimulation by reactive oxygen intermediates. [NIH]

Acidity: The quality of being acid or sour; containing acid (hydrogen ions). [EU]

Acidosis: A pathologic condition resulting from accumulation of acid or depletion of the alkaline reserve (bicarbonate content) in the blood and body tissues, and characterized by an increase in hydrogen ion concentration. [EU]

Acute lymphoblastic leukemia: ALL. A quickly progressing disease in which too many immature white blood cells called lymphoblasts are found in the blood and bone marrow. Also called acute lymphocytic leukemia. [NIH]

Acute lymphocytic leukemia: ALL. A quickly progressing disease in which too many immature white blood cells called lymphoblasts are found in the blood and bone marrow. Also called acute lymphoblastic leukemia. [NIH]

Acute renal: A condition in which the kidneys suddenly stop working. In most cases, kidneys can recover from almost complete loss of function. [NIH]

Adaptability: Ability to develop some form of tolerance to conditions extremely different from those under which a living organism evolved. [NIH]

Adaptation: 1. The adjustment of an organism to its environment, or the process by which it enhances such fitness. 2. The normal ability of the eye to adjust itself to variations in the intensity of light; the adjustment to such variations. 3. The decline in the frequency of firing of a neuron, particularly of a receptor, under conditions of constant stimulation. 4. In dentistry, (a) the proper fitting of a denture, (b) the degree of proximity and interlocking of restorative material to a tooth preparation, (c) the exact adjustment of bands to teeth. 5. In microbiology, the adjustment of bacterial physiology to a new environment. [EU]

Adenocarcinoma: A malignant epithelial tumor with a glandular organization. [NIH]

Adenoma: A benign epithelial tumor with a glandular organization. [NIH]

Adenovirus: A group of viruses that cause respiratory tract and eye infections. Adenoviruses used in gene therapy are altered to carry a specific tumor-fighting gene. [NIH]

Adjustment: The dynamic process wherein the thoughts, feelings, behavior, and biophysiological mechanisms of the individual continually change to adjust to the environment. [NIH]

Adjuvant: A substance which aids another, such as an auxiliary remedy; in immunology, nonspecific stimulator (e.g., BCG vaccine) of the immune response. [EU]

Adrenal Glands: Paired glands situated in the retroperitoneal tissues at the superior pole of each kidney. [NIH]

Adverse Effect: An unwanted side effect of treatment. [NIH]

Aerobic: In biochemistry, reactions that need oxygen to happen or happen when oxygen is present. [NIH]

Aerobic Exercise: A type of physical activity that includes walking, jogging, running, and dancing. Aerobic training improves the efficiency of the aerobic energy-producing systems that can improve cardiorespiratory endurance. [NIH]

Aerosol: A solution of a drug which can be atomized into a fine mist for inhalation therapy. [EU]

Affinity: 1. Inherent likeness or relationship. 2. A special attraction for a specific element, organ, or structure. 3. Chemical affinity; the force that binds atoms in molecules; the tendency of substances to combine by chemical reaction. 4. The strength of noncovalent chemical binding between two substances as measured by the dissociation constant of the complex. 5. In immunology, a thermodynamic expression of the strength of interaction between a single antigen-binding site and a single antigenic determinant (and thus of the stereochemical compatibility between them), most accurately applied to interactions among simple, uniform antigenic determinants such as haptens. Expressed as the association constant (K litres mole -1), which, owing to the heterogeneity of affinities in a population of antibody molecules of a given specificity, actually represents an average value (mean intrinsic association constant). 6. The reciprocal of the dissociation constant. [EU]

Agar: A complex sulfated polymer of galactose units, extracted from Gelidium cartilagineum, Gracilaria confervoides, and related red algae. It is used as a gel in the preparation of solid culture media for microorganisms, as a bulk laxative, in making emulsions, and as a supporting medium for immunodiffusion and immunoelectrophoresis. [NIH]

Aggressiveness: The quality of being aggressive (= characterized by aggression; militant; enterprising; spreading with vigour; chemically active; variable and adaptable). [EU]

Agonist: In anatomy, a prime mover. In pharmacology, a drug that has affinity for and stimulates physiologic activity at cell receptors normally stimulated by naturally occurring substances. [EU]

Airway: A device for securing unobstructed passage of air into and out of the lungs during general anesthesia. [NIH]

Algorithms: A procedure consisting of a sequence of algebraic formulas and/or logical steps to calculate or determine a given task. [NIH]

Alkaline: Having the reactions of an alkali. [EU]

Alkylating Agents: Highly reactive chemicals that introduce alkyl radicals into biologically active molecules and thereby prevent their proper functioning. Many are used as antineoplastic agents, but most are very toxic, with carcinogenic, mutagenic, teratogenic, and immunosuppressant actions. They have also been used as components in poison gases. [NIH]

Alleles: Mutually exclusive forms of the same gene, occupying the same locus on homologous chromosomes, and governing the same biochemical and developmental process. [NIH]

Allergen: An antigenic substance capable of producing immediate-type hypersensitivity (allergy). [EU]

Allo: A female hormone. [NIH]

Allogeneic: Taken from different individuals of the same species. [NIH]

Alloys: A mixture of metallic elements or compounds with other metallic or metalloid elements in varying proportions. [NIH]

Alopecia: Absence of hair from areas where it is normally present. [NIH]

Alpha Particles: Positively charged particles composed of two protons and two neutrons, i.e., helium nuclei, emitted during disintegration of very heavy isotopes; a beam of alpha particles or an alpha ray has very strong ionizing power, but weak penetrability. [NIH]

Alternative medicine: Practices not generally recognized by the medical community as standard or conventional medical approaches and used instead of standard treatments. Alternative medicine includes the taking of dietary supplements, megadose vitamins, and herbal preparations; the drinking of special teas; and practices such as massage therapy, magnet therapy, spiritual healing, and meditation. [NIH]

Aluminum: A metallic element that has the atomic number 13, atomic symbol Al, and atomic weight 26.98. [NIH]

Alveoli: Tiny air sacs at the end of the bronchioles in the lungs. [NIH]

Ambulatory Care: Health care services provided to patients on an ambulatory basis, rather than by admission to a hospital or other health care facility. The services may be a part of a hospital, augmenting its inpatient services, or may be provided at a free-standing facility. [NIH]

Ameloblastoma: An epithelial tumor of the jaw originating from the epithelial rests of Malassez or from other epithelial remnants of the developing period of the enamel. [NIH]

Amifostine: A phosphorothioate proposed as a radiation-protective agent. It causes splenic vasodilation and may block autonomic ganglia. [NIH]

Amino acid: Any organic compound containing an amino (-NH2 and a carboxyl (- COOH) group. The 20 a-amino acids listed in the accompanying table are the amino acids from which proteins are synthesized by formation of peptide bonds during ribosomal translation of messenger RNA; all except glycine, which is not optically active, have the L configuration. Other amino acids occurring in proteins, such as hydroxyproline in collagen, are formed by posttranslational enzymatic modification of amino acids residues in polypeptide chains. There are also several important amino acids, such as the neurotransmitter y-aminobutyric acid, that have no relation to proteins. Abbreviated AA. [EU]

Amino Acid Sequence: The order of amino acids as they occur in a polypeptide chain. This is referred to as the primary structure of proteins. It is of fundamental importance in determining protein conformation. [NIH]

Amplification: The production of additional copies of a chromosomal DNA sequence, found as either intrachromosomal or extrachromosomal DNA. [NIH]

Anaesthesia: Loss of feeling or sensation. Although the term is used for loss of tactile sensibility, or of any of the other senses, it is applied especially to loss of the sensation of pain, as it is induced to permit performance of surgery or other painful procedures. [EU]

Anal: Having to do with the anus, which is the posterior opening of the large bowel. [NIH]

Analgesic: An agent that alleviates pain without causing loss of consciousness. [EU]

Analog: In chemistry, a substance that is similar, but not identical, to another. [NIH]

Analogous: Resembling or similar in some respects, as in function or appearance, but not in origin or development;. [EU]

Anaphylatoxins: The family of peptides C3a, C4a, C5a, and C5a des-arginine produced in the serum during complement activation. They produce smooth muscle contraction, mast cell histamine release, affect platelet aggregation, and act as mediators of the local inflammatory process. The order of anaphylatoxin activity from strongest to weakest is C5a, C3a, C4a, and C5a des-arginine. The latter is the so-called "classical" anaphylatoxin but shows no spasmogenic activity though it contains some chemotactic ability. [NIH]

Anaplastic: A term used to describe cancer cells that divide rapidly and bear little or no resemblance to normal cells. [NIH]

Anatomical: Pertaining to anatomy, or to the structure of the organism. [EU]

Androgenic: Producing masculine characteristics. [EU]

Androgens: A class of sex hormones associated with the development and maintenance of the secondary male sex characteristics, sperm induction, and sexual differentiation. In addition to increasing virility and libido, they also increase nitrogen and water retention and stimulate skeletal growth. [NIH]

Anemia: A reduction in the number of circulating erythrocytes or in the quantity of hemoglobin. [NIH]

Anesthesia: A state characterized by loss of feeling or sensation. This depression of nerve function is usually the result of pharmacologic action and is induced to allow performance of surgery or other painful procedures. [NIH]

Anginal: Pertaining to or characteristic of angina. [EU]

Angiogenesis: Blood vessel formation. Tumor angiogenesis is the growth of blood vessels from surrounding tissue to a solid tumor. This is caused by the release of chemicals by the tumor. [NIH]

Angiogenesis inhibitor: A substance that may prevent the formation of blood vessels. In anticancer therapy, an angiogenesis inhibitor prevents the growth of blood vessels from surrounding tissue to a solid tumor. [NIH]

Angiography: Radiography of blood vessels after injection of a contrast medium. [NIH]

Angiosarcoma: A type of cancer that begins in the lining of blood vessels. [NIH]

Animal model: An animal with a disease either the same as or like a disease in humans. Animal models are used to study the development and progression of diseases and to test new treatments before they are given to humans. Animals with transplanted human cancers or other tissues are called xenograft models. [NIH]

Anionic: Pertaining to or containing an anion. [EU]

Anions: Negatively charged atoms, radicals or groups of atoms which travel to the anode or positive pole during electrolysis. [NIH]

Anoikis: Apoptosis triggered by loss of contact with the extracellular matrix. [NIH]

Anorexia: Lack or loss of appetite for food. Appetite is psychologic, dependent on memory and associations. Anorexia can be brought about by unattractive food, surroundings, or company. [NIH]

Antiandrogens: Drugs used to block the production or interfere with the action of male sex hormones. [NIH]

Antiangiogenic: Having to do with reducing the growth of new blood vessels. [NIH]

Antibacterial: A substance that destroys bacteria or suppresses their growth or reproduction. [EU]

Antibiotic: A drug used to treat infections caused by bacteria and other microorganisms. [NIH]

Antibodies: Immunoglobulin molecules having a specific amino acid sequence by virtue of which they interact only with the antigen that induced their synthesis in cells of the lymphoid series (especially plasma cells), or with an antigen closely related to it. [NIH]

Antibody: A type of protein made by certain white blood cells in response to a foreign substance (antigen). Each antibody can bind to only a specific antigen. The purpose of this binding is to help destroy the antigen. Antibodies can work in several ways, depending on the nature of the antigen. Some antibodies destroy antigens directly. Others make it easier for white blood cells to destroy the antigen. [NIH]

Anticoagulant: A drug that helps prevent blood clots from forming. Also called a blood thinner. [NIH]

Antidote: A remedy for counteracting a poison. [EU]

Antifungal: Destructive to fungi, or suppressing their reproduction or growth; effective against fungal infections. [EU]

Antigen: Any substance which is capable, under appropriate conditions, of inducing a specific immune response and of reacting with the products of that response, that is, with specific antibody or specifically sensitized T-lymphocytes, or both. Antigens may be soluble substances, such as toxins and foreign proteins, or particulate, such as bacteria and tissue cells; however, only the portion of the protein or polysaccharide molecule known as the antigenic determinant (q.v.) combines with antibody or a specific receptor on a lymphocyte. Abbreviated Ag. [EU]

Antigen-Antibody Complex: The complex formed by the binding of antigen and antibody molecules. The deposition of large antigen-antibody complexes leading to tissue damage causes immune complex diseases. [NIH]

Antigen-presenting cell: APC. A cell that shows antigen on its surface to other cells of the immune system. This is an important part of an immune response. [NIH]

Anti-infective: An agent that so acts. [EU]

Anti-inflammatory: Having to do with reducing inflammation. [NIH]

Antimetabolite: A chemical that is very similar to one required in a normal biochemical reaction in cells. Antimetabolites can stop or slow down the reaction. [NIH]

Antineoplastic: Inhibiting or preventing the development of neoplasms, checking the maturation and proliferation of malignant cells. [EU]

Antioxidant: A substance that prevents damage caused by free radicals. Free radicals are highly reactive chemicals that often contain oxygen. They are produced when molecules are split to give products that have unpaired electrons. This process is called oxidation. [NIH]

Antiseptic: A substance that inhibits the growth and development of microorganisms without necessarily killing them. [EU]

Antiviral: Destroying viruses or suppressing their replication. [EU]

Anus: The opening of the rectum to the outside of the body. [NIH]

Anxiety: Persistent feeling of dread, apprehension, and impending disaster. [NIH]

Aorta: The main trunk of the systemic arteries. [NIH]

Aphakia: Absence of crystalline lens totally or partially from field of vision, from any cause except after cataract extraction. Aphakia is mainly congenital or as result of lens dislocation and subluxation. [NIH]

Apoptosis: One of the two mechanisms by which cell death occurs (the other being the pathological process of necrosis). Apoptosis is the mechanism responsible for the physiological deletion of cells and appears to be intrinsically programmed. It is characterized by distinctive morphologic changes in the nucleus and cytoplasm, chromatin cleavage at regularly spaced sites, and the endonucleolytic cleavage of genomic DNA (DNA fragmentation) at internucleosomal sites. This mode of cell death serves as a balance to mitosis in regulating the size of animal tissues and in mediating pathologic processes associated with tumor growth. [NIH]

Approximate: Approximal [EU]

Aqueous: Having to do with water. [NIH]

Archaea: One of the three domains of life (the others being bacteria and Eucarya), formerly called Archaebacteria under the taxon Bacteria, but now considered separate and distinct. They are characterized by: 1) the presence of characteristic tRNAs and ribosomal RNAs; 2) the absence of peptidoglycan cell walls; 3) the presence of ether-linked lipids built from branched-chain subunits; and 4) their occurrence in unusual habitats. While archaea resemble bacteria in morphology and genomic organization, they resemble eukarya in their method of genomic replication. The domain contains at least three kingdoms: crenarchaeota, euryarchaeota, and korarchaeota. [NIH]

Arsenic trioxide: An anticancer drug that induces programmed cell death (apoptosis) in certain cancer cells. [NIH]

Arterial: Pertaining to an artery or to the arteries. [EU]

Arteries: The vessels carrying blood away from the heart. [NIH]

Artery: Vessel-carrying blood from the heart to various parts of the body. [NIH]

Arthrosis: A disease of a joint. [EU]

Articular: Of or pertaining to a joint. [EU]

Artifacts: Any visible result of a procedure which is caused by the procedure itself and not by the entity being analyzed. Common examples include histological structures introduced by tissue processing, radiographic images of structures that are not naturally present in living tissue, and products of chemical reactions that occur during analysis. [NIH]

Asbestos: Fibrous incombustible mineral composed of magnesium and calcium silicates with or without other elements. It is relatively inert chemically and used in thermal insulation and fireproofing. Inhalation of dust causes asbestosis and later lung and gastrointestinal neoplasms. [NIH]

Assay: Determination of the amount of a particular constituent of a mixture, or of the biological or pharmacological potency of a drug. [EU]

Astrocytes: The largest and most numerous neuroglial cells in the brain and spinal cord. Astrocytes (from "star" cells) are irregularly shaped with many long processes, including those with "end feet" which form the glial (limiting) membrane and directly and indirectly contribute to the blood brain barrier. They regulate the extracellular ionic and chemical environment, and "reactive astrocytes" (along with microglia) respond to injury. Astrocytes have high- affinity transmitter uptake systems, voltage-dependent and transmitter-gated ion channels, and can release transmitter, but their role in signaling (as in many other functions) is not well understood. [NIH]

Astrocytoma: A tumor that begins in the brain or spinal cord in small, star-shaped cells called astrocytes. [NIH]

Atmospheric Pressure: The pressure at any point in an atmosphere due solely to the weight of the atmospheric gases above the point concerned. [NIH]

Atrophy: Decrease in the size of a cell, tissue, organ, or multiple organs, associated with a variety of pathological conditions such as abnormal cellular changes, ischemia, malnutrition, or hormonal changes. [NIH]

Attenuated: Strain with weakened or reduced virulence. [NIH]

Attenuation: Reduction of transmitted sound energy or its electrical equivalent. [NIH]

Autologous: Taken from an individual's own tissues, cells, or DNA. [NIH]

Autonomic: Self-controlling; functionally independent. [EU]

Autopsy: Postmortem examination of the body. [NIH]

Autoradiography: A process in which radioactive material within an object produces an image when it is in close proximity to a radiation sensitive emulsion. [NIH]

Autosuggestion: Suggestion coming from the subject himself. [NIH]

Axilla: The underarm or armpit. [NIH]

Axillary: Pertaining to the armpit area, including the lymph nodes that are located there. [NIH]

Axons: Nerve fibers that are capable of rapidly conducting impulses away from the neuron cell body. [NIH]

Bacteria: Unicellular prokaryotic microorganisms which generally possess rigid cell walls, multiply by cell division, and exhibit three principal forms: round or coccal, rodlike or bacillary, and spiral or spirochetal. [NIH]

Bacterial Infections: Infections by bacteria, general or unspecified. [NIH]

Bacterial Physiology: Physiological processes and activities of bacteria. [NIH]

Bacteriophage: A virus whose host is a bacterial cell; A virus that exclusively infects bacteria. It generally has a protein coat surrounding the genome (DNA or RNA). One of the coliphages most extensively studied is the lambda phage, which is also one of the most important. [NIH]

Bacterium: Microscopic organism which may have a spherical, rod-like, or spiral unicellular or non-cellular body. Bacteria usually reproduce through asexual processes. [NIH]

Balloon Dilatation: Nonoperative repair of occluded vessels, ducts, or valves by insertion of a balloon catheter. It is used, among other things, to treat varices, torn retinas, renal and biliary calculi, gastric, bronchial and rectal stenoses, and heart valves, and includes catheterization with Fogarty and Foley catheters. [NIH]

Basal cell carcinoma: A type of skin cancer that arises from the basal cells, small round cells found in the lower part (or base) of the epidermis, the outer layer of the skin. [NIH]

Basal cells: Small, round cells found in the lower part (or base) of the epidermis, the outer layer of the skin. [NIH]

Basal Ganglia: Large subcortical nuclear masses derived from the telencephalon and located in the basal regions of the cerebral hemispheres. [NIH]

Base Sequence: The sequence of purines and pyrimidines in nucleic acids and polynucleotides. It is also called nucleotide or nucleoside sequence. [NIH]

Benign: Not cancerous; does not invade nearby tissue or spread to other parts of the body. [NIH]

Benign tumor: A noncancerous growth that does not invade nearby tissue or spread to other parts of the body. [NIH]

Beta Rays: A stream of positive or negative electrons ejected with high energy from a disintegrating atomic nucleus; most biomedically used isotopes emit negative particles (electrons or negatrons, rather than positrons). Cathode rays are low-energy negative electrons produced in cathode ray tubes, also called television tubes or oscilloscopes. [NIH]

Bile: An emulsifying agent produced in the liver and secreted into the duodenum. Its composition includes bile acids and salts, cholesterol, and electrolytes. It aids digestion of fats in the duodenum. [NIH]

Biliary: Having to do with the liver, bile ducts, and/or gallbladder. [NIH]

Binding Sites: The reactive parts of a macromolecule that directly participate in its specific combination with another molecule. [NIH]

Biochemical: Relating to biochemistry; characterized by, produced by, or involving chemical reactions in living organisms. [EU]

Biological Factors: Compounds made by living organisms that contribute to or influence a phenomenon or process. They have biological or physiological activities. [NIH]

Biological Markers: Measurable and quantifiable biological parameters (e.g., specific enzyme concentration, specific hormone concentration, specific gene phenotype distribution in a population, presence of biological substances) which serve as indices for health- and physiology-related assessments, such as disease risk, psychiatric disorders, environmental exposure and its effects, disease diagnosis, metabolic processes, substance abuse, pregnancy, cell line development, epidemiologic studies, etc. [NIH]

Biological Response Modifiers: Biological or synthetic agents that are capable of eliciting specific and/or non-specific effects on immune responsiveness, thereby ultimately leading to an improvement in overall health of the patient. These agents can be further subcategorized into those that facilitate a normal immune response, those that stimulate the immune response, those that are capable of inducing noncytotoxic immunosuppression, and those that increase the ability of the host to tolerate damage by the cytotoxic modalities of the treatment. [NIH]

Biological therapy: Treatment to stimulate or restore the ability of the immune system to fight infection and disease. Also used to lessen side effects that may be caused by some cancer treatments. Also known as immunotherapy, biotherapy, or biological response modifier (BRM) therapy. [NIH]

Biological Transport: The movement of materials (including biochemical substances and drugs) across cell membranes and epithelial layers, usually by passive diffusion. [NIH]

Biomarkers: Substances sometimes found in an increased amount in the blood, other body fluids, or tissues and that may suggest the presence of some types of cancer. Biomarkers include CA 125 (ovarian cancer), CA 15-3 (breast cancer), CEA (ovarian, lung, breast, pancreas, and GI tract cancers), and PSA (prostate cancer). Also called tumor markers. [NIH]

Biopsy: Removal and pathologic examination of specimens in the form of small pieces of tissue from the living body. [NIH]

Biopsy specimen: Tissue removed from the body and examined under a microscope to determine whether disease is present. [NIH]

Biosynthesis: The building up of a chemical compound in the physiologic processes of a living organism. [EU]

Biotechnology: Body of knowledge related to the use of organisms, cells or cell-derived constituents for the purpose of developing products which are technically, scientifically and clinically useful. Alteration of biologic function at the molecular level (i.e., genetic engineering) is a central focus; laboratory methods used include transfection and cloning technologies, sequence and structure analysis algorithms, computer databases, and gene and protein structure function analysis and prediction. [NIH]

Bivalent: Pertaining to a group of 2 homologous or partly homologous chromosomes during the zygotene stage of prophase to the first metaphase in meiosis. [NIH]

Bladder: The organ that stores urine. [NIH]

Bleomycin: A complex of related glycopeptide antibiotics from Streptomyces verticillus consisting of bleomycin A2 and B2. It inhibits DNA metabolism and is used as an antineoplastic, especially for solid tumors. [NIH]

Blood Coagulation: The process of the interaction of blood coagulation factors that results in an insoluble fibrin clot. [NIH]

Blood Coagulation Factors: Endogenous substances, usually proteins, that are involved in the blood coagulation process. [NIH]

Blood Glucose: Glucose in blood. [NIH]

Blood pressure: The pressure of blood against the walls of a blood vessel or heart chamber. Unless there is reference to another location, such as the pulmonary artery or one of the heart chambers, it refers to the pressure in the systemic arteries, as measured, for example, in the forearm. [NIH]

Blood vessel: A tube in the body through which blood circulates. Blood vessels include a network of arteries, arterioles, capillaries, venules, and veins. [NIH]

Blood-Brain Barrier: Specialized non-fenestrated tightly-joined endothelial cells (tight junctions) that form a transport barrier for certain substances between the cerebral capillaries and the brain tissue. [NIH]

Blot: To transfer DNA, RNA, or proteins to an immobilizing matrix such as nitrocellulose. [NIH]

Body Composition: The relative amounts of various components in the body, such as percent body fat. [NIH]

Body Fluids: Liquid components of living organisms. [NIH]

Body-section: A technique of making radiographs of predetermined layers within objects, the sharp image of the chosen layer and the blurred images of other layers being produced by coordinated motion of any two of an X-ray tube, an object, or a film. [NIH]

Bolus: A single dose of drug usually injected into a blood vessel over a short period of time. Also called bolus infusion. [NIH]

Bolus infusion: A single dose of drug usually injected into a blood vessel over a short period of time. Also called bolus. [NIH]

Bone Marrow: The soft tissue filling the cavities of bones. Bone marrow exists in two types, yellow and red. Yellow marrow is found in the large cavities of large bones and consists mostly of fat cells and a few primitive blood cells. Red marrow is a hematopoietic tissue and is the site of production of erythrocytes and granular leukocytes. Bone marrow is made up of a framework of connective tissue containing branching fibers with the frame being filled with marrow cells. [NIH]

Bone Marrow Transplantation: The transference of bone marrow from one human or animal to another. [NIH]

Bone metastases: Cancer that has spread from the original (primary) tumor to the bone. [NIH]

Bone scan: A technique to create images of bones on a computer screen or on film. A small amount of radioactive material is injected into a blood vessel and travels through the bloodstream; it collects in the bones and is detected by a scanner. [NIH]

Bowel: The long tube-shaped organ in the abdomen that completes the process of digestion. There is both a small and a large bowel. Also called the intestine. [NIH]

Brachytherapy: A collective term for interstitial, intracavity, and surface radiotherapy. It uses small sealed or partly-sealed sources that may be placed on or near the body surface or within a natural body cavity or implanted directly into the tissues. [NIH]

Brain metastases: Cancer that has spread from the original (primary) tumor to the brain. [NIH]

Bromine: A halogen with the atomic symbol Br, atomic number 36, and atomic weight 79.904. It is a volatile reddish-brown liquid that gives off suffocating vapors, is corrosive to the skin, and may cause severe gastroenteritis if ingested. [NIH]

Bronchial: Pertaining to one or more bronchi. [EU]

Buccal: Pertaining to or directed toward the cheek. In dental anatomy, used to refer to the buccal surface of a tooth. [EU]

Cachexia: General ill health, malnutrition, and weight loss, usually associated with chronic disease. [NIH]

Calcium: A basic element found in nearly all organized tissues. It is a member of the alkaline earth family of metals with the atomic symbol Ca, atomic number 20, and atomic weight 40. Calcium is the most abundant mineral in the body and combines with phosphorus to form calcium phosphate in the bones and teeth. It is essential for the normal functioning of nerves and muscles and plays a role in blood coagulation (as factor IV) and in many enzymatic processes. [NIH]

Calcium channel blocker: A drug used to relax the blood vessel and heart muscle, causing pressure inside blood vessels to drop. It also can regulate heart rhythm. [NIH]

Calculi: An abnormal concretion occurring mostly in the urinary and biliary tracts, usually composed of mineral salts. Also called stones. [NIH]

Calibration: Determination, by measurement or comparison with a standard, of the correct value of each scale reading on a meter or other measuring instrument; or determination of the settings of a control device that correspond to particular values of voltage, current, frequency, or other output. [NIH]

Callus: A callosity or hard, thick skin; the bone-like reparative substance that is formed round the edges and fragments of broken bone. [NIH]

Camptothecin: An alkaloid isolated from the stem wood of the Chinese tree, Camptotheca acuminata. This compound selectively inhibits the nuclear enzyme DNA topoisomerase. Several semisynthetic analogs of camptothecin have demonstrated antitumor activity. [NIH]

Cancer vaccine: A vaccine designed to prevent or treat cancer. [NIH]

Candidiasis: Infection with a fungus of the genus Candida. It is usually a superficial infection of the moist cutaneous areas of the body, and is generally caused by C. albicans; it most commonly involves the skin (dermatocandidiasis), oral mucous membranes (thrush, def. 1), respiratory tract (bronchocandidiasis), and vagina (vaginitis). Rarely there is a systemic infection or endocarditis. Called also moniliasis, candidosis, oidiomycosis, and formerly blastodendriosis. [EU]

Candidosis: An infection caused by an opportunistic yeasts that tends to proliferate and become pathologic when the environment is favorable and the host resistance is weakened. [NIH]

Capsules: Hard or soft soluble containers used for the oral administration of medicine. [NIH]

Captopril: A potent and specific inhibitor of peptidyl-dipeptidase A. It blocks the conversion of angiotensin I to angiotensin II, a vasoconstrictor and important regulator of arterial blood pressure. Captopril acts to suppress the renin-angiotensin system and inhibits pressure responses to exogenous angiotensin. [NIH]

Carbohydrate: An aldehyde or ketone derivative of a polyhydric alcohol, particularly of the pentahydric and hexahydric alcohols. They are so named because the hydrogen and oxygen are usually in the proportion to form water, $(CH2O)n$. The most important carbohydrates are the starches, sugars, celluloses, and gums. They are classified into mono-, di-, tri-, poly- and heterosaccharides. [EU]

Carbon Dioxide: A colorless, odorless gas that can be formed by the body and is necessary for the respiration cycle of plants and animals. [NIH]

Carboplatin: An organoplatinum compound that possesses antineoplastic activity. [NIH]

Carcinogen: Any substance that causes cancer. [NIH]

Carcinogenesis: The process by which normal cells are transformed into cancer cells. [NIH]

Carcinogenic: Producing carcinoma. [EU]

Carcinoma: Cancer that begins in the skin or in tissues that line or cover internal organs. [NIH]

Cardiac: Having to do with the heart. [NIH]

Cardiomyopathy: A general diagnostic term designating primary myocardial disease, often of obscure or unknown etiology. [EU]

Cardiorespiratory: Relating to the heart and lungs and their function. [EU]

Cardiovascular: Having to do with the heart and blood vessels. [NIH]

Cardiovascular disease: Any abnormal condition characterized by dysfunction of the heart and blood vessels. CVD includes atherosclerosis (especially coronary heart disease, which can lead to heart attacks), cerebrovascular disease (e.g., stroke), and hypertension (high blood pressure). [NIH]

Carotene: The general name for a group of pigments found in green, yellow, and leafy vegetables, and yellow fruits. The pigments are fat-soluble, unsaturated aliphatic hydrocarbons functioning as provitamins and are converted to vitamin A through enzymatic processes in the intestinal wall. [NIH]

Case report: A detailed report of the diagnosis, treatment, and follow-up of an individual patient. Case reports also contain some demographic information about the patient (for example, age, gender, ethnic origin). [NIH]

Case series: A group or series of case reports involving patients who were given similar treatment. Reports of case series usually contain detailed information about the individual patients. This includes demographic information (for example, age, gender, ethnic origin) and information on diagnosis, treatment, response to treatment, and follow-up after treatment. [NIH]

Caspase: Enzyme released by the cell at a crucial stage in apoptosis in order to shred all cellular proteins. [NIH]

Castration: Surgical removal or artificial destruction of gonads. [NIH]

Catabolism: Any destructive metabolic process by which organisms convert substances into excreted compounds. [EU]

Cataract: An opacity, partial or complete, of one or both eyes, on or in the lens or capsule, especially an opacity impairing vision or causing blindness. The many kinds of cataract are classified by their morphology (size, shape, location) or etiology (cause and time of occurrence). [EU]

Catheter: A flexible tube used to deliver fluids into or withdraw fluids from the body. [NIH]

Catheterization: Use or insertion of a tubular device into a duct, blood vessel, hollow organ, or body cavity for injecting or withdrawing fluids for diagnostic or therapeutic purposes. It differs from intubation in that the tube here is used to restore or maintain patency in obstructions. [NIH]

Cathode: An electrode, usually an incandescent filament of tungsten, which emits electrons in an X-ray tube. [NIH]

Cations: Postively charged atoms, radicals or groups of atoms which travel to the cathode or negative pole during electrolysis. [NIH]

Caudal: Denoting a position more toward the cauda, or tail, than some specified point of reference; same as inferior, in human anatomy. [EU]

Cause of Death: Factors which produce cessation of all vital bodily functions. They can be analyzed from an epidemiologic viewpoint. [NIH]

Cell: The individual unit that makes up all of the tissues of the body. All living things are made up of one or more cells. [NIH]

Cell Count: A count of the number of cells of a specific kind, usually measured per unit volume of sample. [NIH]

Cell Cycle: The complex series of phenomena, occurring between the end of one cell division and the end of the next, by which cellular material is divided between daughter cells. [NIH]

Cell Death: The termination of the cell's ability to carry out vital functions such as metabolism, growth, reproduction, responsiveness, and adaptability. [NIH]

Cell Differentiation: Progressive restriction of the developmental potential and increasing specialization of function which takes place during the development of the embryo and leads to the formation of specialized cells, tissues, and organs. [NIH]

Cell Division: The fission of a cell. [NIH]

Cell membrane: Cell membrane = plasma membrane. The structure enveloping a cell, enclosing the cytoplasm, and forming a selective permeability barrier; it consists of lipids, proteins, and some carbohydrates, the lipids thought to form a bilayer in which integral proteins are embedded to varying degrees. [EU]

Cell proliferation: An increase in the number of cells as a result of cell growth and cell division. [NIH]

Cell Respiration: The metabolic process of all living cells (animal and plant) in which oxygen is used to provide a source of energy for the cell. [NIH]

Cell Survival: The span of viability of a cell characterized by the capacity to perform certain functions such as metabolism, growth, reproduction, some form of responsiveness, and adaptability. [NIH]

Cell Transplantation: Transference of cells within an individual, between individuals of the same species, or between individuals of different species. [NIH]

Central Nervous System: The main information-processing organs of the nervous system, consisting of the brain, spinal cord, and meninges. [NIH]

Central Nervous System Infections: Pathogenic infections of the brain, spinal cord, and meninges. DNA virus infections; RNA virus infections; bacterial infections; mycoplasma infections; Spirochaetales infections; fungal infections; protozoan infections; helminthiasis; and prion diseases may involve the central nervous system as a primary or secondary process. [NIH]

Ceramide: A type of fat produced in the body. It may cause some types of cells to die, and is being studied in cancer treatment. [NIH]

Cerebellum: Part of the metencephalon that lies in the posterior cranial fossa behind the brain stem. It is concerned with the coordination of movement. [NIH]

Cerebral: Of or pertaining of the cerebrum or the brain. [EU]

Cerebral hemispheres: The two halves of the cerebrum, the part of the brain that controls muscle functions of the body and also controls speech, emotions, reading, writing, and learning. The right hemisphere controls muscle movement on the left side of the body, and the left hemisphere controls muscle movement on the right side of the body. [NIH]

Cerebrospinal: Pertaining to the brain and spinal cord. [EU]

Cerebrospinal fluid: CSF. The fluid flowing around the brain and spinal cord. Cerebrospinal fluid is produced in the ventricles in the brain. [NIH]

Cerebrovascular: Pertaining to the blood vessels of the cerebrum, or brain. [EU]

Cerebrum: The largest part of the brain. It is divided into two hemispheres, or halves, called the cerebral hemispheres. The cerebrum controls muscle functions of the body and also controls speech, emotions, reading, writing, and learning. [NIH]

Cervical: Relating to the neck, or to the neck of any organ or structure. Cervical lymph nodes are located in the neck; cervical cancer refers to cancer of the uterine cervix, which is the lower, narrow end (the "neck") of the uterus. [NIH]

Cervix: The lower, narrow end of the uterus that forms a canal between the uterus and vagina. [NIH]

Character: In current usage, approximately equivalent to personality. The sum of the relatively fixed personality traits and habitual modes of response of an individual. [NIH]

Chelating Agents: Organic chemicals that form two or more coordination bonds with a central metal ion. Heterocyclic rings are formed with the central metal atom as part of the ring. Some biological systems form metal chelates, e.g., the iron-binding porphyrin group of hemoglobin and the magnesium-binding chlorophyll of plants. (From Hawley's Condensed Chemical Dictionary, 12th ed) They are used chemically to remove ions from solutions, medicinally against microorganisms, to treat metal poisoning, and in chemotherapy protocols. [NIH]

Chelation: Combination with a metal in complexes in which the metal is part of a ring. [EU]

Chemoembolization: A procedure in which the blood supply to the tumor is blocked surgically or mechanically, and anticancer drugs are administered directly into the tumor. This permits a higher concentration of drug to be in contact with the tumor for a longer period of time. [NIH]

Chemoprevention: The use of drugs, vitamins, or other agents to try to reduce the risk of, or delay the development or recurrence of, cancer. [NIH]

Chemopreventive: Natural or synthetic compound used to intervene in the early precancerous stages of carcinogenesis. [NIH]

Chemoprotective: A quality of some drugs used in cancer treatment. Chemoprotective agents protect healthy tissue from the toxic effects of anticancer drugs. [NIH]

Chemotactic Factors: Chemical substances that attract or repel cells or organisms. The concept denotes especially those factors released as a result of tissue injury, invasion, or immunologic activity, that attract leukocytes, macrophages, or other cells to the site of infection or insult. [NIH]

Chemotherapeutic agent: A drug used to treat cancer. [NIH]

Chemotherapeutics: Noun plural but singular or plural in constructions : chemotherapy. [EU]

Chemotherapy: Treatment with anticancer drugs. [NIH]

Chest wall: The ribs and muscles, bones, and joints that make up the area of the body between the neck and the abdomen. [NIH]

Chlorophyll: Porphyrin derivatives containing magnesium that act to convert light energy in photosynthetic organisms. [NIH]

Cholesterol: The principal sterol of all higher animals, distributed in body tissues, especially the brain and spinal cord, and in animal fats and oils. [NIH]

Choline: A basic constituent of lecithin that is found in many plants and animal organs. It is important as a precursor of acetylcholine, as a methyl donor in various metabolic processes, and in lipid metabolism. [NIH]

Chromatin: The material of chromosomes. It is a complex of DNA, histones, and nonhistone proteins (chromosomal proteins, non-histone) found within the nucleus of a cell. [NIH]

Chromosomal: Pertaining to chromosomes. [EU]

Chromosome: Part of a cell that contains genetic information. Except for sperm and eggs, all human cells contain 46 chromosomes. [NIH]

Chronic: A disease or condition that persists or progresses over a long period of time. [NIH]

Chronic Disease: Disease or ailment of long duration. [NIH]

Chronic Fatigue Syndrome: Fatigue caused by the combined effects of different types of prolonged fatigue. [NIH]

Chronic renal: Slow and progressive loss of kidney function over several years, often resulting in end-stage renal disease. People with end-stage renal disease need dialysis or transplantation to replace the work of the kidneys. [NIH]

Chymotrypsin: A serine endopeptidase secreted by the pancreas as its zymogen, chymotrypsinogen and carried in the pancreatic juice to the duodenum where it is activated by trypsin. It selectively cleaves aromatic amino acids on the carboxyl side. [NIH]

Circadian: Repeated more or less daily, i. e. on a 23- to 25-hour cycle. [NIH]

CIS: Cancer Information Service. The CIS is the National Cancer Institute's link to the public, interpreting and explaining research findings in a clear and understandable manner, and providing personalized responses to specific questions about cancer. Access the CIS by calling 1-800-4-CANCER, or by using the Web site at http://cis.nci.nih.gov. [NIH]

Cisplatin: An inorganic and water-soluble platinum complex. After undergoing hydrolysis, it reacts with DNA to produce both intra and interstrand crosslinks. These crosslinks appear to impair replication and transcription of DNA. The cytotoxicity of cisplatin correlates with cellular arrest in the G2 phase of the cell cycle. [NIH]

Clavicle: A long bone of the shoulder girdle. [NIH]

Cleave: A double-stranded cut in DNA with a restriction endonuclease. [NIH]

Cleft Lip: Congenital defect in the upper lip where the maxillary prominence fails to merge with the merged medial nasal prominences. It is thought to be caused by faulty migration of the mesoderm in the head region. [NIH]

Clinical Medicine: The study and practice of medicine by direct examination of the patient. [NIH]

Clinical Protocols: Precise and detailed plans for the study of a medical or biomedical problem and/or plans for a regimen of therapy. [NIH]

Clinical series: A case series in which the patients receive treatment in a clinic or other medical facility. [NIH]

Clinical study: A research study in which patients receive treatment in a clinic or other medical facility. Reports of clinical studies can contain results for single patients (case reports) or many patients (case series or clinical trials). [NIH]

Clinical trial: A research study that tests how well new medical treatments or other interventions work in people. Each study is designed to test new methods of screening, prevention, diagnosis, or treatment of a disease. [NIH]

Cloning: The production of a number of genetically identical individuals; in genetic engineering, a process for the efficient replication of a great number of identical DNA molecules. [NIH]

Cobalt: A trace element that is a component of vitamin B12. It has the atomic symbol Co, atomic number 27, and atomic weight 58.93. It is used in nuclear weapons, alloys, and pigments. Deficiency in animals leads to anemia; its excess in humans can lead to erythrocytosis. [NIH]

Codeine: An opioid analgesic related to morphine but with less potent analgesic properties and mild sedative effects. It also acts centrally to suppress cough. [NIH]

Cofactor: A substance, microorganism or environmental factor that activates or enhances the action of another entity such as a disease-causing agent. [NIH]

Cognitive restructuring: A method of identifying and replacing fear-promoting, irrational beliefs with more realistic and functional ones. [NIH]

Collagen: A polypeptide substance comprising about one third of the total protein in mammalian organisms. It is the main constituent of skin, connective tissue, and the organic substance of bones and teeth. Different forms of collagen are produced in the body but all consist of three alpha-polypeptide chains arranged in a triple helix. Collagen is differentiated from other fibrous proteins, such as elastin, by the content of proline, hydroxyproline, and hydroxylysine; by the absence of tryptophan; and particularly by the high content of polar groups which are responsible for its swelling properties. [NIH]

Collagen disease: A term previously used to describe chronic diseases of the connective tissue (e.g., rheumatoid arthritis, systemic lupus erythematosus, and systemic sclerosis), but now is thought to be more appropriate for diseases associated with defects in collagen, which is a component of the connective tissue. [NIH]

Colloidal: Of the nature of a colloid. [EU]

Colon: The long, coiled, tubelike organ that removes water from digested food. The remaining material, solid waste called stool, moves through the colon to the rectum and leaves the body through the anus. [NIH]

Colorectal: Having to do with the colon or the rectum. [NIH]

Colorectal Cancer: Cancer that occurs in the colon (large intestine) or the rectum (the end of the large intestine). A number of digestive diseases may increase a person's risk of colorectal cancer, including polyposis and Zollinger-Ellison Syndrome. [NIH]

Combination chemotherapy: Treatment using more than one anticancer drug. [NIH]

Combinatorial: A cut-and-paste process that churns out thousands of potentially valuable compounds at once. [NIH]

Combined Modality Therapy: The treatment of a disease or condition by several different means simultaneously or sequentially. Chemoimmunotherapy, radioimmunotherapy, chemoradiotherapy, cryochemotherapy, and salvage therapy are seen most frequently, but their combinations with each other and surgery are also used. [NIH]

Competency: The capacity of the bacterium to take up DNA from its surroundings. [NIH]

Complement: A term originally used to refer to the heat-labile factor in serum that causes immune cytolysis, the lysis of antibody-coated cells, and now referring to the entire functionally related system comprising at least 20 distinct serum proteins that is the effector not only of immune cytolysis but also of other biologic functions. Complement activation occurs by two different sequences, the classic and alternative pathways. The proteins of the classic pathway are termed 'components of complement' and are designated by the symbols C1 through C9. C1 is a calcium-dependent complex of three distinct proteins C1q, C1r and C1s. The proteins of the alternative pathway (collectively referred to as the properdin system) and complement regulatory proteins are known by semisystematic or trivial names. Fragments resulting from proteolytic cleavage of complement proteins are designated with lower-case letter suffixes, e.g., C3a. Inactivated fragments may be designated with the suffix 'i', e.g. C3bi. Activated components or complexes with biological activity are designated by a bar over the symbol e.g. C1 or C4b,2a. The classic pathway is activated by the binding of C1 to classic pathway activators, primarily antigen-antibody complexes containing IgM, IgG1, IgG3; C1q binds to a single IgM molecule or two adjacent IgG molecules. The alternative pathway can be activated by IgA immune complexes and also by nonimmunologic materials including bacterial endotoxins, microbial polysaccharides, and cell walls. Activation of the classic pathway triggers an enzymatic cascade involving C1, C4, C2 and C3; activation of the alternative pathway triggers a cascade involving C3 and factors B, D and P. Both result in the cleavage of C5 and the formation of the membrane attack complex. Complement activation also results in the formation of many biologically active complement fragments that act as anaphylatoxins, opsonins, or chemotactic factors. [EU]

Complementary and alternative medicine: CAM. Forms of treatment that are used in addition to (complementary) or instead of (alternative) standard treatments. These practices are not considered standard medical approaches. CAM includes dietary supplements, megadose vitamins, herbal preparations, special teas, massage therapy, magnet therapy, spiritual healing, and meditation. [NIH]

Complementary medicine: Practices not generally recognized by the medical community as standard or conventional medical approaches and used to enhance or complement the standard treatments. Complementary medicine includes the taking of dietary supplements, megadose vitamins, and herbal preparations; the drinking of special teas; and practices such as massage therapy, magnet therapy, spiritual healing, and meditation. [NIH]

Complete response: The disappearance of all signs of cancer in response to treatment. This does not always mean the cancer has been cured. [NIH]

Computational Biology: A field of biology concerned with the development of techniques for the collection and manipulation of biological data, and the use of such data to make biological discoveries or predictions. This field encompasses all computational methods and theories applicable to molecular biology and areas of computer-based techniques for solving biological problems including manipulation of models and datasets. [NIH]

Computed tomography: CT scan. A series of detailed pictures of areas inside the body, taken from different angles; the pictures are created by a computer linked to an x-ray machine. Also called computerized tomography and computerized axial tomography (CAT) scan. [NIH]

Computer Simulation: Computer-based representation of physical systems and phenomena such as chemical processes. [NIH]

Computerized axial tomography: A series of detailed pictures of areas inside the body, taken from different angles; the pictures are created by a computer linked to an x-ray machine. Also called CAT scan, computed tomography (CT scan), or computerized tomography. [NIH]

Computerized tomography: A series of detailed pictures of areas inside the body, taken from different angles; the pictures are created by a computer linked to an x-ray machine. Also called computerized axial tomography (CAT) scan and computed tomography (CT scan). [NIH]

Concomitant: Accompanying; accessory; joined with another. [EU]

Concurrent therapy: A treatment that is given at the same time as another. [NIH]

Conduction: The transfer of sound waves, heat, nervous impulses, or electricity. [EU]

Cone: One of the special retinal receptor elements which are presumed to be primarily concerned with perception of light and color stimuli when the eye is adapted to light. [NIH]

Congestion: Excessive or abnormal accumulation of blood in a part. [EU]

Conjugated: Acting or operating as if joined; simultaneous. [EU]

Conjugation: 1. The act of joining together or the state of being conjugated. 2. A sexual process seen in bacteria, ciliate protozoa, and certain fungi in which nuclear material is exchanged during the temporary fusion of two cells (conjugants). In bacterial genetics a form of sexual reproduction in which a donor bacterium (male) contributes some, or all, of its DNA (in the form of a replicated set) to a recipient (female) which then incorporates differing genetic information into its own chromosome by recombination and passes the recombined set on to its progeny by replication. In ciliate protozoa, two conjugants of separate mating types exchange micronuclear material and then separate, each now being a fertilized cell. In certain fungi, the process involves fusion of two gametes, resulting in union of their nuclei and formation of a zygote. 3. In chemistry, the joining together of two compounds to produce another compound, such as the combination of a toxic product with some substance in the body to form a detoxified product, which is then eliminated. [EU]

Conjunctiva: The mucous membrane that lines the inner surface of the eyelids and the anterior part of the sclera. [NIH]

Connective Tissue: Tissue that supports and binds other tissues. It consists of connective tissue cells embedded in a large amount of extracellular matrix. [NIH]

Connective Tissue: Tissue that supports and binds other tissues. It consists of connective tissue cells embedded in a large amount of extracellular matrix. [NIH]

Consciousness: Sense of awareness of self and of the environment. [NIH]

Consolidation: The healing process of a bone fracture. [NIH]

Continuous infusion: The administration of a fluid into a blood vessel, usually over a prolonged period of time. [NIH]

Contracture: A condition of fixed high resistance to passive stretch of a muscle, resulting from fibrosis of the tissues supporting the muscles or the joints, or from disorders of the muscle fibres. [EU]

Contraindications: Any factor or sign that it is unwise to pursue a certain kind of action or treatment, e. g. giving a general anesthetic to a person with pneumonia. [NIH]

Contralateral: Having to do with the opposite side of the body. [NIH]

Contrast Media: Substances used in radiography that allow visualization of certain tissues. [NIH]

Contrast medium: A substance that is introduced into or around a structure and, because of the difference in absorption of x-rays by the contrast medium and the surrounding tissues, allows radiographic visualization of the structure. [EU]

Control group: In a clinical trial, the group that does not receive the new treatment being studied. This group is compared to the group that receives the new treatment, to see if the new treatment works. [NIH]

Controlled clinical trial: A clinical study that includes a comparison (control) group. The comparison group receives a placebo, another treatment, or no treatment at all. [NIH]

Controlled study: An experiment or clinical trial that includes a comparison (control) group. [NIH]

Conventional therapy: A currently accepted and widely used treatment for a certain type of disease, based on the results of past research. Also called conventional treatment. [NIH]

Conventional treatment: A currently accepted and widely used treatment for a certain type of disease, based on the results of past research. Also called conventional therapy. [NIH]

Cooperative group: A group of physicians, hospitals, or both formed to treat a large number of persons in the same way so that new treatment can be evaluated quickly. Clinical trials of new cancer treatments often require many more people than a single physician or hospital can care for. [NIH]

Coordination: Muscular or motor regulation or the harmonious cooperation of muscles or groups of muscles, in a complex action or series of actions. [NIH]

Corneum: The superficial layer of the epidermis containing keratinized cells. [NIH]

Coronary: Encircling in the manner of a crown; a term applied to vessels; nerves, ligaments, etc. The term usually denotes the arteries that supply the heart muscle and, by extension, a pathologic involvement of them. [EU]

Coronary heart disease: A type of heart disease caused by narrowing of the coronary arteries that feed the heart, which needs a constant supply of oxygen and nutrients carried by the blood in the coronary arteries. When the coronary arteries become narrowed or clogged by fat and cholesterol deposits and cannot supply enough blood to the heart, CHD results. [NIH]

Coronary Thrombosis: Presence of a thrombus in a coronary artery, often causing a myocardial infarction. [NIH]

Corpus: The body of the uterus. [NIH]

Cortex: The outer layer of an organ or other body structure, as distinguished from the internal substance. [EU]

Cranial: Pertaining to the cranium, or to the anterior (in animals) or superior (in humans) end of the body. [EU]

Craniocerebral Trauma: Traumatic injuries involving the cranium and intracranial structures (i.e., brain; cranial nerves; meninges; and other structures). Injuries may be classified by whether or not the skull is penetrated (i.e., penetrating vs. nonpenetrating) or whether there is an associated hemorrhage. [NIH]

Crossing-over: The exchange of corresponding segments between chromatids of homologous chromosomes during meiosia, forming a chiasma. [NIH]

Crowns: A prosthetic restoration that reproduces the entire surface anatomy of the visible natural crown of a tooth. It may be partial (covering three or more surfaces of a tooth) or complete (covering all surfaces). It is made of gold or other metal, porcelain, or resin. [NIH]

Curative: Tending to overcome disease and promote recovery. [EU]

Curettage: Removal of tissue with a curette, a spoon-shaped instrument with a sharp edge. [NIH]

Curette: A spoon-shaped instrument with a sharp edge. [NIH]

Cutaneous: Having to do with the skin. [NIH]

Cyclophosphamide: Precursor of an alkylating nitrogen mustard antineoplastic and immunosuppressive agent that must be activated in the liver to form the active aldophosphamide. It is used in the treatment of lymphomas, leukemias, etc. Its side effect, alopecia, has been made use of in defleecing sheep. Cyclophosphamide may also cause sterility, birth defects, mutations, and cancer. [NIH]

Cyst: A sac or capsule filled with fluid. [NIH]

Cysteine: A thiol-containing non-essential amino acid that is oxidized to form cystine. [NIH]

Cystine: A covalently linked dimeric nonessential amino acid formed by the oxidation of cysteine. Two molecules of cysteine are joined together by a disulfide bridge to form cystine. [NIH]

Cytokine: Small but highly potent protein that modulates the activity of many cell types, including T and B cells. [NIH]

Cytokinesis: Division of the rest of cell. [NIH]

Cytoplasm: The protoplasm of a cell exclusive of that of the nucleus; it consists of a continuous aqueous solution (cytosol) and the organelles and inclusions suspended in it (phaneroplasm), and is the site of most of the chemical activities of the cell. [EU]

Cytoprotection: The process by which chemical compounds provide protection to cells against harmful agents. [NIH]

Cytotoxic: Cell-killing. [NIH]

Cytotoxic chemotherapy: Anticancer drugs that kill cells, especially cancer cells. [NIH]

Cytotoxicity: Quality of being capable of producing a specific toxic action upon cells of special organs. [NIH]

Cytotoxins: Substances elaborated by microorganisms, plants or animals that are specifically toxic to individual cells; they may be involved in immunity or may be contained in venoms. [NIH]

Daunorubicin: Very toxic anthracycline aminoglycoside antibiotic isolated from Streptomyces peucetius and others, used in treatment of leukemias and other neoplasms. [NIH]

Degenerative: Undergoing degeneration : tending to degenerate; having the character of or involving degeneration; causing or tending to cause degeneration. [EU]

Deletion: A genetic rearrangement through loss of segments of DNA (chromosomes), bringing sequences, which are normally separated, into close proximity. [NIH]

Dendrites: Extensions of the nerve cell body. They are short and branched and receive stimuli from other neurons. [NIH]

Dendritic: 1. Branched like a tree. 2. Pertaining to or possessing dendrites. [EU]

Dendritic cell: A special type of antigen-presenting cell (APC) that activates T lymphocytes. [NIH]

Density: The logarithm to the base 10 of the opacity of an exposed and processed film. [NIH]

Dental Abutments: Natural teeth or teeth roots used as anchorage for a fixed or removable denture or other prosthesis (such as an implant) serving the same purpose. [NIH]

Dental Caries: Localized destruction of the tooth surface initiated by decalcification of the enamel followed by enzymatic lysis of organic structures and leading to cavity formation. If left unchecked, the cavity may penetrate the enamel and dentin and reach the pulp. The three most prominent theories used to explain the etiology of the disase are that acids produced by bacteria lead to decalcification; that micro-organisms destroy the enamel protein; or that keratolytic micro-organisms produce chelates that lead to decalcification. [NIH]

Dental Hygienists: Persons trained in an accredited school or dental college and licensed by the state in which they reside to provide dental prophylaxis under the direction of a licensed dentist. [NIH]

Dental implant: A small metal pin placed inside the jawbone to mimic the root of a tooth. Dental implants can be used to help anchor a false tooth or teeth, or a crown or bridge. [NIH]

Dental Staff: Personnel who provide dental service to patients in an organized facility, institution or agency. [NIH]

Dentists: Individuals licensed to practice dentistry. [NIH]

Dentition: The teeth in the dental arch; ordinarily used to designate the natural teeth in position in their alveoli. [EU]

Dentures: An appliance used as an artificial or prosthetic replacement for missing teeth and adjacent tissues. It does not include crowns, dental abutments, nor artificial teeth. [NIH]

Deoxyuridine: 2'-Deoxyuridine. An antimetabolite that is converted to deoxyuridine triphosphate during DNA synthesis. Laboratory suppression of deoxyuridine is used to diagnose megaloblastic anemias due to vitamin B12 and folate deficiencies. [NIH]

Deprivation: Loss or absence of parts, organs, powers, or things that are needed. [EU]

Dermatitis: Any inflammation of the skin. [NIH]

Dermis: A layer of vascular connective tissue underneath the epidermis. The surface of the dermis contains sensitive papillae. Embedded in or beneath the dermis are sweat glands, hair follicles, and sebaceous glands. [NIH]

Desensitization: The prevention or reduction of immediate hypersensitivity reactions by administration of graded doses of allergen; called also hyposensitization and immunotherapy. [EU]

Diabetes Mellitus: A heterogeneous group of disorders that share glucose intolerance in common. [NIH]

Diagnostic Imaging: Any visual display of structural or functional patterns of organs or tissues for diagnostic evaluation. It includes measuring physiologic and metabolic responses to physical and chemical stimuli, as well as ultramicroscopy. [NIH]

Diagnostic procedure: A method used to identify a disease. [NIH]

Diaphragm: The musculofibrous partition that separates the thoracic cavity from the abdominal cavity. Contraction of the diaphragm increases the volume of the thoracic cavity aiding inspiration. [NIH]

Diastolic: Of or pertaining to the diastole. [EU]

Diffusion: The tendency of a gas or solute to pass from a point of higher pressure or concentration to a point of lower pressure or concentration and to distribute itself throughout the available space; a major mechanism of biological transport. [NIH]

Digestion: The process of breakdown of food for metabolism and use by the body. [NIH]

Digestive system: The organs that take in food and turn it into products that the body can use to stay healthy. Waste products the body cannot use leave the body through bowel movements. The digestive system includes the salivary glands, mouth, esophagus, stomach, liver, pancreas, gallbladder, small and large intestines, and rectum. [NIH]

Digestive tract: The organs through which food passes when food is eaten. These organs are the mouth, esophagus, stomach, small and large intestines, and rectum. [NIH]

Diploid: Having two sets of chromosomes. [NIH]

Direct: 1. Straight; in a straight line. 2. Performed immediately and without the intervention of subsidiary means. [EU]

Discrete: Made up of separate parts or characterized by lesions which do not become blended; not running together; separate. [NIH]

Disease-Free Survival: Period after successful treatment in which there is no appearance of the symptoms or effects of the disease. [NIH]

Disposition: A tendency either physical or mental toward certain diseases. [EU]

Dissociation: 1. The act of separating or state of being separated. 2. The separation of a molecule into two or more fragments (atoms, molecules, ions, or free radicals) produced by the absorption of light or thermal energy or by solvation. 3. In psychology, a defense mechanism in which a group of mental processes are segregated from the rest of a person's mental activity in order to avoid emotional distress, as in the dissociative disorders (q.v.), or in which an idea or object is segregated from its emotional significance; in the first sense it is roughly equivalent to splitting, in the second, to isolation. 4. A defect of mental integration in which one or more groups of mental processes become separated off from normal consciousness and, thus separated, function as a unitary whole. [EU]

Distal: Remote; farther from any point of reference; opposed to proximal. In dentistry, used to designate a position on the dental arch farther from the median line of the jaw. [EU]

Docetaxel: An anticancer drug that belongs to the family of drugs called mitotic inhibitors. [NIH]

Dorsal: 1. Pertaining to the back or to any dorsum. 2. Denoting a position more toward the back surface than some other object of reference; same as posterior in human anatomy; superior in the anatomy of quadrupeds. [EU]

Dose-limiting: Describes side effects of a drug or other treatment that are serious enough to prevent an increase in dose or level of that treatment. [NIH]

Dose-rate: The strength of a treatment given over a period of time. [NIH]

Dosimeter: In nuclear science and radiotherapy, a device used for the detection and measurement of radiation absorbed dose or any dose-related ionizing radiation received by the individual; a radiation meter intended to measure absorbed dose. [NIH]

Dosimetry: All the methods either of measuring directly, or of measuring indirectly and computing, absorbed dose, absorbed dose rate, exposure, exposure rate, dose equivalent, and the science associated with these methods. [NIH]

Double-blind: Pertaining to a clinical trial or other experiment in which neither the subject nor the person administering treatment knows which treatment any particular subject is receiving. [EU]

Doxorubicin: Antineoplastic antibiotic obtained from Streptomyces peucetics. It is a hydroxy derivative of daunorubicin and is used in treatment of both leukemia and solid tumors. [NIH]

Drive: A state of internal activity of an organism that is a necessary condition before a given stimulus will elicit a class of responses; e.g., a certain level of hunger (drive) must be present before food will elicit an eating response. [NIH]

Drug Interactions: The action of a drug that may affect the activity, metabolism, or toxicity of another drug. [NIH]

Drug Resistance: Diminished or failed response of an organism, disease or tissue to the intended effectiveness of a chemical or drug. It should be differentiated from drug tolerance which is the progressive diminution of the susceptibility of a human or animal to the effects of a drug, as a result of continued administration. [NIH]

Drug Tolerance: Progressive diminution of the susceptibility of a human or animal to the effects of a drug, resulting from its continued administration. It should be differentiated from drug resistance wherein an organism, disease, or tissue fails to respond to the intended effectiveness of a chemical or drug. It should also be differentiated from maximum tolerated dose and no-observed-adverse-effect level. [NIH]

Duct: A tube through which body fluids pass. [NIH]

Duodenum: The first part of the small intestine. [NIH]

Dysphagia: Difficulty in swallowing. [EU]

Edema: Excessive amount of watery fluid accumulated in the intercellular spaces, most commonly present in subcutaneous tissue. [NIH]

Effector: It is often an enzyme that converts an inactive precursor molecule into an active second messenger. [NIH]

Efferent: Nerve fibers which conduct impulses from the central nervous system to muscles and glands. [NIH]

Efficacy: The extent to which a specific intervention, procedure, regimen, or service produces a beneficial result under ideal conditions. Ideally, the determination of efficacy is based on the results of a randomized control trial. [NIH]

Elastic: Susceptible of resisting and recovering from stretching, compression or distortion applied by a force. [EU]

Elasticity: Resistance and recovery from distortion of shape. [NIH]

Elastin: The protein that gives flexibility to tissues. [NIH]

Electrolysis: Destruction by passage of a galvanic electric current, as in disintegration of a chemical compound in solution. [NIH]

Electrolyte: A substance that dissociates into ions when fused or in solution, and thus becomes capable of conducting electricity; an ionic solute. [EU]

Electromyography: Recording of the changes in electric potential of muscle by means of surface or needle electrodes. [NIH]

Electrons: Stable elementary particles having the smallest known negative charge, present in all elements; also called negatrons. Positively charged electrons are called positrons. The numbers, energies and arrangement of electrons around atomic nuclei determine the chemical identities of elements. Beams of electrons are called cathode rays or beta rays, the latter being a high-energy biproduct of nuclear decay. [NIH]

Electrophoresis: An electrochemical process in which macromolecules or colloidal particles with a net electric charge migrate in a solution under the influence of an electric current. [NIH]

Elementary Particles: Individual components of atoms, usually subatomic; subnuclear particles are usually detected only when the atomic nucleus decays and then only transiently, as most of them are unstable, often yielding pure energy without substance, i.e., radiation. [NIH]

Emboli: Bit of foreign matter which enters the blood stream at one point and is carried until it is lodged or impacted in an artery and obstructs it. It may be a blood clot, an air bubble, fat or other tissue, or clumps of bacteria. [NIH]

Embolization: The blocking of an artery by a clot or foreign material. Embolization can be done as treatment to block the flow of blood to a tumor. [NIH]

Embryo: The prenatal stage of mammalian development characterized by rapid morphological changes and the differentiation of basic structures. [NIH]

Embryogenesis: The process of embryo or embryoid formation, whether by sexual (zygotic) or asexual means. In asexual embryogenesis embryoids arise directly from the explant or on intermediary callus tissue. In some cases they arise from individual cells (somatic cell embryoge). [NIH]

Embryology: The study of the development of an organism during the embryonic and fetal stages of life. [NIH]

Empiric: Empirical; depending upon experience or observation alone, without using scientific method or theory. [EU]

Empirical: A treatment based on an assumed diagnosis, prior to receiving confirmatory laboratory test results. [NIH]

Emulsion: A preparation of one liquid distributed in small globules throughout the body of a second liquid. The dispersed liquid is the discontinuous phase, and the dispersion medium is the continuous phase. When oil is the dispersed liquid and an aqueous solution is the continuous phase, it is known as an oil-in-water emulsion, whereas when water or aqueous solution is the dispersed phase and oil or oleaginous substance is the continuous phase, it is known as a water-in-oil emulsion. Pharmaceutical emulsions for which official standards have been promulgated include cod liver oil emulsion, cod liver oil emulsion with malt, liquid petrolatum emulsion, and phenolphthalein in liquid petrolatum emulsion. [EU]

Enamel: A very hard whitish substance which covers the dentine of the anatomical crown of a tooth. [NIH]

Encapsulated: Confined to a specific, localized area and surrounded by a thin layer of tissue. [NIH]

Endocarditis: Exudative and proliferative inflammatory alterations of the endocardium, characterized by the presence of vegetations on the surface of the endocardium or in the endocardium itself, and most commonly involving a heart valve, but sometimes affecting the inner lining of the cardiac chambers or the endocardium elsewhere. It may occur as a primary disorder or as a complication of or in association with another disease. [EU]

Endocytosis: Cellular uptake of extracellular materials within membrane-limited vacuoles or microvesicles. Endosomes play a central role in endocytosis. [NIH]

Endogenous: Produced inside an organism or cell. The opposite is external (exogenous) production. [NIH]

Endometrial: Having to do with the endometrium (the layer of tissue that lines the uterus). [NIH]

Endometrium: The layer of tissue that lines the uterus. [NIH]

Endostatin: A drug that is being studied for its ability to prevent the growth of new blood vessels into a solid tumor. Endostatin belongs to the family of drugs called angiogenesis inhibitors. [NIH]

Endothelial cell: The main type of cell found in the inside lining of blood vessels, lymph vessels, and the heart. [NIH]

Endotoxins: Toxins closely associated with the living cytoplasm or cell wall of certain microorganisms, which do not readily diffuse into the culture medium, but are released upon lysis of the cells. [NIH]

End-stage renal: Total chronic kidney failure. When the kidneys fail, the body retains fluid and harmful wastes build up. A person with ESRD needs treatment to replace the work of the failed kidneys. [NIH]

Energetic: Exhibiting energy : strenuous; operating with force, vigour, or effect. [EU]

Enhancer: Transcriptional element in the virus genome. [NIH]

Enucleation: Removal of the nucleus from an eucaryotic cell. [NIH]

Environmental Exposure: The exposure to potentially harmful chemical, physical, or biological agents in the environment or to environmental factors that may include ionizing radiation, pathogenic organisms, or toxic chemicals. [NIH]

Environmental Health: The science of controlling or modifying those conditions, influences, or forces surrounding man which relate to promoting, establishing, and maintaining health. [NIH]

Enzymatic: Phase where enzyme cuts the precursor protein. [NIH]

Enzyme: A protein that speeds up chemical reactions in the body. [NIH]

Eosinophilia: Abnormal increase in eosinophils in the blood, tissues or organs. [NIH]

Ependymal: It lines the cavities of the brain's ventricles and the spinal cord and slowly divides to create a stem cell. [NIH]

Ependymal tumors: A type of brain tumor that usually begins in the central canal of the spinal cord. Ependymomas may also develop in the cells lining the ventricles of the brain, which produce and store the special fluid (cerebrospinal fluid) that protects the brain and spinal cord. Also called ependymomas. [NIH]

Ependymomas: Brain tumors that usually begin in the central canal of the spinal cord. Ependymomas may also develop in the cells lining the ventricles of the brain, which produce and store the special fluid (cerebrospinal fluid) that protects the brain and spinal cord. Also called ependymal tumors. [NIH]

Epidemiologic Studies: Studies designed to examine associations, commonly, hypothesized causal relations. They are usually concerned with identifying or measuring the effects of risk factors or exposures. The common types of analytic study are case-control studies, cohort studies, and cross-sectional studies. [NIH]

Epidemiological: Relating to, or involving epidemiology. [EU]

Epidermal: Pertaining to or resembling epidermis. Called also epidermic or epidermoid. [EU]

Epidermal Growth Factor: A 6 kD polypeptide growth factor initially discovered in mouse submaxillary glands. Human epidermal growth factor was originally isolated from urine based on its ability to inhibit gastric secretion and called urogastrone. epidermal growth factor exerts a wide variety of biological effects including the promotion of proliferation and differentiation of mesenchymal and epithelial cells. [NIH]

Epidermis: Nonvascular layer of the skin. It is made up, from within outward, of five layers: 1) basal layer (stratum basale epidermidis); 2) spinous layer (stratum spinosum epidermidis); 3) granular layer (stratum granulosum epidermidis); 4) clear layer (stratum lucidum epidermidis); and 5) horny layer (stratum corneum epidermidis). [NIH]

Epidermoid carcinoma: A type of cancer in which the cells are flat and look like fish scales. Also called squamous cell carcinoma. [NIH]

Epidural: The space between the wall of the spinal canal and the covering of the spinal cord.

An epidural injection is given into this space. [NIH]

Epinephrine: The active sympathomimetic hormone from the adrenal medulla in most species. It stimulates both the alpha- and beta- adrenergic systems, causes systemic vasoconstriction and gastrointestinal relaxation, stimulates the heart, and dilates bronchi and cerebral vessels. It is used in asthma and cardiac failure and to delay absorption of local anesthetics. [NIH]

Epithelial: Refers to the cells that line the internal and external surfaces of the body. [NIH]

Epithelial Cells: Cells that line the inner and outer surfaces of the body. [NIH]

Epithelium: One or more layers of epithelial cells, supported by the basal lamina, which covers the inner or outer surfaces of the body. [NIH]

Erectile: The inability to get or maintain an erection for satisfactory sexual intercourse. Also called impotence. [NIH]

Erythema: Redness of the skin produced by congestion of the capillaries. This condition may result from a variety of causes. [NIH]

Erythrocytes: Red blood cells. Mature erythrocytes are non-nucleated, biconcave disks containing hemoglobin whose function is to transport oxygen. [NIH]

Erythroleukemia: Cancer of the blood-forming tissues in which large numbers of immature, abnormal red blood cells are found in the blood and bone marrow. [NIH]

Escalation: Progressive use of more harmful drugs. [NIH]

Esophageal: Having to do with the esophagus, the muscular tube through which food passes from the throat to the stomach. [NIH]

Esophagectomy: An operation to remove a portion of the esophagus. [NIH]

Esophagitis: Inflammation, acute or chronic, of the esophagus caused by bacteria, chemicals, or trauma. [NIH]

Esophagus: The muscular tube through which food passes from the throat to the stomach. [NIH]

Estrogen: One of the two female sex hormones. [NIH]

Estrogen Antagonists: Compounds which inhibit or antagonize the action or biosynthesis of estrogen. [NIH]

Estrogen receptor: ER. Protein found on some cancer cells to which estrogen will attach. [NIH]

Estrogen receptor positive: ER+. Breast cancer cells that have a protein (receptor molecule) to which estrogen will attach. Breast cancer cells that are ER+ need the hormone estrogen to grow and will usually respond to hormone (antiestrogen) therapy that blocks these receptor sites. [NIH]

Etoposide: A semisynthetic derivative of podophyllotoxin that exhibits antitumor activity. Etoposide inhibits DNA synthesis by forming a complex with topoisomerase II and DNA. This complex induces breaks in double stranded DNA and prevents repair by topoisomerase II binding. Accumulated breaks in DNA prevent entry into the mitotic phase of cell division, and lead to cell death. Etoposide acts primarily in the G2 and S phases of the cell cycle. [NIH]

Eukaryote: An organism (or a cell) that carries its genetic material physically constrained within a nuclear membrane, separate from the cytoplasm. [NIH]

Eukaryotic Cells: Cells of the higher organisms, containing a true nucleus bounded by a nuclear membrane. [NIH]

Evaluable disease: Disease that cannot be measured directly by the size of the tumor but can be evaluated by other methods specific to a particular clinical trial. [NIH]

Exhaustion: The feeling of weariness of mind and body. [NIH]

Exogenous: Developed or originating outside the organism, as exogenous disease. [EU]

Exotoxin: Toxic substance excreted by living bacterial cells. [NIH]

Expiration: The act of breathing out, or expelling air from the lungs. [EU]

Expiratory: The volume of air which leaves the breathing organs in each expiration. [NIH]

External radiation: Radiation therapy that uses a machine to aim high-energy rays at the cancer. Also called external-beam radiation. [NIH]

External-beam radiation: Radiation therapy that uses a machine to aim high-energy rays at the cancer. Also called external radiation. [NIH]

Extracellular: Outside a cell or cells. [EU]

Extracellular Matrix: A meshwork-like substance found within the extracellular space and in association with the basement membrane of the cell surface. It promotes cellular proliferation and provides a supporting structure to which cells or cell lysates in culture dishes adhere. [NIH]

Extracellular Matrix Proteins: Macromolecular organic compounds that contain carbon, hydrogen, oxygen, nitrogen, and usually, sulfur. These macromolecules (proteins) form an intricate meshwork in which cells are embedded to construct tissues. Variations in the relative types of macromolecules and their organization determine the type of extracellular matrix, each adapted to the functional requirements of the tissue. The two main classes of macromolecules that form the extracellular matrix are: glycosaminoglycans, usually linked to proteins (proteoglycans), and fibrous proteins (e.g., collagen, elastin, fibronectins and laminin). [NIH]

Extracorporeal: Situated or occurring outside the body. [EU]

Extraction: The process or act of pulling or drawing out. [EU]

Extremity: A limb; an arm or leg (membrum); sometimes applied specifically to a hand or foot. [EU]

Eye Infections: Infection, moderate to severe, caused by bacteria, fungi, or viruses, which occurs either on the external surface of the eye or intraocularly with probable inflammation, visual impairment, or blindness. [NIH]

Facial: Of or pertaining to the face. [EU]

Facial Nerve: The 7th cranial nerve. The facial nerve has two parts, the larger motor root which may be called the facial nerve proper, and the smaller intermediate or sensory root. Together they provide efferent innervation to the muscles of facial expression and to the lacrimal and salivary glands, and convey afferent information for taste from the anterior two-thirds of the tongue and for touch from the external ear. [NIH]

Fallopian tube: The oviduct, a muscular tube about 10 cm long, lying in the upper border of the broad ligament. [NIH]

Family Planning: Programs or services designed to assist the family in controlling reproduction by either improving or diminishing fertility. [NIH]

Fasciitis: Inflammation of the fascia. There are three major types: 1) Eosinophilic fasciitis, an inflammatory reaction with eosinophilia, producing hard thickened skin with an orange-peel configuration suggestive of scleroderma and considered by some a variant of scleroderma; 2) Necrotizing fasciitis, a serious fulminating infection (usually by a beta hemolytic Streptococcus) causing extensive necrosis of superficial fascia; 3)

Nodular/Pseudosarcomatous/Proliferative fasciitis, characterized by a rapid growth of fibroblasts with mononuclear inflammatory cells and proliferating capillaries in soft tissue, often the forearm; it is not malignant but is sometimes mistaken for fibrosarcoma. [NIH]

Fat: Total lipids including phospholipids. [NIH]

Fatigue: The state of weariness following a period of exertion, mental or physical, characterized by a decreased capacity for work and reduced efficiency to respond to stimuli. [NIH]

Femoral: Pertaining to the femur, or to the thigh. [EU]

Femur: The longest and largest bone of the skeleton, it is situated between the hip and the knee. [NIH]

Fentanyl: A narcotic opioid drug that is used in the treatment of pain. [NIH]

Ferritin: An iron-containing protein complex that is formed by a combination of ferric iron with the protein apoferritin. [NIH]

Fetus: The developing offspring from 7 to 8 weeks after conception until birth. [NIH]

Fibrinogen: Plasma glycoprotein clotted by thrombin, composed of a dimer of three non-identical pairs of polypeptide chains (alpha, beta, gamma) held together by disulfide bonds. Fibrinogen clotting is a sol-gel change involving complex molecular arrangements: whereas fibrinogen is cleaved by thrombin to form polypeptides A and B, the proteolytic action of other enzymes yields different fibrinogen degradation products. [NIH]

Fibrinolysis: The natural enzymatic dissolution of fibrin. [NIH]

Fibroblasts: Connective tissue cells which secrete an extracellular matrix rich in collagen and other macromolecules. [NIH]

Fibrosarcoma: A type of soft tissue sarcoma that begins in fibrous tissue, which holds bones, muscles, and other organs in place. [NIH]

Fibrosis: Any pathological condition where fibrous connective tissue invades any organ, usually as a consequence of inflammation or other injury. [NIH]

Fistula: Abnormal communication most commonly seen between two internal organs, or between an internal organ and the surface of the body. [NIH]

Fixation: 1. The act or operation of holding, suturing, or fastening in a fixed position. 2. The condition of being held in a fixed position. 3. In psychiatry, a term with two related but distinct meanings : (1) arrest of development at a particular stage, which like regression (return to an earlier stage), if temporary is a normal reaction to setbacks and difficulties but if protracted or frequent is a cause of developmental failures and emotional problems, and (2) a close and suffocating attachment to another person, especially a childhood figure, such as one's mother or father. Both meanings are derived from psychoanalytic theory and refer to 'fixation' of libidinal energy either in a specific erogenous zone, hence fixation at the oral, anal, or phallic stage, or in a specific object, hence mother or father fixation. 4. The use of a fixative (q.v.) to preserve histological or cytological specimens. 5. In chemistry, the process whereby a substance is removed from the gaseous or solution phase and localized, as in carbon dioxide fixation or nitrogen fixation. 6. In ophthalmology, direction of the gaze so that the visual image of the object falls on the fovea centralis. 7. In film processing, the chemical removal of all undeveloped salts of the film emulsion, leaving only the developed silver to form a permanent image. [EU]

Flatus: Gas passed through the rectum. [NIH]

Fluconazole: Triazole antifungal agent that is used to treat oropharyngeal candidiasis and cryptococcal meningitis in AIDS. [NIH]

Fluorescence: The property of emitting radiation while being irradiated. The radiation emitted is usually of longer wavelength than that incident or absorbed, e.g., a substance can be irradiated with invisible radiation and emit visible light. X-ray fluorescence is used in diagnosis. [NIH]

Fluorine: A nonmetallic, diatomic gas that is a trace element and member of the halogen family. It is used in dentistry as flouride to prevent dental caries. [NIH]

Fluoroscopy: Production of an image when X-rays strike a fluorescent screen. [NIH]

Fluorouracil: A pyrimidine analog that acts as an antineoplastic antimetabolite and also has immunosuppressant. It interferes with DNA synthesis by blocking the thymidylate synthetase conversion of deoxyuridylic acid to thymidylic acid. [NIH]

Folate: A B-complex vitamin that is being studied as a cancer prevention agent. Also called folic acid. [NIH]

Fold: A plication or doubling of various parts of the body. [NIH]

Folic Acid: N-(4-(((2-Amino-1,4-dihydro-4-oxo-6-pteridinyl)methyl)amino)benzoyl)-L-glutamic acid. A member of the vitamin B family that stimulates the hematopoietic system. It is present in the liver and kidney and is found in mushrooms, spinach, yeast, green leaves, and grasses. Folic acid is used in the treatment and prevention of folate deficiencies and megaloblastic anemia. [NIH]

Follicles: Shafts through which hair grows. [NIH]

Forearm: The part between the elbow and the wrist. [NIH]

Fossa: A cavity, depression, or pit. [NIH]

Fovea: The central part of the macula that provides the sharpest vision. [NIH]

Fractionation: Dividing the total dose of radiation therapy into several smaller, equal doses delivered over a period of several days. [NIH]

Free Radicals: Highly reactive molecules with an unsatisfied electron valence pair. Free radicals are produced in both normal and pathological processes. They are proven or suspected agents of tissue damage in a wide variety of circumstances including radiation, damage from environment chemicals, and aging. Natural and pharmacological prevention of free radical damage is being actively investigated. [NIH]

Fungi: A kingdom of eukaryotic, heterotrophic organisms that live as saprobes or parasites, including mushrooms, yeasts, smuts, molds, etc. They reproduce either sexually or asexually, and have life cycles that range from simple to complex. Filamentous fungi refer to those that grow as multicelluar colonies (mushrooms and molds). [NIH]

Fungus: A general term used to denote a group of eukaryotic protists, including mushrooms, yeasts, rusts, moulds, smuts, etc., which are characterized by the absence of chlorophyll and by the presence of a rigid cell wall composed of chitin, mannans, and sometimes cellulose. They are usually of simple morphological form or show some reversible cellular specialization, such as the formation of pseudoparenchymatous tissue in the fruiting body of a mushroom. The dimorphic fungi grow, according to environmental conditions, as moulds or yeasts. [EU]

Gallbladder: The pear-shaped organ that sits below the liver. Bile is concentrated and stored in the gallbladder. [NIH]

Gallium: A rare, metallic element designated by the symbol, Ga, atomic number 31, and atomic weight 69.72. [NIH]

Gamma knife: Radiation therapy in which high-energy rays are aimed at a tumor from many angles in a single treatment session. [NIH]

Gamma Rays: Very powerful and penetrating, high-energy electromagnetic radiation of shorter wavelength than that of x-rays. They are emitted by a decaying nucleus, usually between 0.01 and 10 MeV. They are also called nuclear x-rays. [NIH]

Ganglia: Clusters of multipolar neurons surrounded by a capsule of loosely organized connective tissue located outside the central nervous system. [NIH]

Gas: Air that comes from normal breakdown of food. The gases are passed out of the body through the rectum (flatus) or the mouth (burp). [NIH]

Gastric: Having to do with the stomach. [NIH]

Gastrin: A hormone released after eating. Gastrin causes the stomach to produce more acid. [NIH]

Gastroenteritis: An acute inflammation of the lining of the stomach and intestines, characterized by anorexia, nausea, diarrhoea, abdominal pain, and weakness, which has various causes, including food poisoning due to infection with such organisms as Escherichia coli, Staphylococcus aureus, and Salmonella species; consumption of irritating food or drink; or psychological factors such as anger, stress, and fear. Called also enterogastritis. [EU]

Gastrointestinal: Refers to the stomach and intestines. [NIH]

Gastrointestinal tract: The stomach and intestines. [NIH]

Gels: Colloids with a solid continuous phase and liquid as the dispersed phase; gels may be unstable when, due to temperature or other cause, the solid phase liquifies; the resulting colloid is called a sol. [NIH]

Gemcitabine: An anticancer drug that belongs to the family of drugs called antimetabolites. [NIH]

Gene: The functional and physical unit of heredity passed from parent to offspring. Genes are pieces of DNA, and most genes contain the information for making a specific protein. [NIH]

Gene Conversion: The asymmetrical segregation of genes during replication which leads to the production of non-reciprocal recombinant strands and the apparent conversion of one allele into another. Thus, e.g., the meiotic products of an Aa individual may be AAAa or aaaA instead of AAaa, i.e., the A allele has been converted into the a allele or vice versa. [NIH]

Gene Deletion: A genetic rearrangement through loss of segments of DNA or RNA, bringing sequences which are normally separated into close proximity. This deletion may be detected using cytogenetic techniques and can also be inferred from the phenotype, indicating a deletion at one specific locus. [NIH]

Gene Expression: The phenotypic manifestation of a gene or genes by the processes of gene action. [NIH]

Gene Expression Profiling: The determination of the pattern of genes expressed i.e., transcribed, under specific circumstances or in a specific cell. [NIH]

Gene Therapy: The introduction of new genes into cells for the purpose of treating disease by restoring or adding gene expression. Techniques include insertion of retroviral vectors, transfection, homologous recombination, and injection of new genes into the nuclei of single cell embryos. The entire gene therapy process may consist of multiple steps. The new genes may be introduced into proliferating cells in vivo (e.g., bone marrow) or in vitro (e.g., fibroblast cultures) and the modified cells transferred to the site where the gene expression is required. Gene therapy may be particularly useful for treating enzyme deficiency diseases, hemoglobinopathies, and leukemias and may also prove useful in restoring drug sensitivity, particularly for leukemia. [NIH]

General practitioner: A medical practitioner who does not specialize in a particular branch of medicine or limit his practice to a specific class of diseases. [NIH]

Genetic Code: The specifications for how information, stored in nucleic acid sequence (base sequence), is translated into protein sequence (amino acid sequence). The start, stop, and order of amino acids of a protein is specified by consecutive triplets of nucleotides called codons (codon). [NIH]

Genetic Techniques: Chromosomal, biochemical, intracellular, and other methods used in the study of genetics. [NIH]

Genetics: The biological science that deals with the phenomena and mechanisms of heredity. [NIH]

Genital: Pertaining to the genitalia. [EU]

Genitourinary system: The parts of the body that play a role in reproduction, getting rid of waste products in the form of urine, or both. [NIH]

Genotype: The genetic constitution of the individual; the characterization of the genes. [NIH]

Germ Cells: The reproductive cells in multicellular organisms. [NIH]

Germinoma: The most frequent type of germ-cell tumor in the brain. [NIH]

Giant Cells: Multinucleated masses produced by the fusion of many cells; often associated with viral infections. In AIDS, they are induced when the envelope glycoprotein of the HIV virus binds to the CD4 antigen of uninfected neighboring T4 cells. The resulting syncytium leads to cell death and thus may account for the cytopathic effect of the virus. [NIH]

Gingivitis: Inflammation of the gingivae. Gingivitis associated with bony changes is referred to as periodontitis. Called also oulitis and ulitis. [EU]

Ginseng: An araliaceous genus of plants that contains a number of pharmacologically active agents used as stimulants, sedatives, and tonics, especially in traditional medicine. [NIH]

Gland: An organ that produces and releases one or more substances for use in the body. Some glands produce fluids that affect tissues or organs. Others produce hormones or participate in blood production. [NIH]

Glioblastoma: A malignant form of astrocytoma histologically characterized by pleomorphism of cells, nuclear atypia, microhemorrhage, and necrosis. They may arise in any region of the central nervous system, with a predilection for the cerebral hemispheres, basal ganglia, and commissural pathways. Clinical presentation most frequently occurs in the fifth or sixth decade of life with focal neurologic signs or seizures. [NIH]

Glioblastoma multiforme: A type of brain tumor that forms from glial (supportive) tissue of the brain. It grows very quickly and has cells that look very different from normal cells. Also called grade IV astrocytoma. [NIH]

Glioma: A cancer of the brain that comes from glial, or supportive, cells. [NIH]

Glossectomy: Amputation of the tongue. [NIH]

Glucose: D-Glucose. A primary source of energy for living organisms. It is naturally occurring and is found in fruits and other parts of plants in its free state. It is used therapeutically in fluid and nutrient replacement. [NIH]

Glutathione Peroxidase: An enzyme catalyzing the oxidation of 2 moles of glutathione in the presence of hydrogen peroxide to yield oxidized glutathione and water. EC 1.11.1.9. [NIH]

Glycine: A non-essential amino acid. It is found primarily in gelatin and silk fibroin and used therapeutically as a nutrient. It is also a fast inhibitory neurotransmitter. [NIH]

Glycolysis: The pathway by which glucose is catabolized into two molecules of pyruvic acid with the generation of ATP. [NIH]

Glycoprotein: A protein that has sugar molecules attached to it. [NIH]

Glycosylation: The chemical or biochemical addition of carbohydrate or glycosyl groups to other chemicals, especially peptides or proteins. Glycosyl transferases are used in this biochemical reaction. [NIH]

Gonad: A sex organ, such as an ovary or a testicle, which produces the gametes in most multicellular animals. [NIH]

Gonadal: Pertaining to a gonad. [EU]

Governing Board: The group in which legal authority is vested for the control of health-related institutions and organizations. [NIH]

Gp120: 120-kD HIV envelope glycoprotein which is involved in the binding of the virus to its membrane receptor, the CD4 molecule, found on the surface of certain cells in the body. [NIH]

Grade: The grade of a tumor depends on how abnormal the cancer cells look under a microscope and how quickly the tumor is likely to grow and spread. Grading systems are different for each type of cancer. [NIH]

Grading: A system for classifying cancer cells in terms of how abnormal they appear when examined under a microscope. The objective of a grading system is to provide information about the probable growth rate of the tumor and its tendency to spread. The systems used to grade tumors vary with each type of cancer. Grading plays a role in treatment decisions. [NIH]

Graft: Healthy skin, bone, or other tissue taken from one part of the body and used to replace diseased or injured tissue removed from another part of the body. [NIH]

Graft Rejection: An immune response with both cellular and humoral components, directed against an allogeneic transplant, whose tissue antigens are not compatible with those of the recipient. [NIH]

Grafting: The operation of transfer of tissue from one site to another. [NIH]

Granulocytes: Leukocytes with abundant granules in the cytoplasm. They are divided into three groups: neutrophils, eosinophils, and basophils. [NIH]

Granuloma: A relatively small nodular inflammatory lesion containing grouped mononuclear phagocytes, caused by infectious and noninfectious agents. [NIH]

Growth factors: Substances made by the body that function to regulate cell division and cell survival. Some growth factors are also produced in the laboratory and used in biological therapy. [NIH]

Gynecologic cancer: Cancer of the female reproductive tract, including the cervix, endometrium, fallopian tubes, ovaries, uterus, and vagina. [NIH]

Half-Life: The time it takes for a substance (drug, radioactive nuclide, or other) to lose half of its pharmacologic, physiologic, or radiologic activity. [NIH]

Haploid: An organism with one basic chromosome set, symbolized by n; the normal condition of gametes in diploids. [NIH]

Haptens: Small antigenic determinants capable of eliciting an immune response only when coupled to a carrier. Haptens bind to antibodies but by themselves cannot elicit an antibody response. [NIH]

Headache: Pain in the cranial region that may occur as an isolated and benign symptom or as a manifestation of a wide variety of conditions including subarachnoid hemorrhage;

craniocerebral trauma; central nervous system infections; intracranial hypertension; and other disorders. In general, recurrent headaches that are not associated with a primary disease process are referred to as headache disorders (e.g., migraine). [NIH]

Headache Disorders: Common conditions characterized by persistent or recurrent headaches. Headache syndrome classification systems may be based on etiology (e.g., vascular headache, post-traumatic headaches, etc.), temporal pattern (e.g., cluster headache, paroxysmal hemicrania, etc.), and precipitating factors (e.g., cough headache). [NIH]

Health Education: Education that increases the awareness and favorably influences the attitudes and knowledge relating to the improvement of health on a personal or community basis. [NIH]

Health Physics: The science concerned with problems of radiation protection relevant to reducing or preventing radiation exposure, and the effects of ionizing radiation on humans and their environment. [NIH]

Health Promotion: Encouraging consumer behaviors most likely to optimize health potentials (physical and psychosocial) through health information, preventive programs, and access to medical care. [NIH]

Heart attack: A seizure of weak or abnormal functioning of the heart. [NIH]

Heart Valves: Flaps of tissue that prevent regurgitation of blood from the ventricles to the atria or from the pulmonary arteries or aorta to the ventricles. [NIH]

Hematologic malignancies: Cancers of the blood or bone marrow, including leukemia and lymphoma. Also called hematologic cancers. [NIH]

Hematopoiesis: The development and formation of various types of blood cells. [NIH]

Hematuria: Presence of blood in the urine. [NIH]

Hemoglobin: One of the fractions of glycosylated hemoglobin A1c. Glycosylated hemoglobin is formed when linkages of glucose and related monosaccharides bind to hemoglobin A and its concentration represents the average blood glucose level over the previous several weeks. HbA1c levels are used as a measure of long-term control of plasma glucose (normal, 4 to 6 percent). In controlled diabetes mellitus, the concentration of glycosylated hemoglobin A is within the normal range, but in uncontrolled cases the level may be 3 to 4 times the normal conentration. Generally, complications are substantially lower among patients with Hb levels of 7 percent or less than in patients with HbA1c levels of 9 percent or more. [NIH]

Hemoglobin A: Normal adult human hemoglobin. The globin moiety consists of two alpha and two beta chains. [NIH]

Hemoglobinopathies: A group of inherited disorders characterized by structural alterations within the hemoglobin molecule. [NIH]

Hemolytic: A disease that affects the blood and blood vessels. It destroys red blood cells, cells that cause the blood to clot, and the lining of blood vessels. HUS is often caused by the Escherichia coli bacterium in contaminated food. People with HUS may develop acute renal failure. [NIH]

Hemorrhage: Bleeding or escape of blood from a vessel. [NIH]

Hemostasis: The process which spontaneously arrests the flow of blood from vessels carrying blood under pressure. It is accomplished by contraction of the vessels, adhesion and aggregation of formed blood elements, and the process of blood or plasma coagulation. [NIH]

Hepatic: Refers to the liver. [NIH]

Hepatocellular: Pertaining to or affecting liver cells. [EU]

Hepatocellular carcinoma: A type of adenocarcinoma, the most common type of liver tumor. [NIH]

Hereditary: Of, relating to, or denoting factors that can be transmitted genetically from one generation to another. [NIH]

Heredity: 1. The genetic transmission of a particular quality or trait from parent to offspring. 2. The genetic constitution of an individual. [EU]

Heterodimer: Zippered pair of nonidentical proteins. [NIH]

Heterogeneity: The property of one or more samples or populations which implies that they are not identical in respect of some or all of their parameters, e. g. heterogeneity of variance. [NIH]

Heterotrophic: Pertaining to organisms that are consumers and dependent on other organisms for their source of energy (food). [NIH]

Histology: The study of tissues and cells under a microscope. [NIH]

Histones: Small chromosomal proteins (approx 12-20 kD) possessing an open, unfolded structure and attached to the DNA in cell nuclei by ionic linkages. Classification into the various types (designated histone I, histone II, etc.) is based on the relative amounts of arginine and lysine in each. [NIH]

Homologous: Corresponding in structure, position, origin, etc., as (a) the feathers of a bird and the scales of a fish, (b) antigen and its specific antibody, (c) allelic chromosomes. [EU]

Hormonal: Pertaining to or of the nature of a hormone. [EU]

Hormonal therapy: Treatment of cancer by removing, blocking, or adding hormones. Also called hormone therapy or endocrine therapy. [NIH]

Hormone: A substance in the body that regulates certain organs. Hormones such as gastrin help in breaking down food. Some hormones come from cells in the stomach and small intestine. [NIH]

Hormone therapy: Treatment of cancer by removing, blocking, or adding hormones. Also called endocrine therapy. [NIH]

Hospice: Institution dedicated to caring for the terminally ill. [NIH]

Human papillomavirus: HPV. A virus that causes abnormal tissue growth (warts) and is often associated with some types of cancer. [NIH]

Hybrid: Cross fertilization between two varieties or, more usually, two species of vines, see also crossing. [NIH]

Hydration: Combining with water. [NIH]

Hydrogen: The first chemical element in the periodic table. It has the atomic symbol H, atomic number 1, and atomic weight 1. It exists, under normal conditions, as a colorless, odorless, tasteless, diatomic gas. Hydrogen ions are protons. Besides the common H1 isotope, hydrogen exists as the stable isotope deuterium and the unstable, radioactive isotope tritium. [NIH]

Hydrolysis: The process of cleaving a chemical compound by the addition of a molecule of water. [NIH]

Hydroxylysine: A hydroxylated derivative of the amino acid lysine that is present in certain collagens. [NIH]

Hydroxyproline: A hydroxylated form of the imino acid proline. A deficiency in ascorbic acid can result in impaired hydroxyproline formation. [NIH]

Hydroxyurea: An antineoplastic agent that inhibits DNA synthesis through the inhibition of ribonucleoside diphosphate reductase. [NIH]

Hyperbaric: Characterized by greater than normal pressure or weight; applied to gases under greater than atmospheric pressure, as hyperbaric oxygen, or to a solution of greater specific gravity than another taken as a standard of reference. [EU]

Hyperbaric oxygen: Oxygen that is at an atmospheric pressure higher than the pressure at sea level. Breathing hyperbaric oxygen to enhance the effectiveness of radiation therapy is being studied. [NIH]

Hyperlipidemia: An excess of lipids in the blood. [NIH]

Hypersensitivity: Altered reactivity to an antigen, which can result in pathologic reactions upon subsequent exposure to that particular antigen. [NIH]

Hypersplenism: Condition characterized by splenomegaly, some reduction in the number of circulating blood cells in the presence of a normal or hyperactive bone marrow, and the potential for reversal by splenectomy. [NIH]

Hypertension: Persistently high arterial blood pressure. Currently accepted threshold levels are 140 mm Hg systolic and 90 mm Hg diastolic pressure. [NIH]

Hyperthermia: A type of treatment in which body tissue is exposed to high temperatures to damage and kill cancer cells or to make cancer cells more sensitive to the effects of radiation and certain anticancer drugs. [NIH]

Hypoglycemic: An orally active drug that produces a fall in blood glucose concentration. [NIH]

Hypopharynx: The portion of the pharynx between the inferior portion of the oropharynx and the larynx. [NIH]

Hypotensive: Characterized by or causing diminished tension or pressure, as abnormally low blood pressure. [EU]

Hypothalamus: Ventral part of the diencephalon extending from the region of the optic chiasm to the caudal border of the mammillary bodies and forming the inferior and lateral walls of the third ventricle. [NIH]

Hypoxia: Reduction of oxygen supply to tissue below physiological levels despite adequate perfusion of the tissue by blood. [EU]

Hypoxic: Having too little oxygen. [NIH]

Hysterectomy: Excision of the uterus. [NIH]

Iatrogenic: Resulting from the activity of physicians. Originally applied to disorders induced in the patient by autosuggestion based on the physician's examination, manner, or discussion, the term is now applied to any adverse condition in a patient occurring as the result of treatment by a physician or surgeon, especially to infections acquired by the patient during the course of treatment. [EU]

Idiopathic: Describes a disease of unknown cause. [NIH]

Imaging procedures: Methods of producing pictures of areas inside the body. [NIH]

Immune Complex Diseases: Group of diseases mediated by the deposition of large soluble complexes of antigen and antibody with resultant damage to tissue. Besides serum sickness and the arthus reaction, evidence supports a pathogenic role for immune complexes in many other systemic immunologic diseases including glomerulonephritis, systemic lupus erythematosus and polyarteritis nodosa. [NIH]

Immune function: Production and action of cells that fight disease or infection. [NIH]

Immune response: The activity of the immune system against foreign substances (antigens). [NIH]

Immune system: The organs, cells, and molecules responsible for the recognition and disposal of foreign ("non-self") material which enters the body. [NIH]

Immunization: Deliberate stimulation of the host's immune response. Active immunization involves administration of antigens or immunologic adjuvants. Passive immunization involves administration of immune sera or lymphocytes or their extracts (e.g., transfer factor, immune RNA) or transplantation of immunocompetent cell producing tissue (thymus or bone marrow). [NIH]

Immunoconjugates: Combinations of diagnostic or therapeutic substances linked with specific immune substances such as immunoglobulins, monoclonal antibodies or antigens. Often the diagnostic or therapeutic substance is a radionuclide. These conjugates are useful tools for specific targeting of drugs and radioisotopes in the chemotherapy and radioimmunotherapy of certain cancers. [NIH]

Immunodeficiency: The decreased ability of the body to fight infection and disease. [NIH]

Immunogenic: Producing immunity; evoking an immune response. [EU]

Immunoglobulin: A protein that acts as an antibody. [NIH]

Immunohistochemistry: Histochemical localization of immunoreactive substances using labeled antibodies as reagents. [NIH]

Immunologic: The ability of the antibody-forming system to recall a previous experience with an antigen and to respond to a second exposure with the prompt production of large amounts of antibody. [NIH]

Immunology: The study of the body's immune system. [NIH]

Immunosuppressant: An agent capable of suppressing immune responses. [EU]

Immunosuppression: Deliberate prevention or diminution of the host's immune response. It may be nonspecific as in the administration of immunosuppressive agents (drugs or radiation) or by lymphocyte depletion or may be specific as in desensitization or the simultaneous administration of antigen and immunosuppressive drugs. [NIH]

Immunosuppressive: Describes the ability to lower immune system responses. [NIH]

Immunosuppressive Agents: Agents that suppress immune function by one of several mechanisms of action. Classical cytotoxic immunosuppressants act by inhibiting DNA synthesis. Others may act through activation of suppressor T-cell populations or by inhibiting the activation of helper cells. While immunosuppression has been brought about in the past primarily to prevent rejection of transplanted organs, new applications involving mediation of the effects of interleukins and other cytokines are emerging. [NIH]

Immunosuppressive therapy: Therapy used to decrease the body's immune response, such as drugs given to prevent transplant rejection. [NIH]

Immunotherapy: Manipulation of the host's immune system in treatment of disease. It includes both active and passive immunization as well as immunosuppressive therapy to prevent graft rejection. [NIH]

Immunotoxins: Semisynthetic conjugates of various toxic molecules, including radioactive isotopes and bacterial or plant toxins, with specific immune substances such as immunoglobulins, monoclonal antibodies, and antigens. The antitumor or antiviral immune substance carries the toxin to the tumor or infected cell where the toxin exerts its poisonous effect. [NIH]

Impairment: In the context of health experience, an impairment is any loss or abnormality of psychological, physiological, or anatomical structure or function. [NIH]

Implant radiation: A procedure in which radioactive material sealed in needles, seeds, wires, or catheters is placed directly into or near the tumor. Also called [NIH]

Implantation: The insertion or grafting into the body of biological, living, inert, or radioactive material. [EU]

In situ: In the natural or normal place; confined to the site of origin without invasion of neighbouring tissues. [EU]

In Situ Hybridization: A technique that localizes specific nucleic acid sequences within intact chromosomes, eukaryotic cells, or bacterial cells through the use of specific nucleic acid-labeled probes. [NIH]

In vitro: In the laboratory (outside the body). The opposite of in vivo (in the body). [NIH]

In vivo: In the body. The opposite of in vitro (outside the body or in the laboratory). [NIH]

Incision: A cut made in the body during surgery. [NIH]

Incontinence: Inability to control the flow of urine from the bladder (urinary incontinence) or the escape of stool from the rectum (fecal incontinence). [NIH]

Indolent: A type of cancer that grows slowly. [NIH]

Indolent lymphoma: Lymphoma that grows slowly and has few symptoms. [NIH]

Induction: The act or process of inducing or causing to occur, especially the production of a specific morphogenetic effect in the developing embryo through the influence of evocators or organizers, or the production of anaesthesia or unconsciousness by use of appropriate agents. [EU]

Infarction: A pathological process consisting of a sudden insufficient blood supply to an area, which results in necrosis of that area. It is usually caused by a thrombus, an embolus, or a vascular torsion. [NIH]

Infection: 1. Invasion and multiplication of microorganisms in body tissues, which may be clinically unapparent or result in local cellular injury due to competitive metabolism, toxins, intracellular replication, or antigen-antibody response. The infection may remain localized, subclinical, and temporary if the body's defensive mechanisms are effective. A local infection may persist and spread by extension to become an acute, subacute, or chronic clinical infection or disease state. A local infection may also become systemic when the microorganisms gain access to the lymphatic or vascular system. 2. An infectious disease. [EU]

Infection Control: Programs of disease surveillance, generally within health care facilities, designed to investigate, prevent, and control the spread of infections and their causative microorganisms. [NIH]

Infertility: The diminished or absent ability to conceive or produce an offspring while sterility is the complete inability to conceive or produce an offspring. [NIH]

Infiltration: The diffusion or accumulation in a tissue or cells of substances not normal to it or in amounts of the normal. Also, the material so accumulated. [EU]

Inflammation: A pathological process characterized by injury or destruction of tissues caused by a variety of cytologic and chemical reactions. It is usually manifested by typical signs of pain, heat, redness, swelling, and loss of function. [NIH]

Influenza: An acute viral infection involving the respiratory tract. It is marked by inflammation of the nasal mucosa, the pharynx, and conjunctiva, and by headache and severe, often generalized, myalgia. [NIH]

Information Science: The field of knowledge, theory, and technology dealing with the collection of facts and figures, and the processes and methods involved in their manipulation, storage, dissemination, publication, and retrieval. It includes the fields of communication, publishing, library science and informatics. [NIH]

Infusion: A method of putting fluids, including drugs, into the bloodstream. Also called intravenous infusion. [NIH]

Inhalation: The drawing of air or other substances into the lungs. [EU]

Initiation: Mutation induced by a chemical reactive substance causing cell changes; being a step in a carcinogenic process. [NIH]

Inoperable: Not suitable to be operated upon. [EU]

Inorganic: Pertaining to substances not of organic origin. [EU]

Insight: The capacity to understand one's own motives, to be aware of one's own psychodynamics, to appreciate the meaning of symbolic behavior. [NIH]

Insulin: A protein hormone secreted by beta cells of the pancreas. Insulin plays a major role in the regulation of glucose metabolism, generally promoting the cellular utilization of glucose. It is also an important regulator of protein and lipid metabolism. Insulin is used as a drug to control insulin-dependent diabetes mellitus. [NIH]

Insulin-dependent diabetes mellitus: A disease characterized by high levels of blood glucose resulting from defects in insulin secretion, insulin action, or both. Autoimmune, genetic, and environmental factors are involved in the development of type I diabetes. [NIH]

Insulin-like: Muscular growth factor. [NIH]

Interferon: A biological response modifier (a substance that can improve the body's natural response to disease). Interferons interfere with the division of cancer cells and can slow tumor growth. There are several types of interferons, including interferon-alpha, -beta, and -gamma. These substances are normally produced by the body. They are also made in the laboratory for use in treating cancer and other diseases. [NIH]

Interferon-alpha: One of the type I interferons produced by peripheral blood leukocytes or lymphoblastoid cells when exposed to live or inactivated virus, double-stranded RNA, or bacterial products. It is the major interferon produced by virus-induced leukocyte cultures and, in addition to its pronounced antiviral activity, it causes activation of NK cells. [NIH]

Interleukin-2: Chemical mediator produced by activated T lymphocytes and which regulates the proliferation of T cells, as well as playing a role in the regulation of NK cell activity. [NIH]

Internal radiation: A procedure in which radioactive material sealed in needles, seeds, wires, or catheters is placed directly into or near the tumor. Also called brachytherapy, implant radiation, or interstitial radiation therapy. [NIH]

Interphase: The interval between two successive cell divisions during which the chromosomes are not individually distinguishable and DNA replication occurs. [NIH]

Interstitial: Pertaining to or situated between parts or in the interspaces of a tissue. [EU]

Intervertebral: Situated between two contiguous vertebrae. [EU]

Intestine: A long, tube-shaped organ in the abdomen that completes the process of digestion. There is both a large intestine and a small intestine. Also called the bowel. [NIH]

Intoxication: Poisoning, the state of being poisoned. [EU]

Intracellular: Inside a cell. [NIH]

Intracranial tumors: Tumors that occur in the brain. [NIH]

Intraocular: Within the eye. [EU]

Intrathecal: Describes the fluid-filled space between the thin layers of tissue that cover the brain and spinal cord. Drugs can be injected into the fluid or a sample of the fluid can be removed for testing. [NIH]

Intrathecal chemotherapy: Anticancer drugs that are injected into the fluid-filled space between the thin layers of tissue that cover the brain and spinal cord. [NIH]

Intravascular: Within a vessel or vessels. [EU]

Intravenous: IV. Into a vein. [NIH]

Intrinsic: Situated entirely within or pertaining exclusively to a part. [EU]

Invasive: 1. Having the quality of invasiveness. 2. Involving puncture or incision of the skin or insertion of an instrument or foreign material into the body; said of diagnostic techniques. [EU]

Invasive cervical cancer: Cancer that has spread from the surface of the cervix to tissue deeper in the cervix or to other parts of the body. [NIH]

Involuntary: Reaction occurring without intention or volition. [NIH]

Iodine: A nonmetallic element of the halogen group that is represented by the atomic symbol I, atomic number 53, and atomic weight of 126.90. It is a nutritionally essential element, especially important in thyroid hormone synthesis. In solution, it has anti-infective properties and is used topically. [NIH]

Iodine-131: Radioactive isotope of iodine. [NIH]

Ionization: 1. Any process by which a neutral atom gains or loses electrons, thus acquiring a net charge, as the dissociation of a substance in solution into ions or ion production by the passage of radioactive particles. 2. Iontophoresis. [EU]

Ionizing: Radiation comprising charged particles, e. g. electrons, protons, alpha-particles, etc., having sufficient kinetic energy to produce ionization by collision. [NIH]

Ions: An atom or group of atoms that have a positive or negative electric charge due to a gain (negative charge) or loss (positive charge) of one or more electrons. Atoms with a positive charge are known as cations; those with a negative charge are anions. [NIH]

Ipsilateral: Having to do with the same side of the body. [NIH]

Irinotecan: An anticancer drug that belongs to a family of anticancer drugs called topoisomerase inhibitors. It is a camptothecin analogue. Also called CPT 11. [NIH]

Irradiation: The use of high-energy radiation from x-rays, neutrons, and other sources to kill cancer cells and shrink tumors. Radiation may come from a machine outside the body (external-beam radiation therapy) or from materials called radioisotopes. Radioisotopes produce radiation and can be placed in or near the tumor or in the area near cancer cells. This type of radiation treatment is called internal radiation therapy, implant radiation, interstitial radiation, or brachytherapy. Systemic radiation therapy uses a radioactive substance, such as a radiolabeled monoclonal antibody, that circulates throughout the body. Irradiation is also called radiation therapy, radiotherapy, and x-ray therapy. [NIH]

Ischemia: Deficiency of blood in a part, due to functional constriction or actual obstruction of a blood vessel. [EU]

Isoelectric: Separation of amphoteric substances, dissolved in water, based on their isoelectric behavior. The amphoteric substances are a mixture of proteins to be separated and of auxiliary "carrier ampholytes". [NIH]

Isoelectric Point: The pH in solutions of proteins and related compounds at which the dipolar ions are at a maximum. [NIH]

Isoenzyme: Different forms of an enzyme, usually occurring in different tissues. The isoenzymes of a particular enzyme catalyze the same reaction but they differ in some of their properties. [NIH]

Iteration: Unvarying repetition or unvarying persistence. [NIH]

Kb: A measure of the length of DNA fragments, 1 Kb = 1000 base pairs. The largest DNA fragments are up to 50 kilobases long. [NIH]

Kidney Pelvis: The flattened, funnel-shaped expansion connecting the ureter to the kidney calices. [NIH]

Kinetic: Pertaining to or producing motion. [EU]

Labile: 1. Gliding; moving from point to point over the surface; unstable; fluctuating. 2. Chemically unstable. [EU]

Language Disorders: Conditions characterized by deficiencies of comprehension or expression of written and spoken forms of language. These include acquired and developmental disorders. [NIH]

Large Intestine: The part of the intestine that goes from the cecum to the rectum. The large intestine absorbs water from stool and changes it from a liquid to a solid form. The large intestine is 5 feet long and includes the appendix, cecum, colon, and rectum. Also called colon. [NIH]

Laryngeal: Having to do with the larynx. [NIH]

Laryngoscope: A thin, lighted tube used to examine the larynx (voice box). [NIH]

Larynx: An irregularly shaped, musculocartilaginous tubular structure, lined with mucous membrane, located at the top of the trachea and below the root of the tongue and the hyoid bone. It is the essential sphincter guarding the entrance into the trachea and functioning secondarily as the organ of voice. [NIH]

Laser Surgery: The use of a laser either to vaporize surface lesions or to make bloodless cuts in tissue. It does not include the coagulation of tissue by laser. [NIH]

Latency: The period of apparent inactivity between the time when a stimulus is presented and the moment a response occurs. [NIH]

Lavage: A cleaning of the stomach and colon. Uses a special drink and enemas. [NIH]

Lens: The transparent, double convex (outward curve on both sides) structure suspended between the aqueous and vitreous; helps to focus light on the retina. [NIH]

Lentinus: A genus of fungi of the family Tricholomataceae, order Agaricales. The commonly known shiitake mushrooms are Lentinus edodes (also seen as Lentinula edodes). [NIH]

Lesion: An area of abnormal tissue change. [NIH]

Lethal: Deadly, fatal. [EU]

Leucocyte: All the white cells of the blood and their precursors (myeloid cell series, lymphoid cell series) but commonly used to indicate granulocytes exclusive of lymphocytes. [NIH]

Leucovorin: The active metabolite of folic acid. Leucovorin is used principally as its calcium salt as an antidote to folic acid antagonists which block the conversion of folic acid to folinic acid. [NIH]

Leukemia: Cancer of blood-forming tissue. [NIH]

Leukocytes: White blood cells. These include granular leukocytes (basophils, eosinophils, and neutrophils) as well as non-granular leukocytes (lymphocytes and monocytes). [NIH]

Levo: It is an experimental treatment for heroin addiction that was developed by German scientists around 1948 as an analgesic. Like methadone, it binds with opioid receptors, but it is longer acting. [NIH]

Libido: The psychic drive or energy associated with sexual instinct in the broad sense (pleasure and love-object seeking). It may also connote the psychic energy associated with instincts in general that motivate behavior. [NIH]

Life cycle: The successive stages through which an organism passes from fertilized ovum or spore to the fertilized ovum or spore of the next generation. [NIH]

Ligament: A band of fibrous tissue that connects bones or cartilages, serving to support and strengthen joints. [EU]

Ligands: A RNA simulation method developed by the MIT. [NIH]

Limb perfusion: A technique that may be used to deliver anticancer drugs directly to an arm or leg. The flow of blood to and from the limb is temporarily stopped with a tourniquet, and anticancer drugs are put directly into the blood of the limb. This allows the person to receive a high dose of drugs in the area where the cancer occurred. [NIH]

Limited-stage small cell lung cancer: Cancer found in one lung and in nearby lymph nodes. [NIH]

Linear accelerator: An accelerator in which charged particles are accelerated along a straight path either by means of a traveling electromagnetic field or through a series of small gaps between electrodes that are so connected to an alternating voltage supply of high frequency. [NIH]

Linear Energy Transfer: Rate of energy dissipation along the path of charged particles. In radiobiology and health physics, exposure is measured in kiloelectron volts per micrometer of tissue (keV/micrometer T). [NIH]

Linkage: The tendency of two or more genes in the same chromosome to remain together from one generation to the next more frequently than expected according to the law of independent assortment. [NIH]

Lip: Either of the two fleshy, full-blooded margins of the mouth. [NIH]

Lipid: Fat. [NIH]

Lipid Peroxidation: Peroxidase catalyzed oxidation of lipids using hydrogen peroxide as an electron acceptor. [NIH]

Liposomal: A drug preparation that contains the active drug in very tiny fat particles. This fat-encapsulated drug is absorbed better, and its distribution to the tumor site is improved. [NIH]

Liposome: A spherical particle in an aqueous medium, formed by a lipid bilayer enclosing an aqueous compartment. [EU]

Lithotripsy: The destruction of a calculus of the kidney, ureter, bladder, or gallbladder by physical forces, including crushing with a lithotriptor through a catheter. Focused percutaneous ultrasound and focused hydraulic shock waves may be used without surgery. Lithotripsy does not include the dissolving of stones by acids or litholysis. Lithotripsy by laser is laser lithotripsy. [NIH]

Liver: A large, glandular organ located in the upper abdomen. The liver cleanses the blood and aids in digestion by secreting bile. [NIH]

Liver metastases: Cancer that has spread from the original (primary) tumor to the liver. [NIH]

Liver scan: An image of the liver created on a computer screen or on film. A radioactive substance is injected into a blood vessel and travels through the bloodstream. It collects in the liver, especially in abnormal areas, and can be detected by the scanner. [NIH]

Localization: The process of determining or marking the location or site of a lesion or disease. May also refer to the process of keeping a lesion or disease in a specific location or site. [NIH]

Localized: Cancer which has not metastasized yet. [NIH]

Locoregional: The characteristic of a disease-producing organism to transfer itself, but typically to the same region of the body (a leg, the lungs, .) [EU]

Lomustine: An alkylating agent of value against both hematologic malignancies and solid tumors. [NIH]

Longitudinal study: Also referred to as a "cohort study" or "prospective study"; the analytic method of epidemiologic study in which subsets of a defined population can be identified who are, have been, or in the future may be exposed or not exposed, or exposed in different degrees, to a factor or factors hypothesized to influence the probability of occurrence of a given disease or other outcome. The main feature of this type of study is to observe large numbers of subjects over an extended time, with comparisons of incidence rates in groups that differ in exposure levels. [NIH]

Loop: A wire usually of platinum bent at one end into a small loop (usually 4 mm inside diameter) and used in transferring microorganisms. [NIH]

Loss of Heterozygosity: The loss of one allele at a specific locus, caused by a deletion mutation; or loss of a chromosome from a chromosome pair. It is detected when heterozygous markers for a locus appear monomorphic because one of the alleles was deleted. When this occurs at a tumor suppressor gene locus where one of the alleles is already abnormal, it can result in neoplastic transformation. [NIH]

Lumpectomy: Surgery to remove the tumor and a small amount of normal tissue around it. [NIH]

Lung volume: The amount of air the lungs hold. [NIH]

Lupus: A form of cutaneous tuberculosis. It is seen predominantly in women and typically involves the nasal, buccal, and conjunctival mucosa. [NIH]

Lutetium: Lutetium. An element of the rare earth family of metals. It has the atomic symbol Lu, atomic number 71, and atomic weight 175. [NIH]

Lymph: The almost colorless fluid that travels through the lymphatic system and carries cells that help fight infection and disease. [NIH]

Lymph node: A rounded mass of lymphatic tissue that is surrounded by a capsule of connective tissue. Also known as a lymph gland. Lymph nodes are spread out along lymphatic vessels and contain many lymphocytes, which filter the lymphatic fluid (lymph). [NIH]

Lymphatic: The tissues and organs, including the bone marrow, spleen, thymus, and lymph nodes, that produce and store cells that fight infection and disease. [NIH]

Lymphatic system: The tissues and organs that produce, store, and carry white blood cells that fight infection and other diseases. This system includes the bone marrow, spleen, thymus, lymph nodes and a network of thin tubes that carry lymph and white blood cells. These tubes branch, like blood vessels, into all the tissues of the body. [NIH]

Lymphoblasts: Interferon produced predominantly by leucocyte cells. [NIH]

Lymphocyte: A white blood cell. Lymphocytes have a number of roles in the immune system, including the production of antibodies and other substances that fight infection and diseases. [NIH]

Lymphocyte Depletion: Immunosuppression by reduction of circulating lymphocytes or by T-cell depletion of bone marrow. The former may be accomplished in vivo by thoracic duct drainage or administration of antilymphocyte serum. The latter is performed ex vivo on bone marrow before its transplantation. [NIH]

Lymphoid: Referring to lymphocytes, a type of white blood cell. Also refers to tissue in which lymphocytes develop. [NIH]

Lymphokine: A soluble protein produced by some types of white blood cell that stimulates other white blood cells to kill foreign invaders. [NIH]

Lymphoma: A general term for various neoplastic diseases of the lymphoid tissue. [NIH]

Macrophage: A type of white blood cell that surrounds and kills microorganisms, removes dead cells, and stimulates the action of other immune system cells. [NIH]

Magnetic Resonance Imaging: Non-invasive method of demonstrating internal anatomy based on the principle that atomic nuclei in a strong magnetic field absorb pulses of radiofrequency energy and emit them as radiowaves which can be reconstructed into computerized images. The concept includes proton spin tomographic techniques. [NIH]

Malformation: A morphologic defect resulting from an intrinsically abnormal developmental process. [EU]

Malignant: Cancerous; a growth with a tendency to invade and destroy nearby tissue and spread to other parts of the body. [NIH]

Malignant mesothelioma: A rare type of cancer in which malignant cells are found in the sac lining the chest or abdomen. Exposure to airborne asbestos particles increases one's risk of developing malignant mesothelioma. [NIH]

Malignant tumor: A tumor capable of metastasizing. [NIH]

Malnutrition: A condition caused by not eating enough food or not eating a balanced diet. [NIH]

Mammary: Pertaining to the mamma, or breast. [EU]

Mammography: Radiographic examination of the breast. [NIH]

Mandible: The largest and strongest bone of the face constituting the lower jaw. It supports the lower teeth. [NIH]

Manifest: Being the part or aspect of a phenomenon that is directly observable : concretely expressed in behaviour. [EU]

Masseter Muscle: A masticatory muscle whose action is closing the jaws. [NIH]

Mastectomy: Surgery to remove the breast (or as much of the breast tissue as possible). [NIH]

Matrix metalloproteinase: A member of a group of enzymes that can break down proteins, such as collagen, that are normally found in the spaces between cells in tissues (i.e., extracellular matrix proteins). Because these enzymes need zinc or calcium atoms to work properly, they are called metalloproteinases. Matrix metalloproteinases are involved in wound healing, angiogenesis, and tumor cell metastasis. [NIH]

Maxillary: Pertaining to the maxilla : the irregularly shaped bone that with its fellow forms the upper jaw. [EU]

Mechlorethamine: A vesicant and necrotizing irritant destructive to mucous membranes. It was formerly used as a war gas. The hydrochloride is used as an antineoplastic in Hodgkin's disease and lymphomas. It causes severe gastrointestinal and bone marrow damage. [NIH]

Medial: Lying near the midsaggital plane of the body; opposed to lateral. [NIH]

Median survival time: The point in time from either diagnosis or treatment at which half of the patients with a given disease are found to be, or expected to be, still alive. In a clinical trial, median survival time is one way to measure how effective a treatment is. [NIH]

Mediate: Indirect; accomplished by the aid of an intervening medium. [EU]

Mediator: An object or substance by which something is mediated, such as (1) a structure of the nervous system that transmits impulses eliciting a specific response; (2) a chemical substance (transmitter substance) that induces activity in an excitable tissue, such as nerve or muscle; or (3) a substance released from cells as the result of the interaction of antigen with antibody or by the action of antigen with a sensitized lymphocyte. [EU]

Medical Informatics: The field of information science concerned with the analysis and dissemination of medical data through the application of computers to various aspects of health care and medicine. [NIH]

Medical Oncology: A subspecialty of internal medicine concerned with the study of neoplasms. [NIH]

Medical Records: Recording of pertinent information concerning patient's illness or illnesses. [NIH]

Medicament: A medicinal substance or agent. [EU]

MEDLINE: An online database of MEDLARS, the computerized bibliographic Medical Literature Analysis and Retrieval System of the National Library of Medicine. [NIH]

Medulloblastoma: A malignant brain tumor that begins in the lower part of the brain and can spread to the spine or to other parts of the body. Medulloblastomas are sometimes called primitive neuroectodermal tumors (PNET). [NIH]

Megaloblastic: A large abnormal red blood cell appearing in the blood in pernicious anaemia. [EU]

Meiosis: A special method of cell division, occurring in maturation of the germ cells, by means of which each daughter nucleus receives half the number of chromosomes characteristic of the somatic cells of the species. [NIH]

Melanin: The substance that gives the skin its color. [NIH]

Melanocytes: Epidermal dendritic pigment cells which control long-term morphological color changes by alteration in their number or in the amount of pigment they produce and store in the pigment containing organelles called melanosomes. Melanophores are larger cells which do not exist in mammals. [NIH]

Melanoma: A form of skin cancer that arises in melanocytes, the cells that produce pigment. Melanoma usually begins in a mole. [NIH]

Melphalan: An alkylating nitrogen mustard that is used as an antineoplastic in the form of the levo isomer - melphalan, the racemic mixture - merphalan, and the dextro isomer - medphalan; toxic to bone marrow, but little vesicant action; potential carcinogen. [NIH]

Membrane: A very thin layer of tissue that covers a surface. [NIH]

Memory: Complex mental function having four distinct phases: (1) memorizing or learning, (2) retention, (3) recall, and (4) recognition. Clinically, it is usually subdivided into immediate, recent, and remote memory. [NIH]

Meninges: The three membranes that cover and protect the brain and spinal cord. [NIH]

Meningioma: A type of tumor that occurs in the meninges, the membranes that cover and protect the brain and spinal cord. Meningiomas usually grow slowly. [NIH]

Meningitis: Inflammation of the meninges. When it affects the dura mater, the disease is termed pachymeningitis; when the arachnoid and pia mater are involved, it is called leptomeningitis, or meningitis proper. [EU]

Mental: Pertaining to the mind; psychic. 2. (L. mentum chin) pertaining to the chin. [EU]

Mesenchymal: Refers to cells that develop into connective tissue, blood vessels, and lymphatic tissue. [NIH]

Mesoderm: The middle germ layer of the embryo. [NIH]

Mesothelioma: A benign (noncancerous) or malignant (cancerous) tumor affecting the lining of the chest or abdomen. Exposure to asbestos particles in the air increases the risk of developing malignant mesothelioma. [NIH]

Meta-Analysis: A quantitative method of combining the results of independent studies (usually drawn from the published literature) and synthesizing summaries and conclusions which may be used to evaluate therapeutic effectiveness, plan new studies, etc., with application chiefly in the areas of research and medicine. [NIH]

Metabolite: Any substance produced by metabolism or by a metabolic process. [EU]

Metalloporphyrins: Porphyrins which are combined with a metal ion. The metal is bound equally to all four nitrogen atoms of the pyrrole rings. They possess characteristic absorption spectra which can be utilized for identification or quantitative estimation of porphyrins and porphyrin-bound compounds. [NIH]

Metaphase: The second phase of cell division, in which the chromosomes line up across the equatorial plane of the spindle prior to separation. [NIH]

Metastasis: The spread of cancer from one part of the body to another. Tumors formed from cells that have spread are called "secondary tumors" and contain cells that are like those in the original (primary) tumor. The plural is metastases. [NIH]

Metastatic: Having to do with metastasis, which is the spread of cancer from one part of the body to another. [NIH]

Methionine: A sulfur containing essential amino acid that is important in many body functions. It is a chelating agent for heavy metals. [NIH]

Methotrexate: An antineoplastic antimetabolite with immunosuppressant properties. It is an inhibitor of dihydrofolate reductase and prevents the formation of tetrahydrofolate, necessary for synthesis of thymidylate, an essential component of DNA. [NIH]

Methyltransferase: A drug-metabolizing enzyme. [NIH]

MI: Myocardial infarction. Gross necrosis of the myocardium as a result of interruption of the blood supply to the area; it is almost always caused by atherosclerosis of the coronary arteries, upon which coronary thrombosis is usually superimposed. [NIH]

Microbe: An organism which cannot be observed with the naked eye; e. g. unicellular animals, lower algae, lower fungi, bacteria. [NIH]

Microbiology: The study of microorganisms such as fungi, bacteria, algae, archaea, and viruses. [NIH]

Microorganism: An organism that can be seen only through a microscope. Microorganisms include bacteria, protozoa, algae, and fungi. Although viruses are not considered living organisms, they are sometimes classified as microorganisms. [NIH]

Microtubules: Slender, cylindrical filaments found in the cytoskeleton of plant and animal cells. They are composed of the protein tubulin. [NIH]

Migration: The systematic movement of genes between populations of the same species, geographic race, or variety. [NIH]

Millimeter: A measure of length. A millimeter is approximately 26-times smaller than an inch. [NIH]

Miotic: 1. Pertaining to, characterized by, or producing miosis : contraction of the pupil. 2. An agent that causes the pupil to contract. 3. Meiotic: characterized by cell division. [EU]

Misonidazole: A nitroimidazole that sensitizes normally radio-resistant hypoxic cells to radiation. It may also be directly cytotoxic to hypoxic cells and has been proposed as an antineoplastic. [NIH]

Mitochondrial Swelling: Increase in volume of mitochondria due to an influx of fluid; it occurs in hypotonic solutions due to osmotic pressure and in isotonic solutions as a result of altered permeability of the membranes of respiring mitochondria. [NIH]

Mitosis: A method of indirect cell division by means of which the two daughter nuclei normally receive identical complements of the number of chromosomes of the somatic cells of the species. [NIH]

Mitotic: Cell resulting from mitosis. [NIH]

Mitotic inhibitors: Drugs that kill cancer cells by interfering with cell division (mitostis). [NIH]

Mobility: Capability of movement, of being moved, or of flowing freely. [EU]

Modeling: A treatment procedure whereby the therapist presents the target behavior which the learner is to imitate and make part of his repertoire. [NIH]

Modification: A change in an organism, or in a process in an organism, that is acquired from its own activity or environment. [NIH]

Modified radical mastectomy: Surgery for breast cancer in which the breast, some of the lymph nodes under the arm, the lining over the chest muscles, and sometimes part of the chest wall muscles are removed. [NIH]

Molecular: Of, pertaining to, or composed of molecules : a very small mass of matter. [EU]

Molecule: A chemical made up of two or more atoms. The atoms in a molecule can be the same (an oxygen molecule has two oxygen atoms) or different (a water molecule has two hydrogen atoms and one oxygen atom). Biological molecules, such as proteins and DNA, can be made up of many thousands of atoms. [NIH]

Monitor: An apparatus which automatically records such physiological signs as respiration, pulse, and blood pressure in an anesthetized patient or one undergoing surgical or other procedures. [NIH]

Monoclonal: An antibody produced by culturing a single type of cell. It therefore consists of a single species of immunoglobulin molecules. [NIH]

Monoclonal antibodies: Laboratory-produced substances that can locate and bind to cancer cells wherever they are in the body. Many monoclonal antibodies are used in cancer detection or therapy; each one recognizes a different protein on certain cancer cells. Monoclonal antibodies can be used alone, or they can be used to deliver drugs, toxins, or radioactive material directly to a tumor. [NIH]

Monocyte: A type of white blood cell. [NIH]

Mononuclear: A cell with one nucleus. [NIH]

Morphine: The principal alkaloid in opium and the prototype opiate analgesic and narcotic. Morphine has widespread effects in the central nervous system and on smooth muscle. [NIH]

Morphology: The science of the form and structure of organisms (plants, animals, and other forms of life). [NIH]

Motion Sickness: Sickness caused by motion, as sea sickness, train sickness, car sickness, and air sickness. [NIH]

Motor nerve: An efferent nerve conveying an impulse that excites muscular contraction. [NIH]

Mucins: A secretion containing mucopolysaccharides and protein that is the chief constituent of mucus. [NIH]

Mucolytic: Destroying or dissolving mucin; an agent that so acts : a mucopolysaccharide or glycoprotein, the chief constituent of mucus. [EU]

Mucosa: A mucous membrane, or tunica mucosa. [EU]

Mucositis: A complication of some cancer therapies in which the lining of the digestive system becomes inflamed. Often seen as sores in the mouth. [NIH]

Multicenter study: A clinical trial that is carried out at more than one medical institution. [NIH]

Multiple Myeloma: A malignant tumor of plasma cells usually arising in the bone marrow; characterized by diffuse involvement of the skeletal system, hyperglobulinemia, Bence-Jones proteinuria, and anemia. [NIH]

Multivalent: Pertaining to a group of 5 or more homologous or partly homologous chromosomes during the zygotene stage of prophase to first metaphasis in meiosis. [NIH]

Mutagenesis: Process of generating genetic mutations. It may occur spontaneously or be induced by mutagens. [NIH]

Mutagenic: Inducing genetic mutation. [EU]

Mutagens: Chemical agents that increase the rate of genetic mutation by interfering with the function of nucleic acids. A clastogen is a specific mutagen that causes breaks in chromosomes. [NIH]

Myalgia: Pain in a muscle or muscles. [EU]

Myocardium: The muscle tissue of the heart composed of striated, involuntary muscle known as cardiac muscle. [NIH]

Myopathy: Any disease of a muscle. [EU]

Myopia: That error of refraction in which rays of light entering the eye parallel to the optic axis are brought to a focus in front of the retina, as a result of the eyeball being too long from front to back (axial m.) or of an increased strength in refractive power of the media of the eye (index m.). Called also nearsightedness, because the near point is less distant than it is in emmetropia with an equal amplitude of accommodation. [EU]

N-acetyl: Analgesic agent. [NIH]

Nadir: The lowest point; point of greatest adversity or despair. [EU]

Narcotic: 1. Pertaining to or producing narcosis. 2. An agent that produces insensibility or stupor, applied especially to the opioids, i.e. to any natural or synthetic drug that has morphine-like actions. [EU]

Nasal Cavity: The proximal portion of the respiratory passages on either side of the nasal septum, lined with ciliated mucosa, extending from the nares to the pharynx. [NIH]

Nasal Mucosa: The mucous membrane lining the nasal cavity. [NIH]

Nasal Septum: The partition separating the two nasal cavities in the midplane, composed of cartilaginous, membranous and bony parts. [NIH]

Nasopharynx: The nasal part of the pharynx, lying above the level of the soft palate. [NIH]

Nausea: An unpleasant sensation in the stomach usually accompanied by the urge to vomit. Common causes are early pregnancy, sea and motion sickness, emotional stress, intense pain, food poisoning, and various enteroviruses. [NIH]

Necrosis: A pathological process caused by the progressive degradative action of enzymes that is generally associated with severe cellular trauma. It is characterized by mitochondrial swelling, nuclear flocculation, uncontrolled cell lysis, and ultimately cell death. [NIH]

Neoplasia: Abnormal and uncontrolled cell growth. [NIH]

Neoplasm: A new growth of benign or malignant tissue. [NIH]

Neoplastic: Pertaining to or like a neoplasm (= any new and abnormal growth); pertaining to neoplasia (= the formation of a neoplasm). [EU]

Nerve: A cordlike structure of nervous tissue that connects parts of the nervous system with other tissues of the body and conveys nervous impulses to, or away from, these tissues. [NIH]

Nervous System: The entire nerve apparatus composed of the brain, spinal cord, nerves and ganglia. [NIH]

Networks: Pertaining to a nerve or to the nerves, a meshlike structure of interlocking fibers or strands. [NIH]

Neural: 1. Pertaining to a nerve or to the nerves. 2. Situated in the region of the spinal axis, as the neutral arch. [EU]

Neuroblastoma: Cancer that arises in immature nerve cells and affects mostly infants and children. [NIH]

Neuroectodermal tumor: A tumor of the central or peripheral nervous system. [NIH]

Neurofibroma: A fibrous tumor, usually benign, arising from the nerve sheath or the endoneurium. [NIH]

Neurologic: Having to do with nerves or the nervous system. [NIH]

Neuropathy: A problem in any part of the nervous system except the brain and spinal cord. Neuropathies can be caused by infection, toxic substances, or disease. [NIH]

Neurosurgery: A surgical specialty concerned with the treatment of diseases and disorders of the brain, spinal cord, and peripheral and sympathetic nervous system. [NIH]

Neurotransmitter: Any of a group of substances that are released on excitation from the axon terminal of a presynaptic neuron of the central or peripheral nervous system and travel across the synaptic cleft to either excite or inhibit the target cell. Among the many substances that have the properties of a neurotransmitter are acetylcholine, norepinephrine, epinephrine, dopamine, glycine, y-aminobutyrate, glutamic acid, substance P, enkephalins, endorphins, and serotonin. [EU]

Neutrons: Electrically neutral elementary particles found in all atomic nuclei except light hydrogen; the mass is equal to that of the proton and electron combined and they are unstable when isolated from the nucleus, undergoing beta decay. Slow, thermal, epithermal, and fast neutrons refer to the energy levels with which the neutrons are ejected from heavier nuclei during their decay. [NIH]

Neutropenia: An abnormal decrease in the number of neutrophils, a type of white blood cell. [NIH]

Neutrophils: Granular leukocytes having a nucleus with three to five lobes connected by slender threads of chromatin, and cytoplasm containing fine inconspicuous granules and stainable by neutral dyes. [NIH]

Nifedipine: A potent vasodilator agent with calcium antagonistic action. It is a useful anti-anginal agent that also lowers blood pressure. The use of nifedipine as a tocolytic is being investigated. [NIH]

Nitrogen: An element with the atomic symbol N, atomic number 7, and atomic weight 14. Nitrogen exists as a diatomic gas and makes up about 78% of the earth's atmosphere by volume. It is a constituent of proteins and nucleic acids and found in all living cells. [NIH]

Node-negative: Cancer that has not spread to the lymph nodes. [NIH]

Nonmetastatic: Cancer that has not spread from the primary (original) site to other sites in the body. [NIH]

Non-small cell lung cancer: A group of lung cancers that includes squamous cell carcinoma, adenocarcinoma, and large cell carcinoma. [NIH]

Nuclear: A test of the structure, blood flow, and function of the kidneys. The doctor injects a mildly radioactive solution into an arm vein and uses x-rays to monitor its progress through the kidneys. [NIH]

Nuclear Medicine: A specialty field of radiology concerned with diagnostic, therapeutic, and investigative use of radioactive compounds in a pharmaceutical form. [NIH]

Nuclei: A body of specialized protoplasm found in nearly all cells and containing the chromosomes. [NIH]

Nucleic acid: Either of two types of macromolecule (DNA or RNA) formed by polymerization of nucleotides. Nucleic acids are found in all living cells and contain the information (genetic code) for the transfer of genetic information from one generation to the next. [NIH]

Nucleolus: A small dense body (sub organelle) within the nucleus of eukaryotic cells, visible by phase contrast and interference microscopy in live cells throughout interphase. Contains RNA and protein and is the site of synthesis of ribosomal RNA. [NIH]

Nucleus: A body of specialized protoplasm found in nearly all cells and containing the chromosomes. [NIH]

Nursing Care: Care given to patients by nursing service personnel. [NIH]

Ocular: 1. Of, pertaining to, or affecting the eye. 2. Eyepiece. [EU]

Oliguria: Clinical manifestation of the urinary system consisting of a decrease in the amount of urine secreted. [NIH]

Oncogene: A gene that normally directs cell growth. If altered, an oncogene can promote or allow the uncontrolled growth of cancer. Alterations can be inherited or caused by an environmental exposure to carcinogens. [NIH]

Oncogenic: Chemical, viral, radioactive or other agent that causes cancer; carcinogenic. [NIH]

Oncologist: A doctor who specializes in treating cancer. Some oncologists specialize in a particular type of cancer treatment. For example, a radiation oncologist specializes in treating cancer with radiation. [NIH]

Oncology: The study of cancer. [NIH]

Oncolysis: The destruction of or disposal by absorption of any neoplastic cells. [NIH]

Oncolytic: Pertaining to, characterized by, or causing oncolysis (= the lysis or destruction of tumour cells). [EU]

Oocytes: Female germ cells in stages between the prophase of the first maturation division and the completion of the second maturation division. [NIH]

Opacity: Degree of density (area most dense taken for reading). [NIH]

Operating Rooms: Facilities equipped for performing surgery. [NIH]

Ophthalmology: A surgical specialty concerned with the structure and function of the eye and the medical and surgical treatment of its defects and diseases. [NIH]

Opsin: A protein formed, together with retinene, by the chemical breakdown of meta-rhodopsin. [NIH]

Optic Chiasm: The X-shaped structure formed by the meeting of the two optic nerves. At the optic chiasm the fibers from the medial part of each retina cross to project to the other side of the brain while the lateral retinal fibers continue on the same side. As a result each half of the brain receives information about the contralateral visual field from both eyes. [NIH]

Optic Nerve: The 2nd cranial nerve. The optic nerve conveys visual information from the retina to the brain. The nerve carries the axons of the retinal ganglion cells which sort at the optic chiasm and continue via the optic tracts to the brain. The largest projection is to the lateral geniculate nuclei; other important targets include the superior colliculi and the suprachiasmatic nuclei. Though known as the second cranial nerve, it is considered part of the central nervous system. [NIH]

Oral Health: The optimal state of the mouth and normal functioning of the organs of the mouth without evidence of disease. [NIH]

Oral Hygiene: The practice of personal hygiene of the mouth. It includes the maintenance of oral cleanliness, tissue tone, and general preservation of oral health. [NIH]

Orbit: One of the two cavities in the skull which contains an eyeball. Each eye is located in a bony socket or orbit. [NIH]

Orbital: Pertaining to the orbit (= the bony cavity that contains the eyeball). [EU]

Organ Culture: The growth in aseptic culture of plant organs such as roots or shoots, beginning with organ primordia or segments and maintaining the characteristics of the organ. [NIH]

Organ Preservation: The process by which organs are kept viable outside of the organism from which they were removed (i.e., kept from decay by means of a chemical agent, cooling, or a fluid substitute that mimics the natural state within the organism). [NIH]

Orofacial: Of or relating to the mouth and face. [EU]

Oropharynx: Oral part of the pharynx. [NIH]

Osseointegration: The growth action of bone tissue, as it assimilates surgically implanted devices or prostheses to be used as either replacement parts (e.g., hip) or as anchors (e.g., endosseous dental implants). [NIH]

Osteomyelitis: Inflammation of bone caused by a pyogenic organism. It may remain localized or may spread through the bone to involve the marrow, cortex, cancellous tissue, and periosteum. [EU]

Osteoradionecrosis: Necrosis of bone following radiation injury. [NIH]

Outpatient: A patient who is not an inmate of a hospital but receives diagnosis or treatment in a clinic or dispensary connected with the hospital. [NIH]

Ovarian ablation: Surgery, radiation therapy, or a drug treatment to stop the functioning of the ovaries. Also called ovarian suppression. [NIH]

Ovaries: The pair of female reproductive glands in which the ova, or eggs, are formed. The ovaries are located in the pelvis, one on each side of the uterus. [NIH]

Ovary: Either of the paired glands in the female that produce the female germ cells and secrete some of the female sex hormones. [NIH]

Overall survival: The percentage of subjects in a study who have survived for a defined period of time. Usually reported as time since diagnosis or treatment. Often called the survival rate. [NIH]

Overexpress: An excess of a particular protein on the surface of a cell. [NIH]

Oxidation: The act of oxidizing or state of being oxidized. Chemically it consists in the increase of positive charges on an atom or the loss of negative charges. Most biological oxidations are accomplished by the removal of a pair of hydrogen atoms (dehydrogenation) from a molecule. Such oxidations must be accompanied by reduction of an acceptor molecule. Univalent o. indicates loss of one electron; divalent o., the loss of two electrons. [EU]

Oxidative Stress: A disturbance in the prooxidant-antioxidant balance in favor of the former, leading to potential damage. Indicators of oxidative stress include damaged DNA bases, protein oxidation products, and lipid peroxidation products (Sies, Oxidative Stress, 1991, pxv-xvi). [NIH]

Oxygen Consumption: The oxygen consumption is determined by calculating the difference between the amount of oxygen inhaled and exhaled. [NIH]

Oxygenation: The process of supplying, treating, or mixing with oxygen. No:1245 - oxygenation the process of supplying, treating, or mixing with oxygen. [EU]

P53 gene: A tumor suppressor gene that normally inhibits the growth of tumors. This gene is altered in many types of cancer. [NIH]

Pacemaker: An object or substance that influences the rate at which a certain phenomenon occurs; often used alone to indicate the natural cardiac pacemaker or an artificial cardiac pacemaker. In biochemistry, a substance whose rate of reaction sets the pace for a series of interrelated reactions. [EU]

Paclitaxel: Antineoplastic agent isolated from the bark of the Pacific yew tree, Taxus brevifolia. Paclitaxel stabilizes microtubules in their polymerized form and thus mimics the action of the proto-oncogene proteins c-mos. [NIH]

Palate: The structure that forms the roof of the mouth. It consists of the anterior hard palate and the posterior soft palate. [NIH]

Palladium: A chemical element having an atomic weight of 106.4, atomic number of 46, and the symbol Pd. It is a white, ductile metal resembling platinum, and following it in abundance and importance of applications. It is used in dentistry in the form of gold, silver, and copper alloys. [NIH]

Palliative: 1. Affording relief, but not cure. 2. An alleviating medicine. [EU]

Pancreas: A mixed exocrine and endocrine gland situated transversely across the posterior abdominal wall in the epigastric and hypochondriac regions. The endocrine portion is comprised of the Islets of Langerhans, while the exocrine portion is a compound acinar gland that secretes digestive enzymes. [NIH]

Pancreatic: Having to do with the pancreas. [NIH]

Pancreatic cancer: Cancer of the pancreas, a salivary gland of the abdomen. [NIH]

Pancreatic Juice: The fluid containing digestive enzymes secreted by the pancreas in response to food in the duodenum. [NIH]

Papilla: A small nipple-shaped elevation. [NIH]

Papillary: Pertaining to or resembling papilla, or nipple. [EU]

Papillomavirus: A genus of Papovaviridae causing proliferation of the epithelium, which may lead to malignancy. A wide range of animals are infected including humans, chimpanzees, cattle, rabbits, dogs, and horses. [NIH]

Paralysis: Loss of ability to move all or part of the body. [NIH]

Parietal: 1. Of or pertaining to the walls of a cavity. 2. Pertaining to or located near the parietal bone, as the parietal lobe. [EU]

Parotid: The space that contains the parotid gland, the facial nerve, the external carotid artery, and the retromandibular vein. [NIH]

Partial remission: The shrinking, but not complete disappearance, of a tumor in response to therapy. Also called partial response. [NIH]

Particle: A tiny mass of material. [EU]

Patch: A piece of material used to cover or protect a wound, an injured part, etc.: a patch over the eye. [NIH]

Pathogenesis: The cellular events and reactions that occur in the development of disease. [NIH]

Pathologic: 1. Indicative of or caused by a morbid condition. 2. Pertaining to pathology (= branch of medicine that treats the essential nature of the disease, especially the structural and functional changes in tissues and organs of the body caused by the disease). [EU]

Pathologic Processes: The abnormal mechanisms and forms involved in the dysfunctions of tissues and organs. [NIH]

Pathologist: A doctor who identifies diseases by studying cells and tissues under a microscope. [NIH]

Patient Education: The teaching or training of patients concerning their own health needs. [NIH]

Pelvic: Pertaining to the pelvis. [EU]

Pelvis: The lower part of the abdomen, located between the hip bones. [NIH]

Penis: The external reproductive organ of males. It is composed of a mass of erectile tissue enclosed in three cylindrical fibrous compartments. Two of the three compartments, the corpus cavernosa, are placed side-by-side along the upper part of the organ. The third compartment below, the corpus spongiosum, houses the urethra. [NIH]

Peptide: Any compound consisting of two or more amino acids, the building blocks of proteins. Peptides are combined to make proteins. [NIH]

Peptide T: N-(N-(N(2)-(N-(N-(N-(N-D-Alanyl L-seryl)-L-threonyl)-L-threonyl) L-threonyl)-L-asparaginyl)-L-tyrosyl) L-threonine. Octapeptide sharing sequence homology with HIV envelope protein gp120. It is potentially useful as antiviral agent in AIDS therapy. The core pentapeptide sequence, TTNYT, consisting of amino acids 4-8 in peptide T, is the HIV envelope sequence required for attachment to the CD4 receptor. [NIH]

Perception: The ability quickly and accurately to recognize similarities and differences among presented objects, whether these be pairs of words, pairs of number series, or multiple sets of these or other symbols such as geometric figures. [NIH]

Percutaneous: Performed through the skin, as injection of radiopacque material in radiological examination, or the removal of tissue for biopsy accomplished by a needle. [EU]

Performance status: A measure of how well a patient is able to perform ordinary tasks and carry out daily activities. [NIH]

Perfusion: Bathing an organ or tissue with a fluid. In regional perfusion, a specific area of the body (usually an arm or a leg) receives high doses of anticancer drugs through a blood vessel. Such a procedure is performed to treat cancer that has not spread. [NIH]

Perillyl alcohol: A drug used in cancer prevention that belongs to the family of plant drugs called monoterpenes. [NIH]

Perineal: Pertaining to the perineum. [EU]

Perineural: Around a nerve or group of nerves. [NIH]

Periodontal disease: Disease involving the supporting structures of the teeth (as the gums and periodontal membranes). [NIH]

Periodontal disease: Disease involving the supporting structures of the teeth (as the gums and periodontal membranes). [NIH]

Periodontitis: Inflammation of the periodontal membrane; also called periodontitis simplex. [NIH]

Perioperative: Around the time of surgery; usually lasts from the time of going into the hospital or doctor's office for surgery until the time the patient goes home. [NIH]

Perioperative Care: Interventions to provide care prior to, during, and immediately after surgery. [NIH]

Peripheral blood: Blood circulating throughout the body. [NIH]

Peripheral Nervous System: The nervous system outside of the brain and spinal cord. The peripheral nervous system has autonomic and somatic divisions. The autonomic nervous system includes the enteric, parasympathetic, and sympathetic subdivisions. The somatic nervous system includes the cranial and spinal nerves and their ganglia and the peripheral sensory receptors. [NIH]

Peritoneal: Having to do with the peritoneum (the tissue that lines the abdominal wall and covers most of the organs in the abdomen). [NIH]

Peritoneum: Endothelial lining of the abdominal cavity, the parietal peritoneum covering the inside of the abdominal wall and the visceral peritoneum covering the bowel, the mesentery, and certain of the organs. The portion that covers the bowel becomes the serosal layer of the bowel wall. [NIH]

Petrolatum: A colloidal system of semisolid hydrocarbons obtained from petroleum. It is used as an ointment base, topical protectant, and lubricant. [NIH]

PH: The symbol relating the hydrogen ion (H+) concentration or activity of a solution to that of a given standard solution. Numerically the pH is approximately equal to the negative logarithm of H+ concentration expressed in molarity. pH 7 is neutral; above it alkalinity increases and below it acidity increases. [EU]

Phagocytosis: The engulfing of microorganisms, other cells, and foreign particles by phagocytic cells. [NIH]

Phallic: Pertaining to the phallus, or penis. [EU]

Phantom: Used to absorb and/or scatter radiation equivalently to a patient, and hence to estimate radiation doses and test imaging systems without actually exposing a patient. It may be an anthropomorphic or a physical test object. [NIH]

Pharmacokinetic: The mathematical analysis of the time courses of absorption, distribution, and elimination of drugs. [NIH]

Pharmacologic: Pertaining to pharmacology or to the properties and reactions of drugs. [EU]

Pharynx: The hollow tube about 5 inches long that starts behind the nose and ends at the top of the trachea (windpipe) and esophagus (the tube that goes to the stomach). [NIH]

Phenolphthalein: An acid-base indicator which is colorless in acid solution, but turns pink to red as the solution becomes alkaline. It is used medicinally as a cathartic. [NIH]

Phenotype: The outward appearance of the individual. It is the product of interactions between genes and between the genotype and the environment. This includes the killer phenotype, characteristic of yeasts. [NIH]

Phenylalanine: An aromatic amino acid that is essential in the animal diet. It is a precursor of melanin, dopamine, noradrenalin, and thyroxine. [NIH]

Phosphorus: A non-metallic element that is found in the blood, muscles, nevers, bones, and teeth, and is a component of adenosine triphosphate (ATP; the primary energy source for the body's cells.) [NIH]

Phosphorylated: Attached to a phosphate group. [NIH]

Physical Examination: Systematic and thorough inspection of the patient for physical signs of disease or abnormality. [NIH]

Physiologic: Having to do with the functions of the body. When used in the phrase "physiologic age," it refers to an age assigned by general health, as opposed to calendar age. [NIH]

Physiology: The science that deals with the life processes and functions of organismus, their cells, tissues, and organs. [NIH]

Pigment: A substance that gives color to tissue. Pigments are responsible for the color of skin, eyes, and hair. [NIH]

Pilocarpine: A slowly hydrolyzed muscarinic agonist with no nicotinic effects. Pilocarpine is used as a miotic and in the treatment of glaucoma. [NIH]

Pilot study: The initial study examining a new method or treatment. [NIH]

Pituitary Gland: A small, unpaired gland situated in the sella turcica tissue. It is connected to the hypothalamus by a short stalk. [NIH]

Plants: Multicellular, eukaryotic life forms of the kingdom Plantae. They are characterized by a mainly photosynthetic mode of nutrition; essentially unlimited growth at localized regions of cell divisions (meristems); cellulose within cells providing rigidity; the absence of organs of locomotion; absense of nervous and sensory systems; and an alteration of haploid and diploid generations. [NIH]

Plaque: A clear zone in a bacterial culture grown on an agar plate caused by localized destruction of bacterial cells by a bacteriophage. The concentration of infective virus in a fluid can be estimated by applying the fluid to a culture and counting the number of. [NIH]

Plasma: The clear, yellowish, fluid part of the blood that carries the blood cells. The proteins that form blood clots are in plasma. [NIH]

Plasma cells: A type of white blood cell that produces antibodies. [NIH]

Plasmin: A product of the lysis of plasminogen (profibrinolysin) by plasminogen activators. It is composed of two polypeptide chains, light (B) and heavy (A), with a molecular weight of 75,000. It is the major proteolytic enzyme involved in blood clot retraction or the lysis of fibrin and quickly inactivated by antiplasmins. EC 3.4.21.7. [NIH]

Plasminogen: Precursor of fibrinolysin (plasmin). It is a single-chain beta-globulin of molecular weight 80-90,000 found mostly in association with fibrinogen in plasma; plasminogen activators change it to fibrinolysin. It is used in wound debriding and has been investigated as a thrombolytic agent. [NIH]

Plasminogen Activators: A heterogeneous group of proteolytic enzymes that convert plasminogen to plasmin. They are concentrated in the lysosomes of most cells and in the vascular endothelium, particularly in the vessels of the microcirculation. EC 3.4.21.-. [NIH]

Plasticity: In an individual or a population, the capacity for adaptation: a) through gene changes (genetic plasticity) or b) through internal physiological modifications in response to changes of environment (physiological plasticity). [NIH]

Platinum: Platinum. A heavy, soft, whitish metal, resembling tin, atomic number 78, atomic weight 195.09, symbol Pt. (From Dorland, 28th ed) It is used in manufacturing equipment for laboratory and industrial use. It occurs as a black powder (platinum black) and as a spongy substance (spongy platinum) and may have been known in Pliny's time as "alutiae". [NIH]

Pleura: The thin serous membrane enveloping the lungs and lining the thoracic cavity. [NIH]

Pleural: A circumscribed area of hyaline whorled fibrous tissue which appears on the surface of the parietal pleura, on the fibrous part of the diaphragm or on the pleura in the interlobar fissures. [NIH]

Ploidy: The number of sets of chromosomes in a cell or an organism. For example, haploid means one set and diploid means two sets. [NIH]

Pneumonectomy: An operation to remove an entire lung. [NIH]

Pneumonia: Inflammation of the lungs. [NIH]

Pneumonitis: A disease caused by inhaling a wide variety of substances such as dusts and molds. Also called "farmer's disease". [NIH]

Podophyllotoxin: The main active constituent of the resin from the roots of may apple or mandrake (Podophyllum peltatum and P. emodi). It is a potent spindle poison, toxic if taken internally, and has been used as a cathartic. It is very irritating to skin and mucous membranes, has keratolytic actions, has been used to treat warts and keratoses, and may have antineoplastic properties, as do some of its congeners and derivatives. [NIH]

Poisoning: A condition or physical state produced by the ingestion, injection or inhalation of, or exposure to a deleterious agent. [NIH]

Polypeptide: A peptide which on hydrolysis yields more than two amino acids; called tripeptides, tetrapeptides, etc. according to the number of amino acids contained. [EU]

Polyposis: The development of numerous polyps (growths that protrude from a mucous membrane). [NIH]

Polysaccharide: A type of carbohydrate. It contains sugar molecules that are linked together chemically. [NIH]

Pons: The part of the central nervous system lying between the medulla oblongata and the mesencephalon, ventral to the cerebellum, and consisting of a pars dorsalis and a pars ventralis. [NIH]

Porphyrins: A group of compounds containing the porphin structure, four pyrrole rings connected by methine bridges in a cyclic configuration to which a variety of side chains are attached. The nature of the side chain is indicated by a prefix, as uroporphyrin, hematoporphyrin, etc. The porphyrins, in combination with iron, form the heme component in biologically significant compounds such as hemoglobin and myoglobin. [NIH]

Port: An implanted device through which blood may be withdrawn and drugs may be infused without repeated needle sticks. Also called a port-a-cath. [NIH]

Port-a-cath: An implanted device through which blood may be withdrawn and drugs may be infused without repeated needle sticks. Also called a port. [NIH]

Posterior: Situated in back of, or in the back part of, or affecting the back or dorsal surface of the body. In lower animals, it refers to the caudal end of the body. [EU]

Postnatal: Occurring after birth, with reference to the newborn. [EU]

Postoperative: After surgery. [NIH]

Post-translational: The cleavage of signal sequence that directs the passage of the protein through a cell or organelle membrane. [NIH]

Post-traumatic: Occurring as a result of or after injury. [EU]

Potentiate: A degree of synergism which causes the exposure of the organism to a harmful substance to worsen a disease already contracted. [NIH]

Practicability: A non-standard characteristic of an analytical procedure. It is dependent on the scope of the method and is determined by requirements such as sample throughout and costs. [NIH]

Practice Guidelines: Directions or principles presenting current or future rules of policy for the health care practitioner to assist him in patient care decisions regarding diagnosis, therapy, or related clinical circumstances. The guidelines may be developed by government agencies at any level, institutions, professional societies, governing boards, or by the convening of expert panels. The guidelines form a basis for the evaluation of all aspects of health care and delivery. [NIH]

Precancerous: A term used to describe a condition that may (or is likely to) become cancer. Also called premalignant. [NIH]

Preclinical: Before a disease becomes clinically recognizable. [EU]

Precursor: Something that precedes. In biological processes, a substance from which another, usually more active or mature substance is formed. In clinical medicine, a sign or symptom that heralds another. [EU]

Prednisone: A synthetic anti-inflammatory glucocorticoid derived from cortisone. It is biologically inert and converted to prednisolone in the liver. [NIH]

Premalignant: A term used to describe a condition that may (or is likely to) become cancer. Also called precancerous. [NIH]

Preoperative: Preceding an operation. [EU]

Prevalence: The total number of cases of a given disease in a specified population at a designated time. It is differentiated from incidence, which refers to the number of new cases in the population at a given time. [NIH]

Primary central nervous system lymphoma: Cancer that arises in the lymphoid tissue found in the central nervous system (CNS). The CNS includes the brain and spinal cord. [NIH]

Primary tumor: The original tumor. [NIH]

Primitive neuroectodermal tumors: PNET. A type of bone cancer that forms in the middle (shaft) of large bones. Also called Ewing's sarcoma/primitive neuroectodermal tumor. [NIH]

Probe: An instrument used in exploring cavities, or in the detection and dilatation of strictures, or in demonstrating the potency of channels; an elongated instrument for exploring or sounding body cavities. [NIH]

Procarbazine: An antineoplastic agent used primarily in combination with mechlorethamine, vincristine, and prednisone (the MOPP protocol) in the treatment of Hodgkin's disease. [NIH]

Prodrug: A substance that gives rise to a pharmacologically active metabolite, although not itself active (i. e. an inactive precursor). [NIH]

Progeny: The offspring produced in any generation. [NIH]

Progesterone: Pregn-4-ene-3,20-dione. The principal progestational hormone of the body, secreted by the corpus luteum, adrenal cortex, and placenta. Its chief function is to prepare the uterus for the reception and development of the fertilized ovum. It acts as an antiovulatory agent when administered on days 5-25 of the menstrual cycle. [NIH]

Prognostic factor: A situation or condition, or a characteristic of a patient, that can be used to estimate the chance of recovery from a disease, or the chance of the disease recurring (coming back). [NIH]

Progression: Increase in the size of a tumor or spread of cancer in the body. [NIH]

Progressive: Advancing; going forward; going from bad to worse; increasing in scope or severity. [EU]

Progressive disease: Cancer that is increasing in scope or severity. [NIH]

Projection: A defense mechanism, operating unconsciously, whereby that which is emotionally unacceptable in the self is rejected and attributed (projected) to others. [NIH]

Proline: A non-essential amino acid that is synthesized from glutamic acid. It is an essential component of collagen and is important for proper functioning of joints and tendons. [NIH]

Promoter: A chemical substance that increases the activity of a carcinogenic process. [NIH]

Prone: Having the front portion of the body downwards. [NIH]

Prophase: The first phase of cell division, in which the chromosomes become visible, the nucleus starts to lose its identity, the spindle appears, and the centrioles migrate toward opposite poles. [NIH]

Prophylaxis: An attempt to prevent disease. [NIH]

Prospective study: An epidemiologic study in which a group of individuals (a cohort), all free of a particular disease and varying in their exposure to a possible risk factor, is followed over a specific amount of time to determine the incidence rates of the disease in the exposed and unexposed groups. [NIH]

Prostate: A gland in males that surrounds the neck of the bladder and the urethra. It secretes a substance that liquifies coagulated semen. It is situated in the pelvic cavity behind the lower part of the pubic symphysis, above the deep layer of the triangular ligament, and rests upon the rectum. [NIH]

Prostate gland: A gland in the male reproductive system just below the bladder. It surrounds part of the urethra, the canal that empties the bladder, and produces a fluid that forms part of semen. [NIH]

Prostatectomy: Complete or partial surgical removal of the prostate. Three primary approaches are commonly employed: suprapubic - removal through an incision above the pubis and through the urinary bladder; retropubic - as for suprapubic but without entering the urinary bladder; and transurethral (transurethral resection of prostate). [NIH]

Prostate-Specific Antigen: Kallikrein-like serine proteinase produced by epithelial cells of both benign and malignant prostate tissue. It is an important marker for the diagnosis of prostate cancer. EC 3.4.21.77. [NIH]

Prostatitis: Inflammation of the prostate. [EU]

Prosthesis: An artificial replacement of a part of the body. [NIH]

Protease: Proteinase (= any enzyme that catalyses the splitting of interior peptide bonds in a protein). [EU]

Protein Binding: The process in which substances, either endogenous or exogenous, bind to proteins, peptides, enzymes, protein precursors, or allied compounds. Specific protein-binding measures are often used as assays in diagnostic assessments. [NIH]

Protein C: A vitamin-K dependent zymogen present in the blood, which, upon activation by thrombin and thrombomodulin exerts anticoagulant properties by inactivating factors Va and VIIIa at the rate-limiting steps of thrombin formation. [NIH]

Protein Conformation: The characteristic 3-dimensional shape of a protein, including the secondary, supersecondary (motifs), tertiary (domains) and quaternary structure of the peptide chain. Quaternary protein structure describes the conformation assumed by multimeric proteins (aggregates of more than one polypeptide chain). [NIH]

Protein S: The vitamin K-dependent cofactor of activated protein C. Together with protein C, it inhibits the action of factors VIIIa and Va. A deficiency in protein S can lead to recurrent venous and arterial thrombosis. [NIH]

Proteins: Polymers of amino acids linked by peptide bonds. The specific sequence of amino acids determines the shape and function of the protein. [NIH]

Proteinuria: The presence of protein in the urine, indicating that the kidneys are not working properly. [NIH]

Proteolytic: 1. Pertaining to, characterized by, or promoting proteolysis. 2. An enzyme that promotes proteolysis (= the splitting of proteins by hydrolysis of the peptide bonds with formation of smaller polypeptides). [EU]

Proteome: The protein complement of an organism coded for by its genome. [NIH]

Protocol: The detailed plan for a clinical trial that states the trial's rationale, purpose, drug or vaccine dosages, length of study, routes of administration, who may participate, and other aspects of trial design. [NIH]

Protons: Stable elementary particles having the smallest known positive charge, found in the nuclei of all elements. The proton mass is less than that of a neutron. A proton is the nucleus of the light hydrogen atom, i.e., the hydrogen ion. [NIH]

Proto-Oncogene Proteins: Products of proto-oncogenes. Normally they do not have oncogenic or transforming properties, but are involved in the regulation or differentiation of cell growth. They often have protein kinase activity. [NIH]

Proto-Oncogene Proteins c-mos: Cellular proteins encoded by the c-mos genes. They function in the cell cycle to maintain maturation promoting factor in the active state and have protein-serine/threonine kinase activity. Oncogenic transformation can take place when c-mos proteins are expressed at the wrong time. [NIH]

Protozoa: A subkingdom consisting of unicellular organisms that are the simplest in the animal kingdom. Most are free living. They range in size from submicroscopic to macroscopic. Protozoa are divided into seven phyla: Sarcomastigophora, Labyrinthomorpha, Apicomplexa, Microspora, Ascetospora, Myxozoa, and Ciliophora. [NIH]

Psychiatric: Pertaining to or within the purview of psychiatry. [EU]

Psychiatry: The medical science that deals with the origin, diagnosis, prevention, and treatment of mental disorders. [NIH]

Psychoactive: Those drugs which alter sensation, mood, consciousness or other psychological or behavioral functions. [NIH]

Public Policy: A course or method of action selected, usually by a government, from among alternatives to guide and determine present and future decisions. [NIH]

Publishing: "The business or profession of the commercial production and issuance of literature" (Webster's 3d). It includes the publisher, publication processes, editing and editors. Production may be by conventional printing methods or by electronic publishing. [NIH]

Pulmonary: Relating to the lungs. [NIH]

Pulse: The rhythmical expansion and contraction of an artery produced by waves of pressure caused by the ejection of blood from the left ventricle of the heart as it contracts. [NIH]

Purifying: Respiratory equipment whose function is to remove contaminants from otherwise wholesome air. [NIH]

Purines: A series of heterocyclic compounds that are variously substituted in nature and are known also as purine bases. They include adenine and guanine, constituents of nucleic acids, as well as many alkaloids such as caffeine and theophylline. Uric acid is the metabolic end product of purine metabolism. [NIH]

Pyogenic: Producing pus; pyopoietic (= liquid inflammation product made up of cells and a thin fluid called liquor puris). [EU]

Pyrimidines: A family of 6-membered heterocyclic compounds occurring in nature in a wide variety of forms. They include several nucleic acid constituents (cytosine, thymine, and uracil) and form the basic structure of the barbiturates. [NIH]

Quality of Health Care: The levels of excellence which characterize the health service or health care provided based on accepted standards of quality. [NIH]

Quality of Life: A generic concept reflecting concern with the modification and enhancement of life attributes, e.g., physical, political, moral and social environment. [NIH]

Race: A population within a species which exhibits general similarities within itself, but is both discontinuous and distinct from other populations of that species, though not sufficiently so as to achieve the status of a taxon. [NIH]

Racemic: Optically inactive but resolvable in the way of all racemic compounds. [NIH]

Radiation: Emission or propagation of electromagnetic energy (waves/rays), or the waves/rays themselves; a stream of electromagnetic particles (electrons, neutrons, protons, alpha particles) or a mixture of these. The most common source is the sun. [NIH]

Radiation oncologist: A doctor who specializes in using radiation to treat cancer. [NIH]

Radiation Oncology: A subspecialty of medical oncology and radiology concerned with the radiotherapy of cancer. [NIH]

Radiation therapy: The use of high-energy radiation from x-rays, gamma rays, neutrons, and other sources to kill cancer cells and shrink tumors. Radiation may come from a machine outside the body (external-beam radiation therapy), or it may come from radioactive material placed in the body in the area near cancer cells (internal radiation therapy, implant radiation, or brachytherapy). Systemic radiation therapy uses a radioactive substance, such as a radiolabeled monoclonal antibody, that circulates throughout the body. Also called radiotherapy. [NIH]

Radical prostatectomy: Surgery to remove the entire prostate. The two types of radical prostatectomy are retropubic prostatectomy and perineal prostatectomy. [NIH]

Radicular: Having the character of or relating to a radicle or root. [NIH]

Radiculopathy: Disease involving a spinal nerve root (see spinal nerve roots) which may result from compression related to intervertebral disk displacement; spinal cord injuries; spinal diseases; and other conditions. Clinical manifestations include radicular pain, weakness, and sensory loss referable to structures innervated by the involved nerve root. [NIH]

Radioactive: Giving off radiation. [NIH]

Radioactivity: The quality of emitting or the emission of corpuscular or electromagnetic radiations consequent to nuclear disintegration, a natural property of all chemical elements of atomic number above 83, and possible of induction in all other known elements. [EU]

Radiobiology: That part of biology which deals with the effects of radiation on living organisms. [NIH]

Radiography: Examination of any part of the body for diagnostic purposes by means of roentgen rays, recording the image on a sensitized surface (such as photographic film). [NIH]

Radioimmunotherapy: Radiotherapy where cytotoxic radionuclides are linked to antibodies in order to deliver toxins directly to tumor targets. Therapy with targeted radiation rather than antibody-targeted toxins (immunotoxins) has the advantage that adjacent tumor cells, which lack the appropriate antigenic determinants, can be destroyed by radiation cross-fire. Radioimmunotherapy is sometimes called targeted radiotherapy, but this latter term can also refer to radionuclides linked to non-immune molecules (radiotherapy). [NIH]

Radioisotope: An unstable element that releases radiation as it breaks down. Radioisotopes can be used in imaging tests or as a treatment for cancer. [NIH]

Radiolabeled: Any compound that has been joined with a radioactive substance. [NIH]

Radiological: Pertaining to radiodiagnostic and radiotherapeutic procedures, and interventional radiology or other planning and guiding medical radiology. [NIH]

Radiology: A specialty concerned with the use of x-ray and other forms of radiant energy in the diagnosis and treatment of disease. [NIH]

Radionuclide Imaging: Process whereby a radionuclide is injected or measured (through tissue) from an external source, and a display is obtained from any one of several rectilinear scanner or gamma camera systems. The image obtained from a moving detector is called a scan, while the image obtained from a stationary camera device is called a scintiphotograph. [NIH]

Radiopharmaceutical: Any medicinal product which, when ready for use, contains one or more radionuclides (radioactive isotopes) included for a medicinal purpose. [NIH]

Radiosensitization: The use of a drug that makes tumor cells more sensitive to radiation therapy. [NIH]

Radiosensitizers: Drugs that make tumor cells more sensitive to radiation. [NIH]

Radiotherapy Dosage: The total amount of radiation absorbed by tissues as a result of radiotherapy. [NIH]

Random Allocation: A process involving chance used in therapeutic trials or other research endeavor for allocating experimental subjects, human or animal, between treatment and control groups, or among treatment groups. It may also apply to experiments on inanimate objects. [NIH]

Randomization: Also called random allocation. Is allocation of individuals to groups, e.g., for experimental and control regimens, by chance. Within the limits of chance variation, random allocation should make the control and experimental groups similar at the start of an investigation and ensure that personal judgment and prejudices of the investigator do not influence allocation. [NIH]

Randomized: Describes an experiment or clinical trial in which animal or human subjects are assigned by chance to separate groups that compare different treatments. [NIH]

Randomized clinical trial: A study in which the participants are assigned by chance to separate groups that compare different treatments; neither the researchers nor the participants can choose which group. Using chance to assign people to groups means that the groups will be similar and that the treatments they receive can be compared objectively. At the time of the trial, it is not known which treatment is best. It is the patient's choice to be in a randomized trial. [NIH]

Reactive Oxygen Species: Reactive intermediate oxygen species including both radicals and non-radicals. These substances are constantly formed in the human body and have been shown to kill bacteria and inactivate proteins, and have been implicated in a number of diseases. Scientific data exist that link the reactive oxygen species produced by inflammatory phagocytes to cancer development. [NIH]

Receptor: A molecule inside or on the surface of a cell that binds to a specific substance and causes a specific physiologic effect in the cell. [NIH]

Recombinant: A cell or an individual with a new combination of genes not found together in either parent; usually applied to linked genes. [EU]

Recombination: The formation of new combinations of genes as a result of segregation in crosses between genetically different parents; also the rearrangement of linked genes due to crossing-over. [NIH]

Reconstitution: 1. A type of regeneration in which a new organ forms by the rearrangement of tissues rather than from new formation at an injured surface. 2. The restoration to original form of a substance previously altered for preservation and storage, as the restoration to a liquid state of blood serum or plasma that has been dried and stored. [EU]

Rectal: By or having to do with the rectum. The rectum is the last 8 to 10 inches of the large intestine and ends at the anus. [NIH]

Rectum: The last 8 to 10 inches of the large intestine. [NIH]

Recur: To occur again. Recurrence is the return of cancer, at the same site as the original (primary) tumor or in another location, after the tumor had disappeared. [NIH]

Recurrence: The return of a sign, symptom, or disease after a remission. [NIH]

Red blood cells: RBCs. Cells that carry oxygen to all parts of the body. Also called erythrocytes. [NIH]

Reductase: Enzyme converting testosterone to dihydrotestosterone. [NIH]

Refer: To send or direct for treatment, aid, information, de decision. [NIH]

Reflux: The term used when liquid backs up into the esophagus from the stomach. [NIH]

Refraction: A test to determine the best eyeglasses or contact lenses to correct a refractive error (myopia, hyperopia, or astigmatism). [NIH]

Refractory: Not readily yielding to treatment. [EU]

Regeneration: The natural renewal of a structure, as of a lost tissue or part. [EU]

Regimen: A treatment plan that specifies the dosage, the schedule, and the duration of treatment. [NIH]

Regional cancer: Refers to cancer that has grown beyond the original (primary) tumor to nearby lymph nodes or organs and tissues. [NIH]

Regional lymph node: In oncology, a lymph node that drains lymph from the region around a tumor. [NIH]

Relapse: The return of signs and symptoms of cancer after a period of improvement. [NIH]

Reliability: Used technically, in a statistical sense, of consistency of a test with itself, i. e. the extent to which we can assume that it will yield the same result if repeated a second time. [NIH]

Remission: A decrease in or disappearance of signs and symptoms of cancer. In partial remission, some, but not all, signs and symptoms of cancer have disappeared. In complete remission, all signs and symptoms of cancer have disappeared, although there still may be cancer in the body. [NIH]

Renal Artery: A branch of the abdominal aorta which supplies the kidneys, adrenal glands and ureters. [NIH]

Renal pelvis: The area at the center of the kidney. Urine collects here and is funneled into the ureter, the tube that connects the kidney to the bladder. [NIH]

Renin: An enzyme which is secreted by the kidney and is formed from prorenin in plasma and kidney. The enzyme cleaves the Leu-Leu bond in angiotensinogen to generate angiotensin I. EC 3.4.23.15. (Formerly EC 3.4.99.19). [NIH]

Renin-Angiotensin System: A system consisting of renin, angiotensin-converting enzyme, and angiotensin II. Renin, an enzyme produced in the kidney, acts on angiotensinogen, an alpha-2 globulin produced by the liver, forming angiotensin I. The converting enzyme contained in the lung acts on angiotensin I in the plasma converting it to angiotensin II, the most powerful directly pressor substance known. It causes contraction of the arteriolar smooth muscle and has other indirect actions mediated through the adrenal cortex. [NIH]

Renovascular: Of or pertaining to the blood vessels of the kidneys. [EU]

Reproductive system: In women, this system includes the ovaries, the fallopian tubes, the uterus (womb), the cervix, and the vagina (birth canal). The reproductive system in men includes the prostate, the testes, and the penis. [NIH]

Research Support: Financial support of research activities. [NIH]

Resected: Surgical removal of part of an organ. [NIH]

Resection: Removal of tissue or part or all of an organ by surgery. [NIH]

Respiration: The act of breathing with the lungs, consisting of inspiration, or the taking into the lungs of the ambient air, and of expiration, or the expelling of the modified air which contains more carbon dioxide than the air taken in (Blakiston's Gould Medical Dictionary, 4th ed.). This does not include tissue respiration (= oxygen consumption) or cell respiration (= cell respiration). [NIH]

Response rate: The percentage of patients whose cancer shrinks or disappears after treatment. [NIH]

Retina: The ten-layered nervous tissue membrane of the eye. It is continuous with the optic nerve and receives images of external objects and transmits visual impulses to the brain. Its outer surface is in contact with the choroid and the inner surface with the vitreous body. The outer-most layer is pigmented, whereas the inner nine layers are transparent. [NIH]

Retinal: 1. Pertaining to the retina. 2. The aldehyde of retinol, derived by the oxidative enzymatic splitting of absorbed dietary carotene, and having vitamin A activity. In the retina, retinal combines with opsins to form visual pigments. One isomer, 11-cis retinal combines with opsin in the rods (scotopsin) to form rhodopsin, or visual purple. Another, all-trans retinal (trans-r.); visual yellow; xanthopsin) results from the bleaching of rhodopsin by light, in which the 11-cis form is converted to the all-trans form. Retinal also combines with opsins in the cones (photopsins) to form the three pigments responsible for colour vision. Called also retinal, and retinene1. [EU]

Retinal Detachment: Separation of the inner layers of the retina (neural retina) from the pigment epithelium. Retinal detachment occurs more commonly in men than in women, in eyes with degenerative myopia, in aging and in aphakia. It may occur after an uncomplicated cataract extraction, but it is seen more often if vitreous humor has been lost during surgery. (Dorland, 27th ed; Newell, Ophthalmology: Principles and Concepts, 7th ed, p310-12). [NIH]

Retinal Ganglion Cells: Cells of the innermost nuclear layer of the retina, the ganglion cell layer, which project axons through the optic nerve to the brain. They are quite variable in size and in the shapes of their dendritic arbors, which are generally confined to the inner plexiform layer. [NIH]

Retinoblastoma: An eye cancer that most often occurs in children younger than 5 years. It occurs in hereditary and nonhereditary (sporadic) forms. [NIH]

Retinol: Vitamin A. It is essential for proper vision and healthy skin and mucous membranes. Retinol is being studied for cancer prevention; it belongs to the family of drugs called retinoids. [NIH]

Retreatment: The therapy of the same disease in a patient, with the same agent or procedure repeated after initial treatment, or with an additional or alternate measure or follow-up. It does not include therapy which requires more than one administration of a therapeutic agent or regimen. Retreatment is often used with reference to a different modality when the original one was inadequate, harmful, or unsuccessful. [NIH]

Retrograde: 1. Moving backward or against the usual direction of flow. 2. Degenerating, deteriorating, or catabolic. [EU]

Retroperitoneal: Having to do with the area outside or behind the peritoneum (the tissue that lines the abdominal wall and covers most of the organs in the abdomen). [NIH]

Retropubic: A potential space between the urinary bladder and the symphisis and body of the pubis. [NIH]

Retropubic prostatectomy: Surgery to remove the prostate through an incision made in the abdominal wall. [NIH]

Retrospective: Looking back at events that have already taken place. [NIH]

Retrospective study: A study that looks backward in time, usually using medical records and interviews with patients who already have or had a disease. [NIH]

Retroviral vector: RNA from a virus that is used to insert genetic material into cells. [NIH]

Retrovirus: A member of a group of RNA viruses, the RNA of which is copied during viral replication into DNA by reverse transcriptase. The viral DNA is then able to be integrated into the host chromosomal DNA. [NIH]

Rhabdomyosarcoma: A malignant tumor of muscle tissue. [NIH]

Rheumatism: A group of disorders marked by inflammation or pain in the connective tissue structures of the body. These structures include bone, cartilage, and fat. [NIH]

Rheumatoid: Resembling rheumatism. [EU]

Rheumatoid arthritis: A form of arthritis, the cause of which is unknown, although infection, hypersensitivity, hormone imbalance and psychologic stress have been suggested as possible causes. [NIH]

Rhodopsin: A photoreceptor protein found in retinal rods. It is a complex formed by the binding of retinal, the oxidized form of retinol, to the protein opsin and undergoes a series of complex reactions in response to visible light resulting in the transmission of nerve impulses to the brain. [NIH]

Ribonucleoside Diphosphate Reductase: An enzyme of the oxidoreductase class that catalyzes the formation of 2'-deoxyribonucleotides from the corresponding ribonucleotides using NADPH as the ultimate electron donor. The deoxyribonucleoside diphosphates are used in DNA synthesis. (From Dorland, 27th ed) EC 1.17.4.1. [NIH]

Ribosome: A granule of protein and RNA, synthesized in the nucleolus and found in the cytoplasm of cells. Ribosomes are the main sites of protein synthesis. Messenger RNA attaches to them and there receives molecules of transfer RNA bearing amino acids. [NIH]

Rickettsiae: One of a group of obligate intracellular parasitic microorganisms, once regarded as intermediate in their properties between bacteria and viruses but now classified as bacteria in the order Rickettsiales, which includes 17 genera and 3 families: Rickettsiace. [NIH]

Risk factor: A habit, trait, condition, or genetic alteration that increases a person's chance of developing a disease. [NIH]

Risk patient: Patient who is at risk, because of his/her behaviour or because of the type of person he/she is. [EU]

Rods: One type of specialized light-sensitive cells (photoreceptors) in the retina that provide side vision and the ability to see objects in dim light (night vision). [NIH]

Ruthenium: A hard, brittle, grayish-white rare earth metal with an atomic symbol Ru, atomic number 44, and atomic weight 101.07. It is used as a catalyst and hardener for platinum and palladium. [NIH]

Saliva: The clear, viscous fluid secreted by the salivary glands and mucous glands of the mouth. It contains mucins, water, organic salts, and ptylin. [NIH]

Salivary: The duct that convey saliva to the mouth. [NIH]

Salivary Gland Neoplasms: Tumors or cancer of the salivary glands. [NIH]

Salivary glands: Glands in the mouth that produce saliva. [NIH]

Salvage Therapy: A therapeutic approach, involving chemotherapy, radiation therapy, or surgery, after initial regimens have failed to lead to improvement in a patient's condition. Salvage therapy is most often used for neoplastic diseases. [NIH]

Saponins: Sapogenin glycosides. A type of glycoside widely distributed in plants. Each consists of a sapogenin as the aglycon moiety, and a sugar. The sapogenin may be a steroid or a triterpene and the sugar may be glucose, galactose, a pentose, or a methylpentose. Sapogenins are poisonous towards the lower forms of life and are powerful hemolytics when injected into the blood stream able to dissolve red blood cells at even extreme dilutions. [NIH]

Sarcoma: A connective tissue neoplasm formed by proliferation of mesodermal cells; it is usually highly malignant. [NIH]

Scans: Pictures of structures inside the body. Scans often used in diagnosing, staging, and monitoring disease include liver scans, bone scans, and computed tomography (CT) or computerized axial tomography (CAT) scans and magnetic resonance imaging (MRI) scans. In liver scanning and bone scanning, radioactive substances that are injected into the bloodstream collect in these organs. A scanner that detects the radiation is used to create pictures. In CT scanning, an x-ray machine linked to a computer is used to produce detailed pictures of organs inside the body. MRI scans use a large magnet connected to a computer to create pictures of areas inside the body. [NIH]

Scatter: The extent to which relative success and failure are divergently manifested in qualitatively different tests. [NIH]

Schizoid: Having qualities resembling those found in greater degree in schizophrenics; a person of schizoid personality. [NIH]

Schizophrenia: A mental disorder characterized by a special type of disintegration of the personality. [NIH]

Schizotypal Personality Disorder: A personality disorder in which there are oddities of thought (magical thinking, paranoid ideation, suspiciousness), perception (illusions, depersonalization), speech (digressive, vague, overelaborate), and behavior (inappropriate affect in social interactions, frequently social isolation) that are not severe enough to characterize schizophrenia. [NIH]

Schwannoma: A tumor of the peripheral nervous system that begins in the nerve sheath (protective covering). It is almost always benign, but rare malignant schwannomas have been reported. [NIH]

Scleroderma: A chronic disorder marked by hardening and thickening of the skin. Scleroderma can be localized or it can affect the entire body (systemic). [NIH]

Sclerosis: A pathological process consisting of hardening or fibrosis of an anatomical structure, often a vessel or a nerve. [NIH]

Screening: Checking for disease when there are no symptoms. [NIH]

Scrotum: In males, the external sac that contains the testicles. [NIH]

Second cancer: Refers to a new primary cancer that is caused by previous cancer treatment, or a new primary cancer in a person with a history of cancer. [NIH]

Secondary tumor: Cancer that has spread from the organ in which it first appeared to another organ. For example, breast cancer cells may spread (metastasize) to the lungs and cause the growth of a new tumor. When this happens, the disease is called metastatic breast cancer, and the tumor in the lungs is called a secondary tumor. Also called secondary cancer. [NIH]

Secretion: 1. The process of elaborating a specific product as a result of the activity of a gland; this activity may range from separating a specific substance of the blood to the elaboration of a new chemical substance. 2. Any substance produced by secretion. [EU]

Secretory: Secreting; relating to or influencing secretion or the secretions. [NIH]

Sedative: 1. Allaying activity and excitement. 2. An agent that allays excitement. [EU]

Segmentation: The process by which muscles in the intestines move food and wastes through the body. [NIH]

Segregation: The separation in meiotic cell division of homologous chromosome pairs and their contained allelomorphic gene pairs. [NIH]

Seizures: Clinical or subclinical disturbances of cortical function due to a sudden, abnormal, excessive, and disorganized discharge of brain cells. Clinical manifestations include abnormal motor, sensory and psychic phenomena. Recurrent seizures are usually referred to as epilepsy or "seizure disorder." [NIH]

Selective estrogen receptor modulator: SERM. A drug that acts like estrogen on some tissues, but blocks the effect of estrogen on other tissues. Tamoxifen and raloxifene are SERMs. [NIH]

Selenium: An element with the atomic symbol Se, atomic number 34, and atomic weight 78.96. It is an essential micronutrient for mammals and other animals but is toxic in large amounts. Selenium protects intracellular structures against oxidative damage. It is an essential component of glutathione peroxidase. [NIH]

Sella Turcica: A bony prominence situated on the upper surface of the body of the sphenoid bone. It houses the pituitary gland. [NIH]

Semen: The thick, yellowish-white, viscid fluid secretion of male reproductive organs discharged upon ejaculation. In addition to reproductive organ secretions, it contains spermatozoa and their nutrient plasma. [NIH]

Seminal vesicles: Glands that help produce semen. [NIH]

Seminoma: A type of cancer of the testicles. [NIH]

Semisynthetic: Produced by chemical manipulation of naturally occurring substances. [EU]

Sensitization: 1. Administration of antigen to induce a primary immune response; priming; immunization. 2. Exposure to allergen that results in the development of hypersensitivity. 3. The coating of erythrocytes with antibody so that they are subject to lysis by complement in the presence of homologous antigen, the first stage of a complement fixation test. [EU]

Sensor: A device designed to respond to physical stimuli such as temperature, light, magnetism or movement and transmit resulting impulses for interpretation, recording, movement, or operating control. [NIH]

Sensory loss: A disease of the nerves whereby the myelin or insulating sheath of myelin on the nerves does not stay intact and the messages from the brain to the muscles through the nerves are not carried properly. [NIH]

Septic: Produced by or due to decomposition by microorganisms; putrefactive. [EU]

Sequence Homology: The degree of similarity between sequences. Studies of amino acid and nucleotide sequences provide useful information about the genetic relatedness of certain species. [NIH]

Sequencing: The determination of the order of nucleotides in a DNA or RNA chain. [NIH]

Serine: A non-essential amino acid occurring in natural form as the L-isomer. It is synthesized from glycine or threonine. It is involved in the biosynthesis of purines, pyrimidines, and other amino acids. [NIH]

Serous: Having to do with serum, the clear liquid part of blood. [NIH]

Serum: The clear liquid part of the blood that remains after blood cells and clotting proteins have been removed. [NIH]

Sex Characteristics: Those characteristics that distinguish one sex from the other. The primary sex characteristics are the ovaries and testes and their related hormones. Secondary sex characteristics are those which are masculine or feminine but not directly related to reproduction. [NIH]

Sexually Transmitted Diseases: Diseases due to or propagated by sexual contact. [NIH]

Sharpness: The apparent blurring of the border between two adjacent areas of a radiograph having different optical densities. [NIH]

Shock: The general bodily disturbance following a severe injury; an emotional or moral upset occasioned by some disturbing or unexpected experience; disruption of the circulation, which can upset all body functions: sometimes referred to as circulatory shock. [NIH]

Shunt: A surgically created diversion of fluid (e.g., blood or cerebrospinal fluid) from one area of the body to another area of the body. [NIH]

Side effect: A consequence other than the one(s) for which an agent or measure is used, as the adverse effects produced by a drug, especially on a tissue or organ system other than the one sought to be benefited by its administration. [EU]

Sigmoid: 1. Shaped like the letter S or the letter C. 2. The sigmoid colon. [EU]

Sigmoid Colon: The lower part of the colon that empties into the rectum. [NIH]

Signs and Symptoms: Clinical manifestations that can be either objective when observed by a physician, or subjective when perceived by the patient. [NIH]

Silicon: A trace element that constitutes about 27.6% of the earth's crust in the form of silicon dioxide. It does not occur free in nature. Silicon has the atomic symbol Si, atomic number 14, and atomic weight 28.09. [NIH]

Silicon Dioxide: Silica. Transparent, tasteless crystals found in nature as agate, amethyst, chalcedony, cristobalite, flint, sand, quartz, and tridymite. The compound is insoluble in water or acids except hydrofluoric acid. [NIH]

Skeletal: Having to do with the skeleton (boney part of the body). [NIH]

Skeleton: The framework that supports the soft tissues of vertebrate animals and protects many of their internal organs. The skeletons of vertebrates are made of bone and/or cartilage. [NIH]

Skin graft: Skin that is moved from one part of the body to another. [NIH]

Skull: The skeleton of the head including the bones of the face and the bones enclosing the brain. [NIH]

Skull Base: The inferior region of the skull consisting of an internal (cerebral), and an external (basilar) surface. [NIH]

Small cell lung cancer: A type of lung cancer in which the cells appear small and round when viewed under the microscope. Also called oat cell lung cancer. [NIH]

Small intestine: The part of the digestive tract that is located between the stomach and the large intestine. [NIH]

Smooth muscle: Muscle that performs automatic tasks, such as constricting blood vessels. [NIH]

Social Environment: The aggregate of social and cultural institutions, forms, patterns, and processes that influence the life of an individual or community. [NIH]

Social Support: Support systems that provide assistance and encouragement to individuals with physical or emotional disabilities in order that they may better cope. Informal social support is usually provided by friends, relatives, or peers, while formal assistance is provided by churches, groups, etc. [NIH]

Soft tissue: Refers to muscle, fat, fibrous tissue, blood vessels, or other supporting tissue of the body. [NIH]

Soft tissue sarcoma: A sarcoma that begins in the muscle, fat, fibrous tissue, blood vessels, or other supporting tissue of the body. [NIH]

Solid tumor: Cancer of body tissues other than blood, bone marrow, or the lymphatic system. [NIH]

Somatic: 1. Pertaining to or characteristic of the soma or body. 2. Pertaining to the body wall in contrast to the viscera. [EU]

Somatostatin: A polypeptide hormone produced in the hypothalamus, and other tissues and organs. It inhibits the release of human growth hormone, and also modulates important physiological functions of the kidney, pancreas, and gastrointestinal tract. Somatostatin receptors are widely expressed throughout the body. Somatostatin also acts as a neurotransmitter in the central and peripheral nervous systems. [NIH]

Sonogram: A computer picture of areas inside the body created by bouncing sound waves off organs and other tissues. Also called ultrasonogram or ultrasound. [NIH]

Sound wave: An alteration of properties of an elastic medium, such as pressure, particle displacement, or density, that propagates through the medium, or a superposition of such alterations. [NIH]

Specialist: In medicine, one who concentrates on 1 special branch of medical science. [NIH]

Species: A taxonomic category subordinate to a genus (or subgenus) and superior to a subspecies or variety, composed of individuals possessing common characters distinguishing them from other categories of individuals of the same taxonomic level. In taxonomic nomenclature, species are designated by the genus name followed by a Latin or Latinized adjective or noun. [EU]

Specificity: Degree of selectivity shown by an antibody with respect to the number and types of antigens with which the antibody combines, as well as with respect to the rates and the extents of these reactions. [NIH]

Spectrometer: An apparatus for determining spectra; measures quantities such as wavelengths and relative amplitudes of components. [NIH]

Spectroscopic: The recognition of elements through their emission spectra. [NIH]

Spectrum: A charted band of wavelengths of electromagnetic vibrations obtained by refraction and diffraction. By extension, a measurable range of activity, such as the range of bacteria affected by an antibiotic (antibacterial s.) or the complete range of manifestations of a disease. [EU]

Speech Disorders: Acquired or developmental conditions marked by an impaired ability to comprehend or generate spoken forms of language. [NIH]

Speech pathologist: A specialist who evaluates and treats people with communication and swallowing problems. Also called a speech therapist. [NIH]

Sperm: The fecundating fluid of the male. [NIH]

Spermatic: A cord-like structure formed by the vas deferens and the blood vessels, nerves and lymphatics of the testis. [NIH]

Sphincter: A ringlike band of muscle fibres that constricts a passage or closes a natural orifice; called also musculus sphincter. [EU]

Spinal cord: The main trunk or bundle of nerves running down the spine through holes in the spinal bone (the vertebrae) from the brain to the level of the lower back. [NIH]

Spinal Nerve Roots: The paired bundles of nerve fibers entering and leaving the spinal cord at each segment. The dorsal and ventral nerve roots join to form the mixed segmental spinal nerves. The dorsal roots are generally afferent, formed by the central projections of the spinal (dorsal root) ganglia sensory cells, and the ventral roots efferent, comprising the axons of spinal motor and autonomic preganglionic neurons. There are, however, some exceptions to this afferent/efferent rule. [NIH]

Spinous: Like a spine or thorn in shape; having spines. [NIH]

Spleen: An organ that is part of the lymphatic system. The spleen produces lymphocytes, filters the blood, stores blood cells, and destroys old blood cells. It is located on the left side of the abdomen near the stomach. [NIH]

Splenectomy: An operation to remove the spleen. [NIH]

Splenomegaly: Enlargement of the spleen. [NIH]

Sporadic: Neither endemic nor epidemic; occurring occasionally in a random or isolated manner. [EU]

Sputum: The material expelled from the respiratory passages by coughing or clearing the throat. [NIH]

Squamous: Scaly, or platelike. [EU]

Squamous cell carcinoma: Cancer that begins in squamous cells, which are thin, flat cells resembling fish scales. Squamous cells are found in the tissue that forms the surface of the skin, the lining of the hollow organs of the body, and the passages of the respiratory and digestive tracts. Also called epidermoid carcinoma. [NIH]

Squamous cell carcinoma: Cancer that begins in squamous cells, which are thin, flat cells resembling fish scales. Squamous cells are found in the tissue that forms the surface of the skin, the lining of the hollow organs of the body, and the passages of the respiratory and digestive tracts. Also called epidermoid carcinoma. [NIH]

Squamous cells: Flat cells that look like fish scales under a microscope. These cells cover internal and external surfaces of the body. [NIH]

Staging: Performing exams and tests to learn the extent of the cancer within the body, especially whether the disease has spread from the original site to other parts of the body. [NIH]

Standard therapy: A currently accepted and widely used treatment for a certain type of cancer, based on the results of past research. [NIH]

Stasis: A word termination indicating the maintenance of (or maintaining) a constant level; preventing increase or multiplication. [EU]

Steel: A tough, malleable, iron-based alloy containing up to, but no more than, two percent carbon and often other metals. It is used in medicine and dentistry in implants and instrumentation. [NIH]

Stem cell transplantation: A method of replacing immature blood-forming cells that were destroyed by cancer treatment. The stem cells are given to the person after treatment to help the bone marrow recover and continue producing healthy blood cells. [NIH]

Stem Cells: Relatively undifferentiated cells of the same lineage (family type) that retain the ability to divide and cycle throughout postnatal life to provide cells that can become specialized and take the place of those that die or are lost. [NIH]

Stenosis: Narrowing or stricture of a duct or canal. [EU]

Stent: A device placed in a body structure (such as a blood vessel or the gastrointestinal tract) to provide support and keep the structure open. [NIH]

Stereotactic: Radiotherapy that treats brain tumors by using a special frame affixed directly to the patient's cranium. By aiming the X-ray source with respect to the rigid frame, technicians can position the beam extremely precisely during each treatment. [NIH]

Stereotactic radiosurgery: A radiation therapy technique involving a rigid head frame that is attached to the skull; high-dose radiation is administered through openings in the head frame to the tumor while decreasing the amount of radiation given to normal brain tissue. This procedure does not involve surgery. Also called stereotaxic radiosurgery and stereotactic radiation therapy. [NIH]

Sterility: 1. The inability to produce offspring, i.e., the inability to conceive (female s.) or to induce conception (male s.). 2. The state of being aseptic, or free from microorganisms. [EU]

Sternum: Breast bone. [NIH]

Steroid: A group name for lipids that contain a hydrogenated cyclopentanoperhydrophenanthrene ring system. Some of the substances included in this group are progesterone, adrenocortical hormones, the gonadal hormones, cardiac aglycones, bile acids, sterols (such as cholesterol), toad poisons, saponins, and some of the carcinogenic hydrocarbons. [EU]

Stimulants: Any drug or agent which causes stimulation. [NIH]

Stimulus: That which can elicit or evoke action (response) in a muscle, nerve, gland or other excitable issue, or cause an augmenting action upon any function or metabolic process. [NIH]

Stomach: An organ of digestion situated in the left upper quadrant of the abdomen between the termination of the esophagus and the beginning of the duodenum. [NIH]

Stomatitis: Inflammation of the oral mucosa, due to local or systemic factors which may involve the buccal and labial mucosa, palate, tongue, floor of the mouth, and the gingivae. [EU]

Stool: The waste matter discharged in a bowel movement; feces. [NIH]

Strand: DNA normally exists in the bacterial nucleus in a helix, in which two strands are coiled together. [NIH]

Streptavidin: A 60kD extracellular protein of Streptomyces avidinii with four high-affinity biotin binding sites. Unlike AVIDIN, streptavidin has a near neutral isoelectric point and is free of carbohydrate side chains. [NIH]

Stress: Forcibly exerted influence; pressure. Any condition or situation that causes strain or tension. Stress may be either physical or psychologic, or both. [NIH]

Stress management: A set of techniques used to help an individual cope more effectively with difficult situations in order to feel better emotionally, improve behavioral skills, and often to enhance feelings of control. Stress management may include relaxation exercises, assertiveness training, cognitive restructuring, time management, and social support. It can be delivered either on a one-to-one basis or in a group format. [NIH]

Stricture: The abnormal narrowing of a body opening. Also called stenosis. [NIH]

Stroke: Sudden loss of function of part of the brain because of loss of blood flow. Stroke may be caused by a clot (thrombosis) or rupture (hemorrhage) of a blood vessel to the brain. [NIH]

Subacute: Somewhat acute; between acute and chronic. [EU]

Subarachnoid: Situated or occurring between the arachnoid and the pia mater. [EU]

Subclinical: Without clinical manifestations; said of the early stage(s) of an infection or other disease or abnormality before symptoms and signs become apparent or detectable by clinical examination or laboratory tests, or of a very mild form of an infection or other disease or abnormality. [EU]

Subcutaneous: Beneath the skin. [NIH]

Submandibular: Four to six lymph glands, located between the lower jaw and the submandibular salivary gland. [NIH]

Submaxillary: Four to six lymph glands, located between the lower jaw and the submandibular salivary gland. [NIH]

Subspecies: A category intermediate in rank between species and variety, based on a smaller number of correlated characters than are used to differentiate species and generally conditioned by geographical and/or ecological occurrence. [NIH]

Substance P: An eleven-amino acid neurotransmitter that appears in both the central and peripheral nervous systems. It is involved in transmission of pain, causes rapid contractions of the gastrointestinal smooth muscle, and modulates inflammatory and immune responses. [NIH]

Subtraction Technique: Combination or superimposition of two images for demonstrating differences between them (e.g., radiograph with contrast vs. one without, radionuclide images using different radionuclides, radiograph vs. radionuclide image) and in the preparation of audiovisual materials (e.g., offsetting identical images, coloring of vessels in angiograms). [NIH]

Sulfur: An element that is a member of the chalcogen family. It has an atomic symbol S, atomic number 16, and atomic weight 32.066. It is found in the amino acids cysteine and methionine. [NIH]

Supplementation: Adding nutrients to the diet. [NIH]

Suppression: A conscious exclusion of disapproved desire contrary with repression, in which the process of exclusion is not conscious. [NIH]

Suppressive: Tending to suppress : effecting suppression; specifically : serving to suppress activity, function, symptoms. [EU]

Supraclavicular: The depression above the clavicle and lateral to the sternomastoid muscle. [NIH]

Surgical Instruments: Hand-held tools or implements used by health professionals for the performance of surgical tasks. [NIH]

Survival Rate: The proportion of survivors in a group, e.g., of patients, studied and followed over a period, or the proportion of persons in a specified group alive at the beginning of a time interval who survive to the end of the interval. It is often studied using life table methods. [NIH]

Suspensions: Colloids with liquid continuous phase and solid dispersed phase; the term is used loosely also for solid-in-gas (aerosol) and other colloidal systems; water-insoluble drugs may be given as suspensions. [NIH]

Sympathetic Nervous System: The thoracolumbar division of the autonomic nervous system. Sympathetic preganglionic fibers originate in neurons of the intermediolateral column of the spinal cord and project to the paravertebral and prevertebral ganglia, which in turn project to target organs. The sympathetic nervous system mediates the body's response to stressful situations, i.e., the fight or flight reactions. It often acts reciprocally to the parasympathetic system. [NIH]

Symphysis: A secondary cartilaginous joint. [NIH]

Symptomatic: Having to do with symptoms, which are signs of a condition or disease. [NIH]

Symptomatic treatment: Therapy that eases symptoms without addressing the cause of disease. [NIH]

Syncytium: A living nucleated tissue without apparent cellular structure; a tissue composed of a mass of nucleated protoplasm without cell boundaries. [NIH]

Synergistic: Acting together; enhancing the effect of another force or agent. [EU]

Systemic: Affecting the entire body. [NIH]

Systemic therapy: Treatment that uses substances that travel through the bloodstream, reaching and affecting cells all over the body. [NIH]

Systolic: Indicating the maximum arterial pressure during contraction of the left ventricle of the heart. [EU]

Tamoxifen: A first generation selective estrogen receptor modulator (SERM). It acts as an agonist for bone tissue and cholesterol metabolism but is an estrogen antagonist in mammary and uterine. [NIH]

Technetium: The first artificially produced element and a radioactive fission product of uranium. The stablest isotope has a mass number 99 and is used diagnostically as a radioactive imaging agent. Technetium has the atomic symbol Tc, atomic number 43, and atomic weight 98.91. [NIH]

Teletherapy: Radiotherapy with a souce-skin distance that is large compared to the dimensions of the irradiated tissue being treated. [NIH]

Temozolomide: An anticancer drug that belongs to the family of drugs called alkylating agents. [NIH]

Temporal: One of the two irregular bones forming part of the lateral surfaces and base of the skull, and containing the organs of hearing. [NIH]

Testicle: The male gonad where, in adult life, spermatozoa develop; the testis. [NIH]

Testicular: Pertaining to a testis. [EU]

Testis: Either of the paired male reproductive glands that produce the male germ cells and the male hormones. [NIH]

Tetanus: A disease caused by tetanospasmin, a powerful protein toxin produced by Clostridium tetani. Tetanus usually occurs after an acute injury, such as a puncture wound or laceration. Generalized tetanus, the most common form, is characterized by tetanic muscular contractions and hyperreflexia. Localized tetanus presents itself as a mild condition with manifestations restricted to muscles near the wound. It may progress to the generalized form. [NIH]

Therapeutics: The branch of medicine which is concerned with the treatment of diseases, palliative or curative. [NIH]

Thermal: Pertaining to or characterized by heat. [EU]

Thigh: A leg; in anatomy, any elongated process or part of a structure more or less comparable to a leg. [NIH]

Thoracic: Having to do with the chest. [NIH]

Thorax: A part of the trunk between the neck and the abdomen; the chest. [NIH]

Threonine: An essential amino acid occurring naturally in the L-form, which is the active form. It is found in eggs, milk, gelatin, and other proteins. [NIH]

Threshold: For a specified sensory modality (e. g. light, sound, vibration), the lowest level (absolute threshold) or smallest difference (difference threshold, difference limen) or intensity of the stimulus discernible in prescribed conditions of stimulation. [NIH]

Thrombin: An enzyme formed from prothrombin that converts fibrinogen to fibrin. (Dorland, 27th ed) EC 3.4.21.5. [NIH]

Thrombolytic: 1. Dissolving or splitting up a thrombus. 2. A thrombolytic agent. [EU]

Thrombomodulin: A cell surface glycoprotein of endothelial cells that binds thrombin and serves as a cofactor in the activation of protein C and its regulation of blood coagulation. [NIH]

Thrombosis: The formation or presence of a blood clot inside a blood vessel. [NIH]

Thrush: A disease due to infection with species of fungi of the genus Candida. [NIH]

Thymidine: A chemical compound found in DNA. Also used as treatment for mucositis. [NIH]

Thyroid: A gland located near the windpipe (trachea) that produces thyroid hormone, which helps regulate growth and metabolism. [NIH]

Tissue: A group or layer of cells that are alike in type and work together to perform a specific function. [NIH]

Tissue Culture: Maintaining or growing of tissue, organ primordia, or the whole or part of an organ in vitro so as to preserve its architecture and/or function (Dorland, 28th ed). Tissue culture includes both organ culture and cell culture. [NIH]

Tolerance: 1. The ability to endure unusually large doses of a drug or toxin. 2. Acquired drug tolerance; a decreasing response to repeated constant doses of a drug or the need for increasing doses to maintain a constant response. [EU]

Tomography: Imaging methods that result in sharp images of objects located on a chosen plane and blurred images located above or below the plane. [NIH]

Tone: 1. The normal degree of vigour and tension; in muscle, the resistance to passive elongation or stretch; tonus. 2. A particular quality of sound or of voice. 3. To make permanent, or to change, the colour of silver stain by chemical treatment, usually with a heavy metal. [EU]

Tooth Preparation: Procedures carried out with regard to the teeth or tooth structures preparatory to specified dental therapeutic and surgical measures. [NIH]

Topoisomerase inhibitors: A family of anticancer drugs. The topoisomerase enzymes are responsible for the arrangement and rearrangement of DNA in the cell and for cell growth and replication. Inhibiting these enzymes may kill cancer cells or stop their growth. [NIH]

Tourniquet: A device, band or elastic tube applied temporarily to press upon an artery to stop bleeding; a device to compress a blood vessel in order to stop bleeding. [NIH]

Toxic: Having to do with poison or something harmful to the body. Toxic substances usually cause unwanted side effects. [NIH]

Toxicity: The quality of being poisonous, especially the degree of virulence of a toxic microbe or of a poison. [EU]

Toxicology: The science concerned with the detection, chemical composition, and pharmacologic action of toxic substances or poisons and the treatment and prevention of toxic manifestations. [NIH]

Toxin: A poison; frequently used to refer specifically to a protein produced by some higher plants, certain animals, and pathogenic bacteria, which is highly toxic for other living organisms. Such substances are differentiated from the simple chemical poisons and the vegetable alkaloids by their high molecular weight and antigenicity. [EU]

Trace element: Substance or element essential to plant or animal life, but present in extremely small amounts. [NIH]

Tracer: A substance (such as a radioisotope) used in imaging procedures. [NIH]

Trachea: The cartilaginous and membranous tube descending from the larynx and branching into the right and left main bronchi. [NIH]

Transcriptase: An enzyme which catalyses the synthesis of a complementary mRNA molecule from a DNA template in the presence of a mixture of the four ribonucleotides (ATP, UTP, GTP and CTP). [NIH]

Transcription Factors: Endogenous substances, usually proteins, which are effective in the initiation, stimulation, or termination of the genetic transcription process. [NIH]

Transcutaneous: Transdermal. [EU]

Transdermal: Entering through the dermis, or skin, as in administration of a drug applied to the skin in ointment or patch form. [EU]

Transduction: The transfer of genes from one cell to another by means of a viral (in the case of bacteria, a bacteriophage) vector or a vector which is similar to a virus particle (pseudovirion). [NIH]

Transfection: The uptake of naked or purified DNA into cells, usually eukaryotic. It is analogous to bacterial transformation. [NIH]

Transferases: Transferases are enzymes transferring a group, for example, the methyl group or a glycosyl group, from one compound (generally regarded as donor) to another compound (generally regarded as acceptor). The classification is based on the scheme "donor:acceptor group transferase". (Enzyme Nomenclature, 1992) EC 2. [NIH]

Translation: The process whereby the genetic information present in the linear sequence of ribonucleotides in mRNA is converted into a corresponding sequence of amino acids in a protein. It occurs on the ribosome and is unidirectional. [NIH]

Translational: The cleavage of signal sequence that directs the passage of the protein through a cell or organelle membrane. [NIH]

Translocation: The movement of material in solution inside the body of the plant. [NIH]

Transmitter: A chemical substance which effects the passage of nerve impulses from one cell to the other at the synapse. [NIH]

Transplantation: Transference of a tissue or organ, alive or dead, within an individual, between individuals of the same species, or between individuals of different species. [NIH]

Transrectal ultrasound: A procedure used to examine the prostate. An instrument is inserted into the rectum, and sound waves bounce off the prostate. These sound waves create echoes, which a computer uses to create a picture called a sonogram. [NIH]

Transurethral: Performed through the urethra. [EU]

Transurethral resection: Surgery performed with a special instrument inserted through the urethra. Also called TUR. [NIH]

Transurethral Resection of Prostate: Resection of the prostate using a cystoscope passed through the urethra. [NIH]

Trauma: Any injury, wound, or shock, must frequently physical or structural shock, producing a disturbance. [NIH]

Treatment Failure: A measure of the quality of health care by assessment of unsuccessful results of management and procedures used in combating disease, in individual cases or series. [NIH]

Treatment Outcome: Evaluation undertaken to assess the results or consequences of management and procedures used in combating disease in order to determine the efficacy, effectiveness, safety, practicability, etc., of these interventions in individual cases or series. [NIH]

Trismus: Spasmodic contraction of the masseter muscle resulting in forceful jaw closure. This may be seen with a variety of diseases, including tetanus, as a complication of radiation therapy, trauma, or in association with neoplastic conditions. [NIH]

Trivalent: Having a valence of three. [EU]

Trypsin: A serine endopeptidase that is formed from trypsinogen in the pancreas. It is converted into its active form by enteropeptidase in the small intestine. It catalyzes hydrolysis of the carboxyl group of either arginine or lysine. EC 3.4.21.4. [NIH]

Tryptophan: An essential amino acid that is necessary for normal growth in infants and for nitrogen balance in adults. It is a precursor serotonin and niacin. [NIH]

Tumor marker: A substance sometimes found in an increased amount in the blood, other body fluids, or tissues and which may mean that a certain type of cancer is in the body. Examples of tumor markers include CA 125 (ovarian cancer), CA 15-3 (breast cancer), CEA (ovarian, lung, breast, pancreas, and gastrointestinal tract cancers), and PSA (prostate cancer). Also called biomarker. [NIH]

Tumor suppressor gene: Genes in the body that can suppress or block the development of cancer. [NIH]

Tumour: 1. Swelling, one of the cardinal signs of inflammations; morbid enlargement. 2. A new growth of tissue in which the multiplication of cells is uncontrolled and progressive; called also neoplasm. [EU]

Tunica: A rather vague term to denote the lining coat of hollow organs, tubes, or cavities. [NIH]

Tyrosine: A non-essential amino acid. In animals it is synthesized from phenylalanine. It is also the precursor of epinephrine, thyroid hormones, and melanin. [NIH]

Ultrasonography: The visualization of deep structures of the body by recording the reflections of echoes of pulses of ultrasonic waves directed into the tissues. Use of ultrasound for imaging or diagnostic purposes employs frequencies ranging from 1.6 to 10 megahertz. [NIH]

Unresectable: Unable to be surgically removed. [NIH]

Uracil: An anticancer drug that belongs to the family of drugs called alkylating agents. [NIH]

Uranium: A radioactive element of the actinide series of metals. It has an atomic symbol U, atomic number 92, and atomic weight 238.03. U-235 is used as the fissionable fuel in nuclear weapons and as fuel in nuclear power reactors. [NIH]

Ureter: One of a pair of thick-walled tubes that transports urine from the kidney pelvis to the bladder. [NIH]

Urethra: The tube through which urine leaves the body. It empties urine from the bladder. [NIH]

Urinary: Having to do with urine or the organs of the body that produce and get rid of urine. [NIH]

Urinary tract: The organs of the body that produce and discharge urine. These include the kidneys, ureters, bladder, and urethra. [NIH]

Urinate: To release urine from the bladder to the outside. [NIH]

Urine: Fluid containing water and waste products. Urine is made by the kidneys, stored in the bladder, and leaves the body through the urethra. [NIH]

Urodynamic: Measures of the bladder's ability to hold and release urine. [NIH]

Urogenital: Pertaining to the urinary and genital apparatus; genitourinary. [EU]

Urogenital Diseases: Diseases of the urogenital tract. [NIH]

Urolithiasis: Stones in the urinary system. [NIH]

Urologic Diseases: Diseases of the urinary tract in both male and female. It does not include the male genitalia for which urogenital diseases is used for general discussions of diseases of both the urinary tract and the genitalia. [NIH]

Uterus: The small, hollow, pear-shaped organ in a woman's pelvis. This is the organ in which a fetus develops. Also called the womb. [NIH]

Vaccination: Administration of vaccines to stimulate the host's immune response. This includes any preparation intended for active immunological prophylaxis. [NIH]

Vaccines: Suspensions of killed or attenuated microorganisms (bacteria, viruses, fungi, protozoa, or rickettsiae), antigenic proteins derived from them, or synthetic constructs, administered for the prevention, amelioration, or treatment of infectious and other diseases. [NIH]

Vacuoles: Any spaces or cavities within a cell. They may function in digestion, storage, secretion, or excretion. [NIH]

Vagina: The muscular canal extending from the uterus to the exterior of the body. Also called the birth canal. [NIH]

Vaginal: Of or having to do with the vagina, the birth canal. [NIH]

Vaginitis: Inflammation of the vagina characterized by pain and a purulent discharge. [NIH]

Valves: Flap-like structures that control the direction of blood flow through the heart. [NIH]

Varices: Stretched veins such as those that form in the esophagus from cirrhosis. [NIH]

Vas Deferens: The excretory duct of the testes that carries spermatozoa. It rises from the scrotum and joins the seminal vesicles to form the ejaculatory duct. [NIH]

Vascular: Pertaining to blood vessels or indicative of a copious blood supply. [EU]

Vasodilation: Physiological dilation of the blood vessels without anatomic change. For dilation with anatomic change, dilatation, pathologic or aneurysm (or specific aneurysm) is used. [NIH]

Vasodilator: An agent that widens blood vessels. [NIH]

Vector: Plasmid or other self-replicating DNA molecule that transfers DNA between cells in nature or in recombinant DNA technology. [NIH]

Vein: Vessel-carrying blood from various parts of the body to the heart. [NIH]

Venoms: Poisonous animal secretions forming fluid mixtures of many different enzymes, toxins, and other substances. These substances are produced in specialized glands and secreted through specialized delivery systems (nematocysts, spines, fangs, etc.) for disabling prey or predator. [NIH]

Venous: Of or pertaining to the veins. [EU]

Ventral: 1. Pertaining to the belly or to any venter. 2. Denoting a position more toward the belly surface than some other object of reference; same as anterior in human anatomy. [EU]

Ventricle: One of the two pumping chambers of the heart. The right ventricle receives oxygen-poor blood from the right atrium and pumps it to the lungs through the pulmonary artery. The left ventricle receives oxygen-rich blood from the left atrium and pumps it to the body through the aorta. [NIH]

Vertebrae: A bony unit of the segmented spinal column. [NIH]

Vertebral: Of or pertaining to a vertebra. [EU]

Vesicoureteral: An abnormal condition in which urine backs up into the ureters, and occasionally into the kidneys, raising the risk of infection. [NIH]

Veterinary Medicine: The medical science concerned with the prevention, diagnosis, and treatment of diseases in animals. [NIH]

Vinblastine: An anticancer drug that belongs to the family of plant drugs called vinca alkaloids. It is a mitotic inhibitor. [NIH]

Vinca Alkaloids: A class of alkaloids from the genus of apocyanaceous woody herbs including periwinkles. They are some of the most useful antineoplastic agents. [NIH]

Vincristine: An anticancer drug that belongs to the family of plant drugs called vinca alkaloids. [NIH]

Vinorelbine: An anticancer drug that belongs to the family of plant drugs called vinca alkaloids. [NIH]

Viral: Pertaining to, caused by, or of the nature of virus. [EU]

Viral vector: A type of virus used in cancer therapy. The virus is changed in the laboratory and cannot cause disease. Viral vectors produce tumor antigens (proteins found on a tumor cell) and can stimulate an antitumor immune response in the body. Viral vectors may also be used to carry genes that can change cancer cells back to normal cells. [NIH]

Virulence: The degree of pathogenicity within a group or species of microorganisms or viruses as indicated by case fatality rates and/or the ability of the organism to invade the tissues of the host. [NIH]

Virus: Submicroscopic organism that causes infectious disease. In cancer therapy, some viruses may be made into vaccines that help the body build an immune response to, and kill, tumor cells. [NIH]

Viscosity: A physical property of fluids that determines the internal resistance to shear forces. [EU]

Visual Acuity: Acuteness or clearness of vision, especially of form vision, which is dependent mainly on the sharpness of the retinal focus. [NIH]

Visual field: The entire area that can be seen when the eye is forward, including peripheral vision. [NIH]

Vitreous: Glasslike or hyaline; often used alone to designate the vitreous body of the eye (corpus vitreum). [EU]

Vitreous Humor: The transparent, colorless mass of gel that lies behind the lens and in front of the retina and fills the center of the eyeball. [NIH]

Vitro: Descriptive of an event or enzyme reaction under experimental investigation occurring outside a living organism. Parts of an organism or microorganism are used together with artificial substrates and/or conditions. [NIH]

Vivo: Outside of or removed from the body of a living organism. [NIH]

Void: To urinate, empty the bladder. [NIH]

Volition: Voluntary activity without external compulsion. [NIH]

Vulva: The external female genital organs, including the clitoris, vaginal lips, and the opening to the vagina. [NIH]

Warts: Benign epidermal proliferations or tumors; some are viral in origin. [NIH]

White blood cell: A type of cell in the immune system that helps the body fight infection and disease. White blood cells include lymphocytes, granulocytes, macrophages, and others. [NIH]

Windpipe: A rigid tube, 10 cm long, extending from the cricoid cartilage to the upper border of the fifth thoracic vertebra. [NIH]

Withdrawal: 1. A pathological retreat from interpersonal contact and social involvement, as may occur in schizophrenia, depression, or schizoid avoidant and schizotypal personality disorders. 2. (DSM III-R) A substance-specific organic brain syndrome that follows the cessation of use or reduction in intake of a psychoactive substance that had been regularly used to induce a state of intoxication. [EU]

Womb: A hollow, thick-walled, muscular organ in which the impregnated ovum is developed into a child. [NIH]

Wound Healing: Restoration of integrity to traumatized tissue. [NIH]

Xenograft: The cells of one species transplanted to another species. [NIH]

Xerostomia: Decreased salivary flow. [NIH]

X-ray: High-energy radiation used in low doses to diagnose diseases and in high doses to treat cancer. [NIH]

X-ray therapy: The use of high-energy radiation from x-rays to kill cancer cells and shrink tumors. Radiation may come from a machine outside the body (external-beam radiation therapy) or from materials called radioisotopes. Radioisotopes produce radiation and can be placed in or near the tumor or in the area near cancer cells. This type of radiation treatment is called internal radiation therapy, implant radiation, interstitial radiation, or brachytherapy. Systemic radiation therapy uses a radioactive substance, such as a radiolabeled monoclonal antibody, that circulates throughout the body. X-ray therapy is also called radiation therapy, radiotherapy, and irradiation. [NIH]

Yeasts: A general term for single-celled rounded fungi that reproduce by budding. Brewers' and bakers' yeasts are Saccharomyces cerevisiae; therapeutic dried yeast is dried yeast. [NIH]

Yttrium: An element of the rare earth family of metals. It has the atomic symbol Y, atomic number 39, and atomic weight 88.91. In conjunction with other rare earths, yttrium is used as a phosphor in television receivers and is a component of the yttrium-aluminum garnet (YAG) lasers. [NIH]

Zygote: The fertilized ovum. [NIH]

Zymogen: Inactive form of an enzyme which can then be converted to the active form, usually by excision of a polypeptide, e. g. trypsinogen is the zymogen of trypsin. [NIH]

INDEX

Printed in the United States
78471LV00001B/171

9 780497 009274